Brain and Spinal Tumors - Primary and Secondary

Edited by Lee Roy Morgan
and Feyzi Birol Sarica

Published in London, United Kingdom

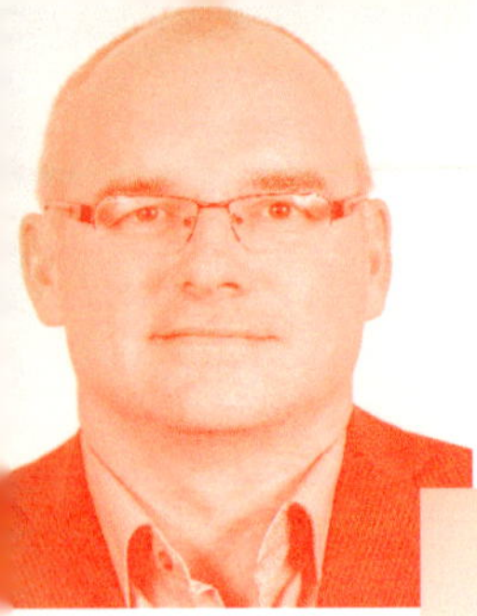
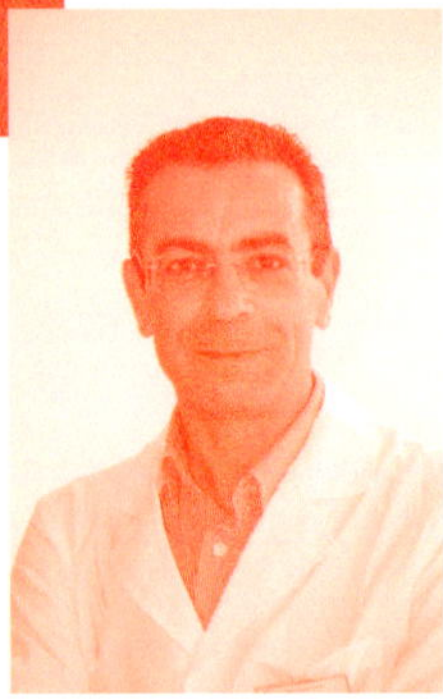
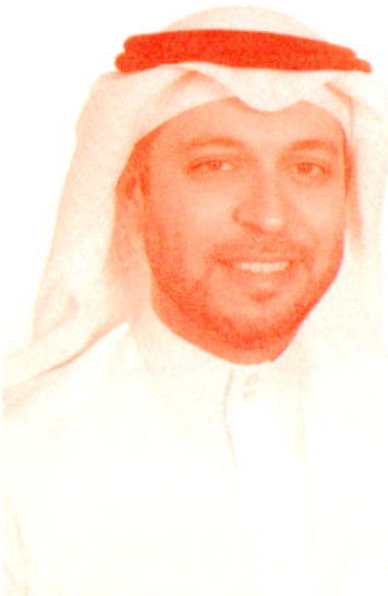
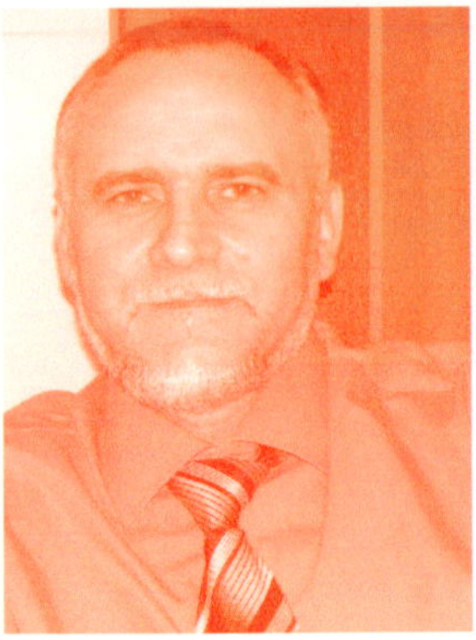
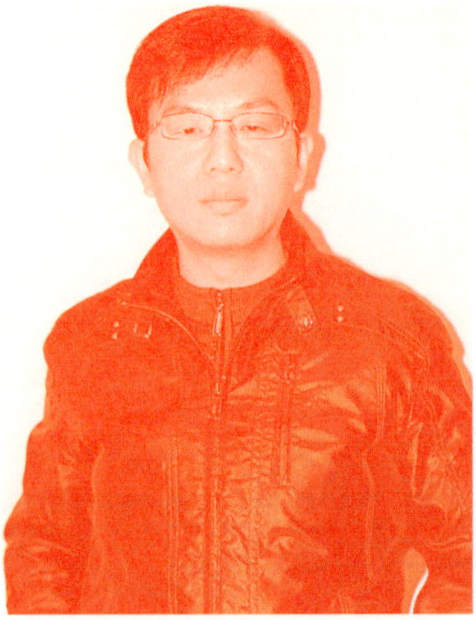
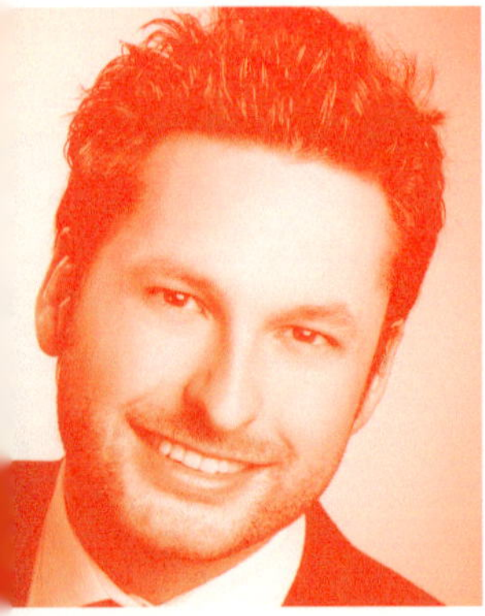
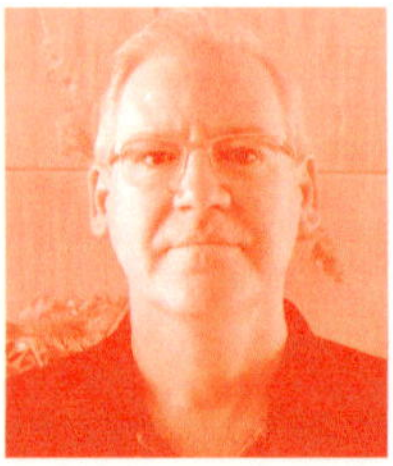

IntechOpen

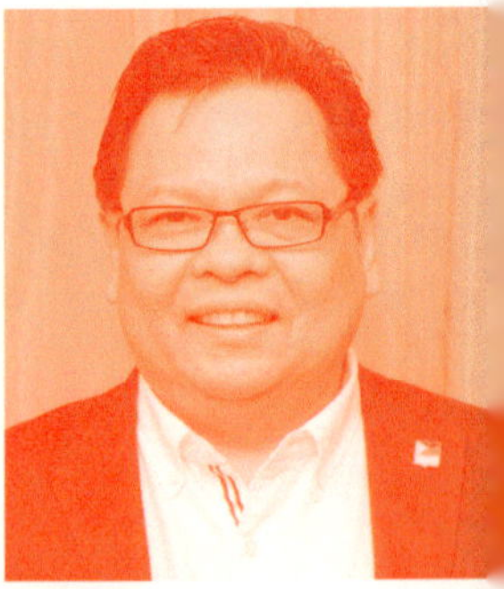
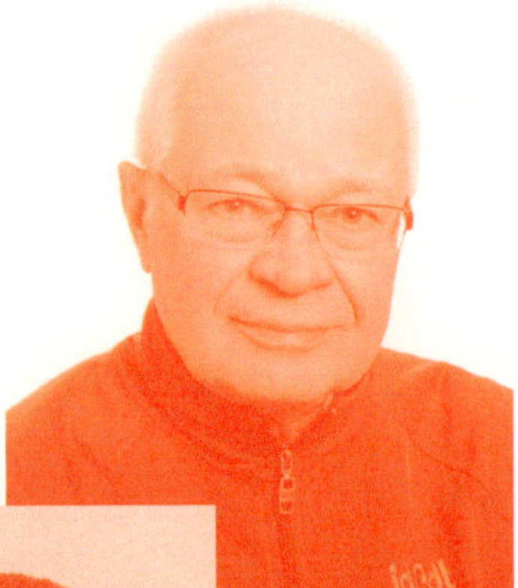
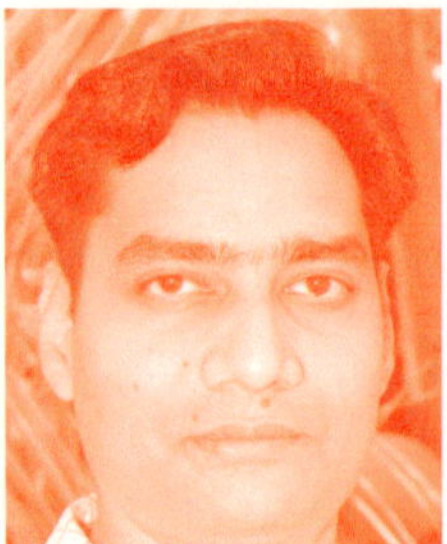
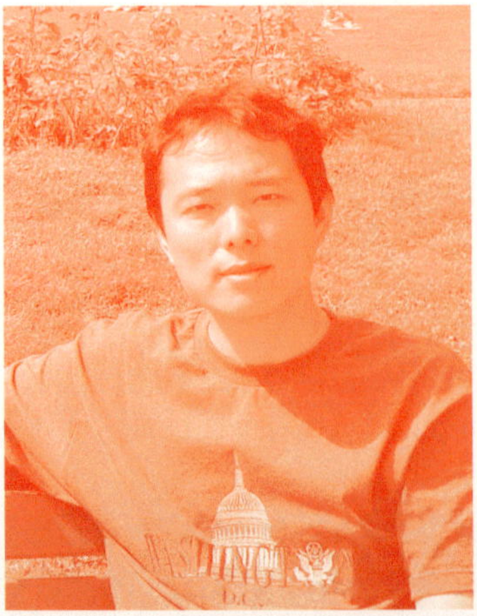
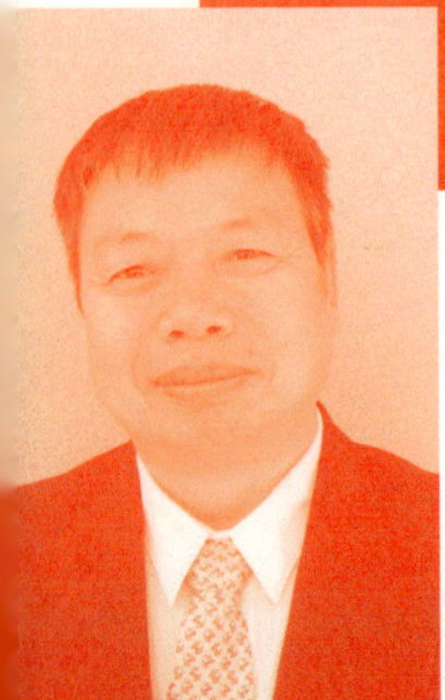
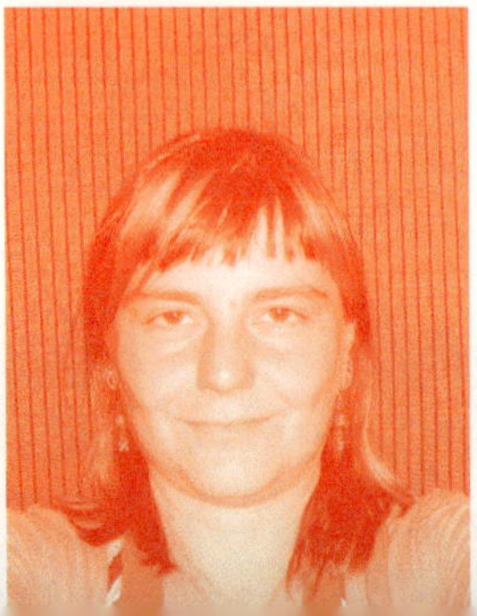

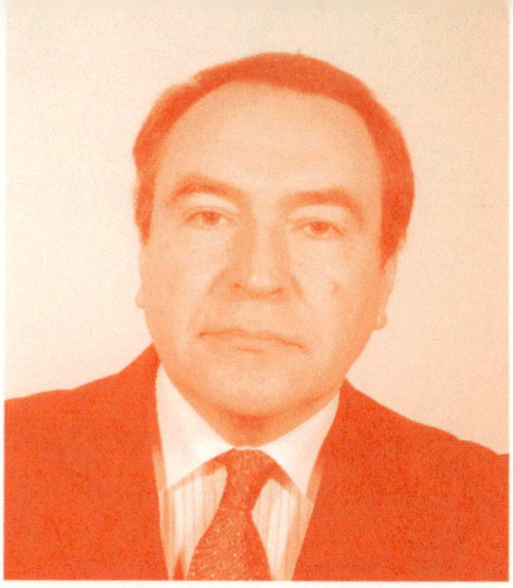
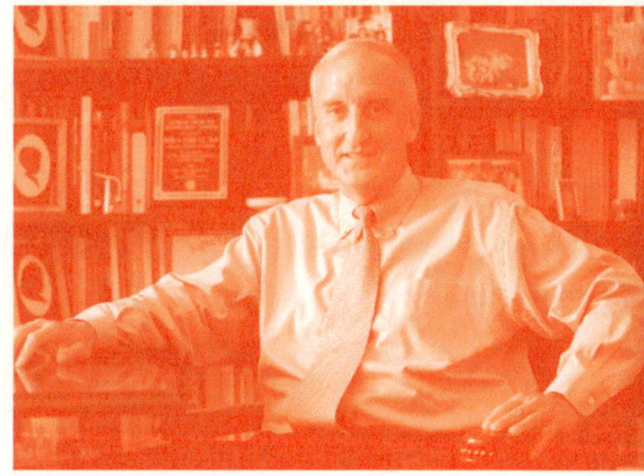
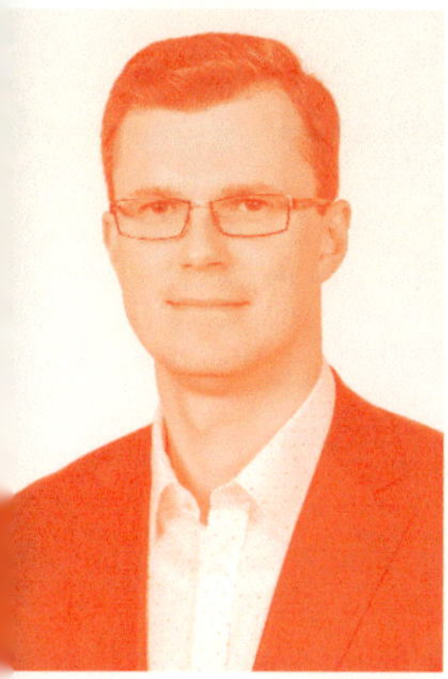
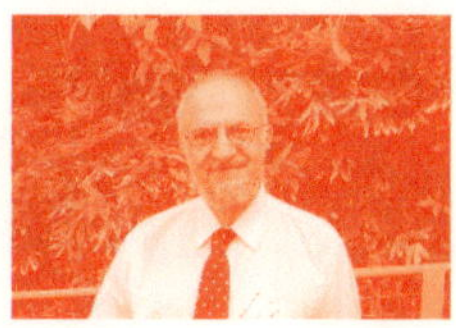
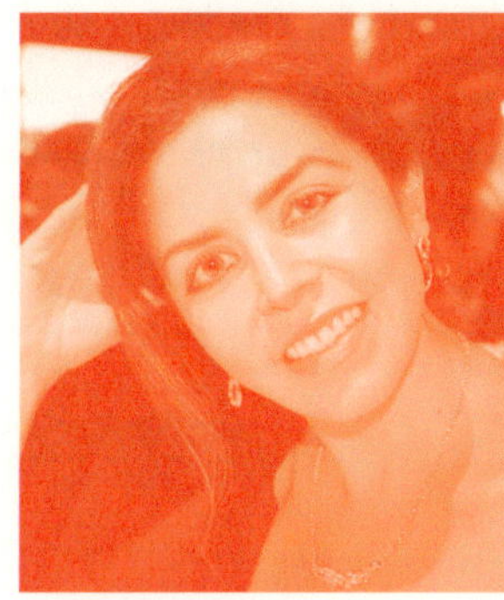

Supporting open minds since 2005

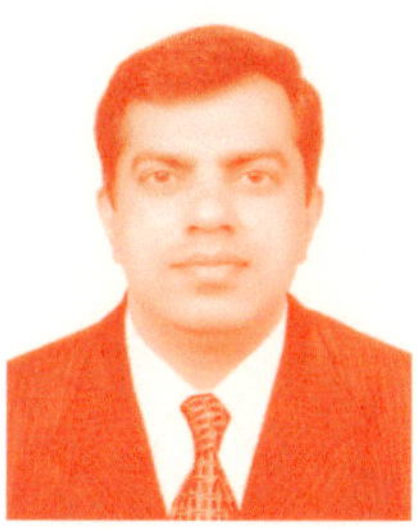
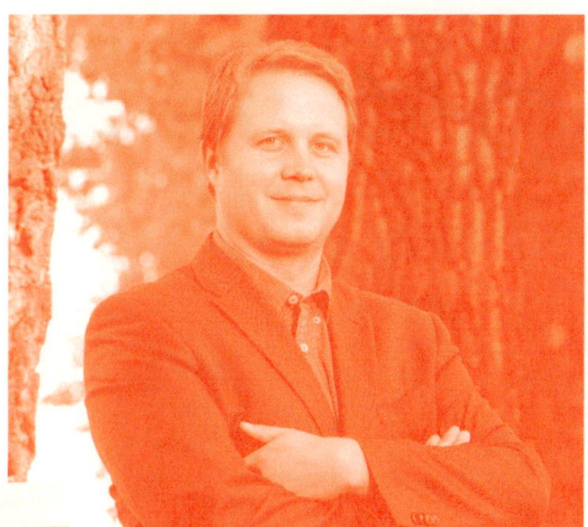
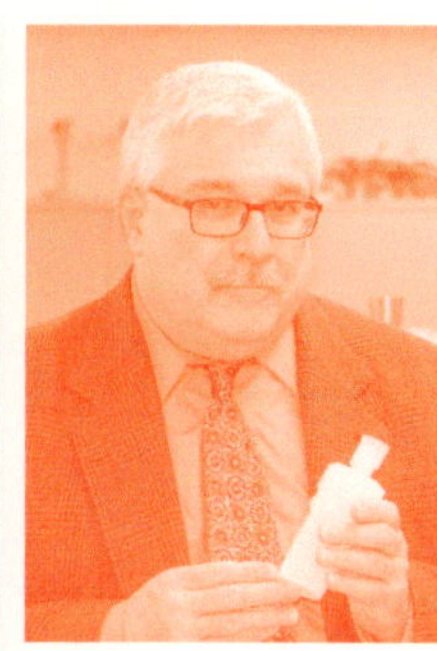
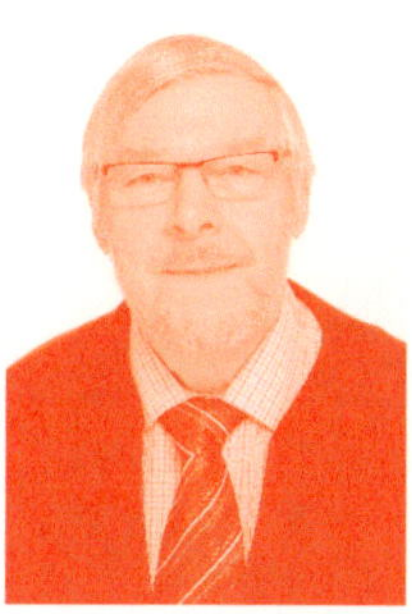
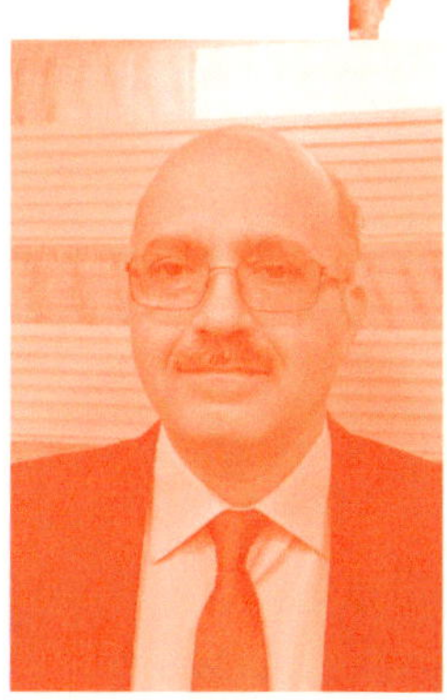
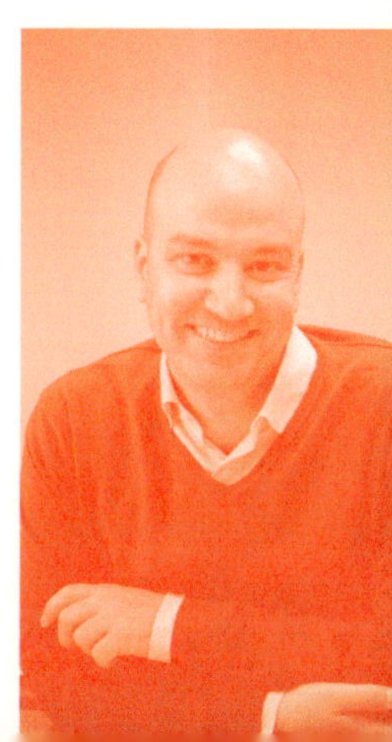
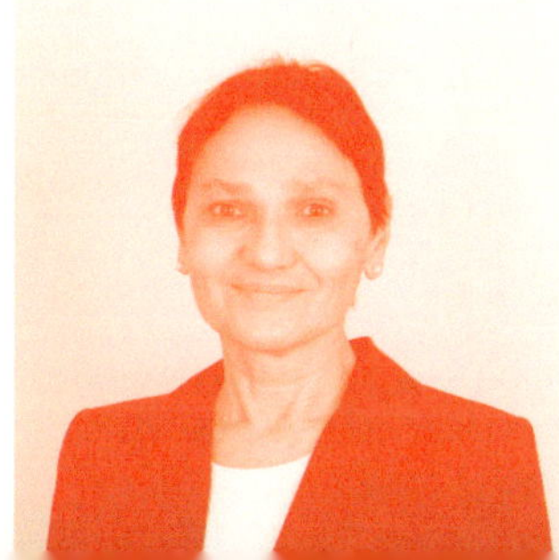

Brain and Spinal Tumors - Primary and Secondary
http://dx.doi.org/10.5772/intechopen.77682
Edited by Lee Roy Morgan and Feyzi Birol Sarica

Contributors
Jerzy Trojan, Saleh Rasras, Marcus Ware, Brody Stewart, Caleb Stewart, Andrew Rodgers, Meenu Gupta, Mushtaq Ahmad, Scott Turner, Breno Nery, Rodrigo Antônio Fernandes Costa, Eduardo Quaggio, Ricardo Araújo, Bernardo Barbosa, Diogo Melo, Carolina Nery, Fred Bernardes Filho, George Peter Stevens, Kensuke Tateishi, Tetsuya Yamamoto, Meral Kurt, Candan Demiröz Abakay, Ali Altay, Meredith Morgan, Feyzi Birol Sarica, Steven DiBiase, Jason Naziri, Vamsi Yerramneni, Ramanadha Reddy, Tirumal Yerragunta, Vasundhara S Rangan, Michael E. Ivan, Alexa Semonche, Daniel Eichberg, Philip Friedlander

First published in London, United Kingdom, 2020 by IntechOpen
IntechOpen is the global imprint of INTECHOPEN LIMITED, registered in England and Wales, registration number: 11086078, 7th floor, 10 Lower Thames Street, London, EC3R 6AF, United Kingdom
Printed in Croatia

British Library Cataloguing-in-Publication Data
A catalogue record for this book is available from the British Library

Additional hard and PDF copies can be obtained from orders@intechopen.com

Brain and Spinal Tumors - Primary and Secondary
Edited by Lee Roy Morgan and Feyzi Birol Sarica
p. cm.
Print ISBN 978-1-78984-157-2
Online ISBN 978-1-78984-158-9
eBook (PDF) ISBN 978-1-83962-794-1

For EU product safety concerns:
IN TECH d.o.o., Prolaz Marije Krucifikse Kozulić 3, 51000 Rijeka, Croatia, info@intechopen.com or visit our website at intechopen.com.

Meet the editors

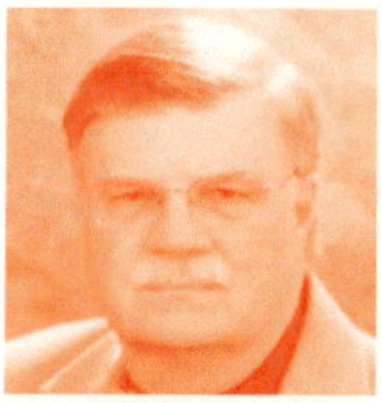

Dr. Lee Roy Morgan is a clinical pharmacologist and oncologist whose research interests are focused on the development of new and novel agents and devices that penetrate the CNS and spine and are effective therapies as treatment for both primary and metastatic malignancies involving the CNS. Dr. Morgan received his PhD degree in Organic Chemistry from Tulane University, New Orleans, Louisiana, USA, in 1960. He completed postdoctoral studies at Imperial College, University of London, in 1961. In 1971 He received his MD degree from Louisiana State University Medical School, New Orleans. From 1961 to 1986, he was Professor and Chairman, Department of Pharmacology, Louisiana State University Medical Center, New Orleans, Louisiana, USA. He founded DEKK-TEC, Inc., New Orleans, Louisiana, in 1983 and is CEO and Medical Director. In addition, he is Adjunct Professor of Medicine, Tulane University School of Medicine and Adjunct Research Professor of Chemistry, University of New Orleans, both in New Orleans, Louisiana, USA. He has published over 200 research articles and book chapters. Dr. Morgan is married with four children and seven grandchildren.

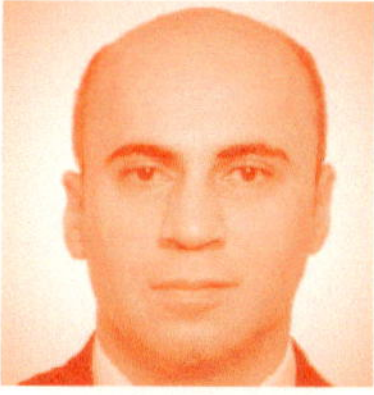

Feyzi Birol Sarıca, born in 1971 in Germany, graduated from the Medicine Faculty of Ankara University in 1997 and received the title medical doctor. In 2005, he gave his expert thesis called "Prognostic Factors in Supratentorial Glial Tumors" at the Neurosurgery Clinic of Ankara Numune Education and Research Hospital and received the title of neurosurgeon by the Turkish Board of Certification. He worked first as a neurosurgeon and lecturer in Adana Education and Research Hospital of Medicine Faculty of Baskent University between 2006 and 2015. He then worked at the Kudret International Hospital in Ankara in 2016. He started work as assistant professor at the Department of Neurosurgery of Medicine Faculty of Giresun University in 2017. He took the title of associate professor in March 2018. He is currently serving as the Chairman of the Giresun University Neurosurgery Department. He has participated in cerebrovascular surgery, hydrocephalus and spinal dysraphism, skull base surgery, and gamma-knife radiosurgery training courses. He is interested in general neurosurgery as well as neurooncology and cerebrovascular surgery.

Contents

Preface

Management of primary and metastatic malignancies involving the central nervous system (CNS) (brain and spine) remains a challenge. Although there have been significant improvements in responses to tumor target-directed therapies in recent years, surgery and radiation remain our primary approaches to the management of CNS malignancies. Advanced unresectable primary and secondary tumors of the CNS are commonly "resistant to systemic therapies" because of the lack of knowledge regarding the best mechanism(s) for drugs to penetrate the blood–brain barrier.

Since the book *New Approaches to the Management of Primary and Secondary CNS Tumors* (IntechOpen) was published in 2017, significant progress has been made: Phase I neurooncology trials for new drugs have increased worldwide, several drugs have been approved as target-specific immunotherapies for the management of brain and spinal malignancies, and new pathways for cancer cells to enter the CNS have been identified.

In addition, major advances in the management of CNS malignancies through molecular and imaging analyses, magnetic devices, and tumor-targeted immunotherapies with/without stereotactic radiosurgery are now available, many of which are discussed in this book. Moreover, the US FDA and other worldwide Orphan Designated Drug and Device programs are inducing incentives for the pharmaceutical and device industries to become more involved in the management of CNS malignancies.

There is light at the end of the tunnel!

Every chapter in *Brain and Spinal Tumors—Primary and Secondary* reviews development of new approaches through neurooncological collaborations, in-depth discussions, and/or reviews of diagnostic and therapeutic concepts that will improve the management of patients with neurooncology challenges.

Metastatic tumors involving the brain and spine are "increasing in occurrence" because drugs are effective versus periphery malignancies (lung, breast, etc.), but are not as effective versus brain and spine malignancies (primary and secondary). Overall, long-term responses for malignancies involving the CNS still remain depressing.

There remains a paucity of useful anticancer therapeutic tools for pediatric and adolescent oncology patients with tumors involving the CNS, who are otherwise healthy, but are seldom referred for clinical trials with novel new agents because they are <18 years of age. However, without new therapies, the management and support for the pediatric and adolescent age groups with primary and secondary CNS malignancies will remain inadequate; these are areas of oncology for which more clinical research efforts are badly needed.

However, in spite of the above deficiencies, the authors who have written chapters are "weaving their webs and establishing their roles in neurooncology." It is the editors' hopes that all readers are also pursuing their dreams and able to accomplish their goals. Only through new research endeavors and concepts are there possibilities of eradicating malignancies involving the CNS.

Each of us has been given the wisdom to reach our goals—just think about where we have been and where we are now—please do not stop!

In summary, it is an honor and pleasure to be an editor of *Brain and Spinal Tumors—Primary and Secondary'* and assist in bringing together dozens of clinicians and scientist-researchers to describe their research contributions that will benefit the neurooncology community's need for new advancements to improve the management of malignancies of the CNS.

Lee Roy Morgan, MD, PhD,
CEO,
DEKK-TEC, Inc.,
New Orleans, LA, United States

Feyzi Birol Sarica
Associate Professor,
Giresun University Faculty of Medicine,
Turkey

Section 1

Principles of Neuropharmacology and Experimental Therapeutics

Chapter 1

Principles of Neuropharmacodynamics: As Applied to Neuro-Oncology

Andrew H. Rodgers

Abstract

The blood-brain barrier (BBB) is a highly selective semi-permeable membrane that separates the cerebral blood circulation from the brain and extracellular fluid in the central nervous system (CNS). The BBB is composed of endothelial cells, astrocyte end-feet and pericytes embedded in the capillary basement membrane. This system allows the passage of water, some gases and lipid-soluble molecules by passive diffusion, as well as, selective molecules such as glucose and amino acids. This review discusses pharmacodynamic concepts and methods that allow drugs to penetrate the BBB structure and enter the CNS and spinal nervous systems (SNS).

Keywords: blood-brain barrier (BBB)

1. Introduction

The blood-brain barrier (BBB) was discovered over 100 years ago by Paul Ehrlich during his studies on the brain [1]. Ehrlich's early observations that water soluble dyes stained all organs of animals except for their brains and components of the central nervous system (CNS) was the key to our present day understanding of the BBB system. Subsequently, other researchers observed that dyes injected into the blood stream did not enter the brain hence a barrier existed between the two compartments [1].

The BBB differs from normal membranes in that it possesses tight junctions between an endothelial cell/astrocyte wall with no pores to allow for transport unless materials are lipophilic, water, and/or an actively transported. The BBB is also lipophilic, free of aqueous electrolytes and highly electrical resistant. However, the BBB compartment can be traversed by lipophilic substances through passive diffusion, while other molecules that are substrates for transferases cross by direct transport [1, 2].

The BBB prevents most systemic therapies from penetrating the brain; however, when cancer cells do penetrate the BBB from a peripheral origin, they generate neo-vascularization or cancer associated "vascular mimicry" structures (new blood vessels associated with tumor-generated penetrate breaks in the BBB) which can connect intracranial metastatic cancer cell colonies with the cerebral blood circulation [3]. If undesirable or toxic materials pass through the BBB into the CNS, a protective mechanism—the P-glycoprotein (P-gP) transfer system will transport toxic materials out of the CNS [4].

IntechOpen

Thus, developing new drugs that can exploit the cancer associated CNS "neo-angiogenic" vascularization that are not substrates for the P-gP system is of major interest and would be very useful in managing CNS and SNS malignancies.

Figure 1 shows a simplified diagram describing the BBB in relation to the brain (CNS) or spinal nervous system (SNS), the cerebral circulation and tumors growing in the CNS or SNS (**Figure 2**).

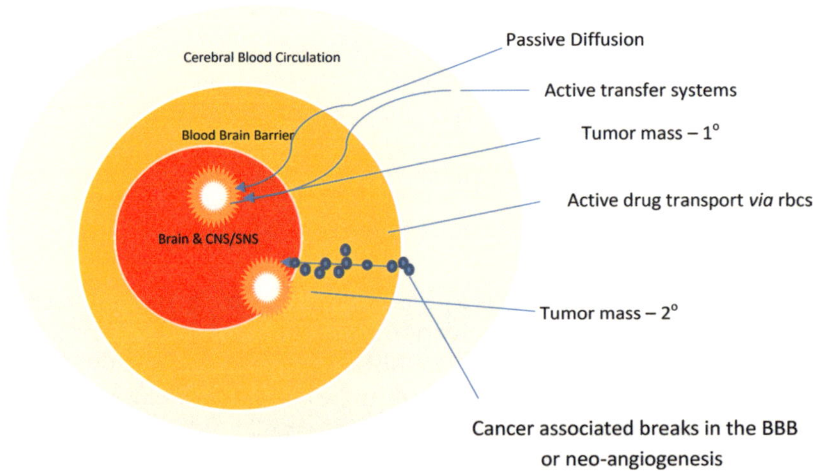

Figure 1.
Depicts three modes of drug transport to primary and secondary brain cancer tumors—direct passive permeability, active transport/transfer, and transport in association with RBCs (modified from Ref. [5]).

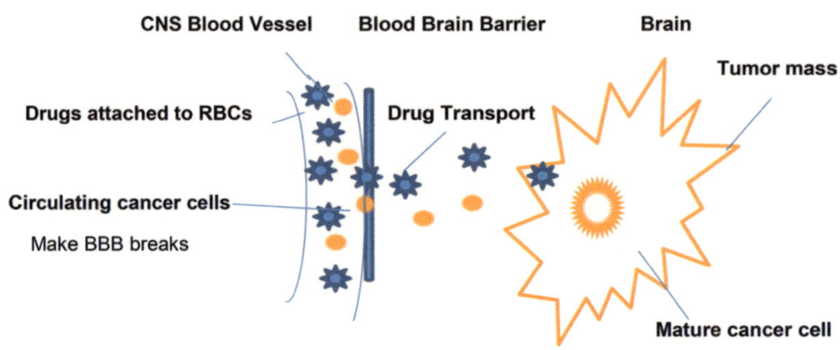

Figure 2.
Describes breaks in the BBB and neoangiogenesis that can be initiated by both metastatic and primary cancers in the CNS, allowing RBCs with drugs to cross the BBB and penetrate the CNS and tumor masses (modified from Ref. [5]).

2. Extravascular transport of cancer cells into the CNS

Not all cancer cells infiltrate the CNS or SNS by breaching the BBB. A recent report by Yao et al. describes how acute lymphocytic leukemia (ALL) cells possess a6 integrin receptors that bind to laminin, a glycoprotein molecule that covers the surfaces of the meninges, its nerve sheaths and blood vessels [6]. Tiny blood vessels pass directly from the bone marrow through the vertebrae to the meninges tissue that line the spinal cord, brain and the cerebral spinal fluid (CSF) circulation. ALL cells can attach to the outside of blood vessels and nerves in the bone marrow and migrate over the scaffolding proteins. Thus, ALL cells can slide into the CNS and

SNS via the scaffolding of the cerebral vascular circulation [6]. Other types of cancer may be able to do the same.

The next step is to design new agents to block the a6 integrin receptor [6].

3. Principles for selecting a drug for brain and spinal nervous systems—primary and secondary

Most therapy regimens for CNS and SNS cancers involve empirical protocols [7]. However, with the advent of tumor targeted and gene mutation designed immunotherapies, there are more selective therapeutic approaches to the management of cancers [8].

However, if a tumor lacks a specific tumor target antigen, genetic mutation or receptor glycoprotein, then a more individualized (personalized) approach is possible. Through in vitro sensitivity studies, cytotoxicity parameters (IC_{50}) vs. selected drugs can be identified for each individual tumor [9]. Obtaining tumor tissue for tumor molecular profiling can now be easily accomplished using liquid biopsy techniques and stem cell cultures [9, 13].

In addition, since drugs penetrate the tumors in the CNS and SNS by lipophilic and/or selective transport mechanism(s), the partition coefficient, *P* value, is also helpful in appreciating whether a drug has a chance of penetrating the lipid rich BBB membrane or if a more selective transportation system is required.

The log *P* value is an accurate and important molecular characteristic that defines lipophilicity and the ability of a drug to diffuse across the lipophilic BBB. This is can be easily measured by dissolving the drug in n-octanol and shaking with equal volumes of water. The concentration of drug is then measured in both phases and the ratio of concentration in n-octanol/water evaluated according to **Eq. 1** [10].

$$log\ P_{oct/wat} = log\left(\frac{[solute]_{octanol}}{[solute]_{water}^{un-ionized}}\right) \tag{1}$$

The estimation of drug penetrating through the BBB (log BB) is the concentration of drug in the brain divided by concentration in the blood [11].

Very lipophilic compounds also tend to be highly protein bound. For a drug to diffuse from the plasma (at pH 7.4) across the BBB (log BB) into the CSF, the ideal octanol-water partition coefficient is usually 1–10 and corresponds to a log *P* of 0–1 [12]. Others recommend higher values—log $P \leq 5$ [11].

In addition, when selecting a drug, the maximum concentration of drug in the plasma initially (C_{max}) and the total drug concentration available after a single treatment—area under the curve (AUC), will be of assistance to predict if sufficient concentration of the drug is present [13].

Thus, the combination of log *P*, AUC and an $IC_{10}/_{50}$ values will be of assistance with the selection for a potentially active/useful drug for a specific individual with cancer (**Table 1**).

The above introductory information provides the general principles which govern the entry of anti-cancer cells—passively or actively, into the CNS and SNS that must be considered. Plus, after entering the brain, chemicals and drugs must not be substrates for P-glycoprotein (P-gP) transfer systems; or at least not before they can penetrate cancer cells and perform their anti-cancer effects.

Compound	Structure	Calculated log *P*	Calculated BB[11]	Actual BB[12]
Cis-platinum	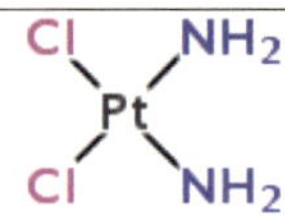	−2.83	0.09	0.05–1
Cytarabine	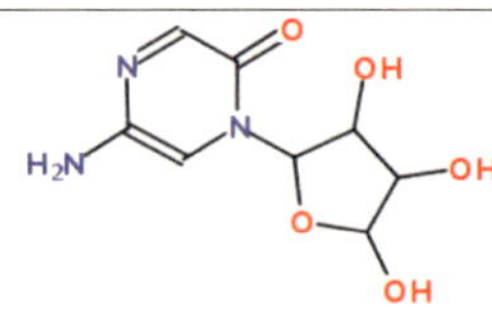	−2.77	0.1	1
Pentostatin	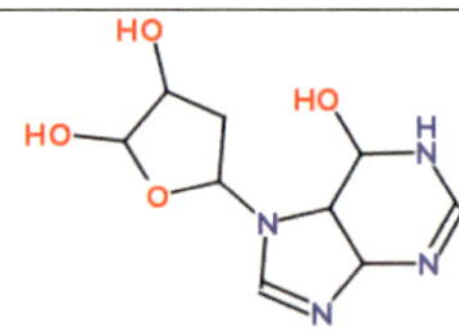	−2.35	0.13	0.1–0.13
Temozolomide	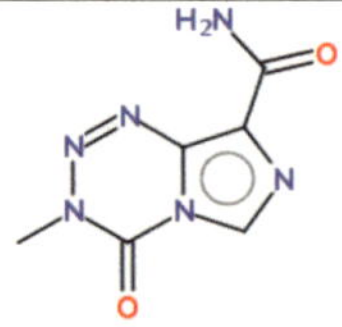	−1.9	0.18	0.19
Cladribine	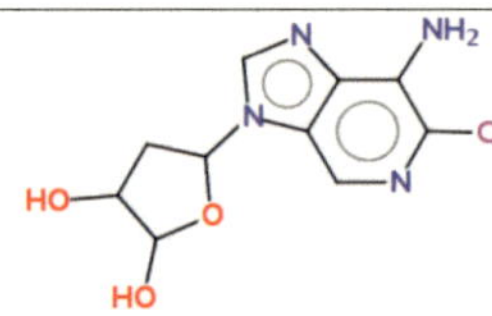	−0.38	0.64	0.25
Dacarbazine	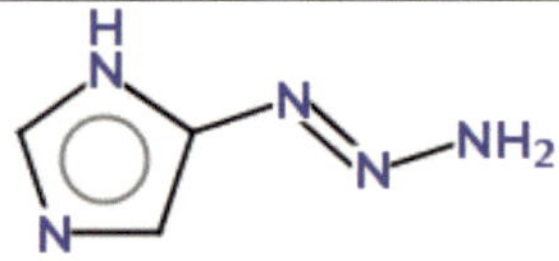	−0.35	0.69	0.14
Melphalan	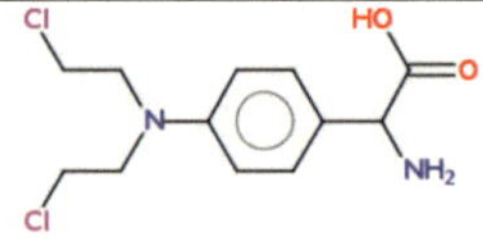	−0.01	0.86	0.01–0.1
Busulfan	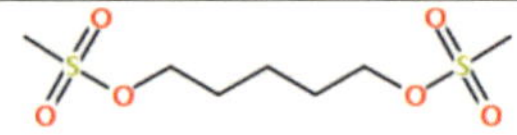	0.08	0.9	1
Topotecan	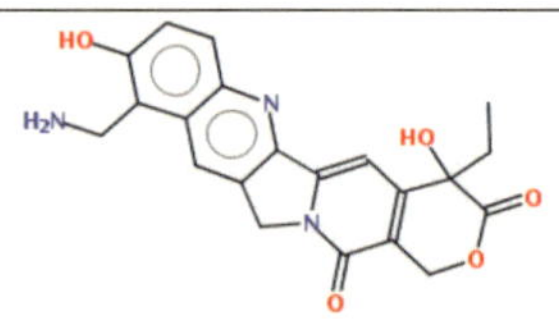	1.41	≥1	0.42
Carmustine	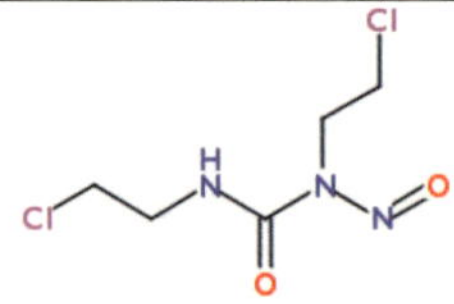	1.67	≥1	0.15–0.9
Lomustine	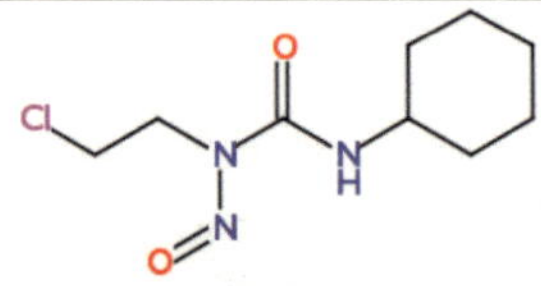	2.96	≥1	>0.5

Compound	Structure	Calculated log *P*	Calculated BB[11]	Actual BB[12]
DM-PEN	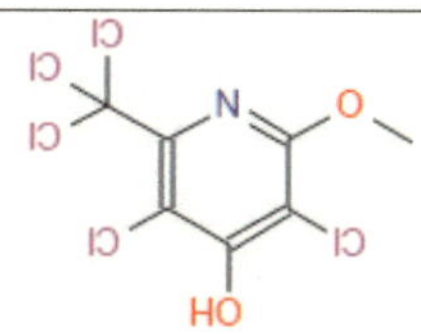	4.32	≥1	TBD
Penclomedine (PEN)	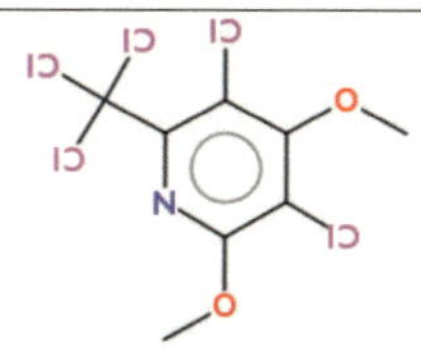	4.59	≥1	TBD
DMCHOCPEN	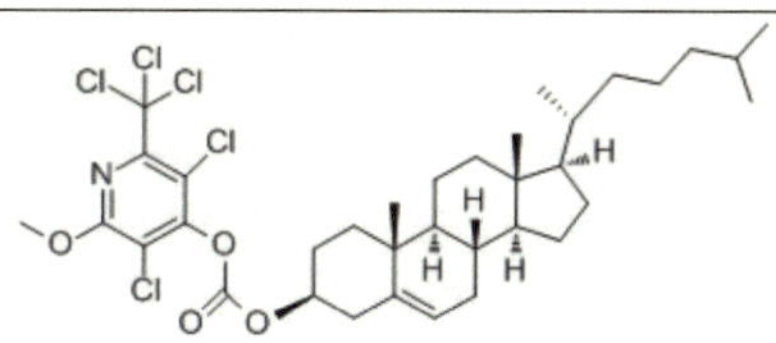	9.68	≥1	TBD

Note: Not shown in **Table 1** *is etoposide which has a low BB value of 0.05 and it is pumped out of the brain by the P-gP pump [14].*

Table 1.
Calculated and structure related activities for drugs with CNS activity [5].

4. Emerging technologies for crossing the brain blood barrier designing new agents

The medicinal chemists and molecular pathologists are constantly designing new agents for neuro-oncology. The goals are always the same—continue to develop new integrative drug designs vs. compliment specific receptors in the BBB or on vessels through which cancer cells penetrate the BBB.

5. Exosomes to deliver treatments across the blood-brain barrier

Matthew Wood et al. claim that exosomes can cross the blood-brain barrier and deliver siRNAs, antisense oligonucleotides, chemotherapeutic agents and proteins specifically to cells—normal and malignant in the brain [15]. Exosomes are cell-derived matrix-bound encapsulated vesicles that contain drugs [15]. They are naturally or synthetically generated, able to cross the blood-brain barrier and deliver poorly solubilized drugs into the CNS and directly to brain cancer, as well as other diseases. Again, they must be able to pass the BBB.

6. Nanoparticles

Nanoparticle drug delivery systems contain drugs bound to nanoparticles which are capable of traversing the blood-brain barrier [16]. Human serum albumin (HSA) is most widely used vehicle to design nanoparticles. The main benefits of HSA nanoparticles are that they are well tolerated with minimal side effects, as well as the albumin functional groups can be utilized for surface modification that allows for specific cell uptake. Nanoparticles have been shown to transverse the blood-brain barrier carrying host drugs into the brain [16]. To enhance the effectiveness of nanoparticles to cross the blood-brain barrier, attempts have been made to coat the nanoparticles with polysorbate to make them more permeable [16]. Polysorbate 80 coated nanoparticles containing doxorubicin delivered up to 6 μg/g concentrations of the drug into the brain after intravenous injections of 5 mg/kg of the drug/nanoparticles [16]. No detectable drug was observed when given alone or with the uncoated nanoparticles. This technology continues to have promise in neuro-oncology.

7. Prodrugs

CNS prodrugs are derivatized forms of active drugs that are unable to cross the BBB. Designing active molecules that are derivatized with lipids, amino acids, esters, salts, etc., can improve the former molecules' ability to penetrate the BBB more efficiently [14]. In situ in the CNS the prodrugs are metabolized or degenerated after crossing the BBB, releasing the active form of the drug [14].

There are still major drawbacks to the use of prodrugs to treat tumors in the CNS. First, the prodrug may be able to pass through the BBB; however, it may be transported out of the CNS by the P-gP transport system without ever releasing the active drug. Second, the sheer size of these derivatized molecules makes it very difficult to pass through the BBB.

Nevertheless, this is a very promising area for new research endeavors [14].

8. Peptide masking

Similar to the prodrug concept, another method to improve drug CNS bioavailability is through derivatizing drugs with peptides and amino acids that have select transfer pathways through the BBB and into the brain [17].

One example is through the use of cholesterol [13]. Although the brain synthesizes its own cholesterol for support and metabolism, cholesteryl derivatized drugs behave like lipids and penetrate the BBB secondary to be lipophilic [13]. This type of masking works well and aids in traversing the blood-brain barrier. Also, a "target molecule" could be attached to the drug that helps it pass through the barrier and then once inside the brain released. If the drug is not transported out of the brain, then it is available for therapeutic use [13].

However, drawbacks to the above exist as well. Once the drug is in the brain there is a point where it needs to be degraded to prevent toxic changes in the brain tissue. Also the drug may not be transported out of the brain and could become toxic with increased concentration. There must always be a mechanism for the removal of the active form of the drug from the brain [13].

9. Receptor-mediated permeators

Drugs that increase the permeability of the BBB are described as receptor-mediated permeators (RMP) [18]. By decreasing the restrictiveness of the BBB, it is much easier for a molecule to pass through the barrier. RMPs increase the permeability of the blood-brain barrier temporarily by increasing the osmotic pressure in the blood which loosen the junctions between the endothelial cells and pericytes. By loosening the junctions, drugs can pass through the BBB and be available as therapy vs. cancer cells. These drugs must be administered in a very controlled environment because of the risk associated with their use [18].

First, a major concern is that the brain can be flooded with the drugs that are in the blood that are usually blocked by the BBB. Secondly, when the tight junctions loosen, the homeostasis of the brain can also be compromised, which can result in seizures and other dysfunctional events in the brain.

10. Microbubble-enhanced focused ultrasound

Microbubbles are small "bubbles" of mono-lipids that are able to pass through the BBB. One obstacle to this, however is that these microbubbles are large, which often prevents their diffusion through the BBB and into the brain. This can be counteracted by focused ultrasound. Ultrasound increases the permeability of the BBB by causing interference in the tight junctions in the BBB. In combination with ultrasound therapy, a very specific area of diffusion will develop, because microbubbles can only diffuse where the ultrasound has disrupted the barrier [19, 20].

The hypothesis and usefulness of this combination is the possibility of loading a microbubble with an active drug to diffuse through the barrier and target a specific area in the brain or spine. There are several important factors that make this a viable solution for drug delivery. The first is that the loaded microbubble must not be substantially greater than the unloaded bubble. This ensures that the diffusion will be similar and the ultrasound disruption will be sufficient to induce diffusion. A second factor is that the stability of the loaded micro-bubble must be stable. This means that the drug is fully retained in the bubble and there is no leakage.

Lastly, it must be determined how the drug is to be released from the microbubble in the CNS once it passes through the BBB. Studies have documented the effectiveness of employing microbubble technology to get drugs to specific sites in the brain in animal models and humans [19, 20].

The author hopes that the concepts discussed herein will be useful to stimulate research ideas that ultimately may lead to new treatments and approaches to the management of CNS and SNS tumors—primary and secondary.

Acknowledgements

This review was supported by the following grants—NCI/SBIR grants—R43/44CA132257; R43CA203351; LACATS—U54 M104940-1.

Author details

Andrew H. Rodgers
University of New Orleans, Emeritus Adjunct, United States of America

*Address all correspondence to: ahrodgers@gmail.com

References

[1] Ribatti D, Nico B, Crivellato E, Artico M. Development of the blood-brain barrier: A historical point of view. Anatomical Record. Part B, New Anatomist. 2006;**289**:3-8

[2] Aleynik A, Gernavage M, Mourad KS, Sherman Y, Liu L, Gubenko K, et al. Stem cell delivery of therapies for brain disorders. Clinical and Translational Medicine. 2014;**3**:24. DOI: 10.1186/2001-1326-3-24

[3] Wrobel JK, Toborek M. Blood–brain barrier remodeling during brain metastasis formation. Molecular Medicine. 2016;**22**:32-40

[4] Schinkel AH. P-glycoprotein, a gatekeeper in the blood–brain barrier. Advanced Drug Delivery Reviews. 1999;**36**:2-3

[5] Rodgers AH, Morgan LR. NeuroPharmacology: As applied to designing new chemotherapeutic agents. Chapter 1. In: Morgan LR, editor. New Approaches to the Management of Primary and Secondary CNS Tumors. Croatia: InTech Publishing; 2017. pp. 3-19

[6] Yao H, Price TT, Cantelli G, Ngo B, Warner MJ, Olivere L, et al. Nature, leukemia hijacks a neural mechanism to invade the central nervous system. Nature. 2018;**560**:55-60

[7] Primary CNS Lymphoma Treatment (PDQ®): Health Professional Version. https://www.ncbi.nlm.nih.gov/pubmedhealth/PMH0032829/

[8] Farkona S, Diamandis EP, Blasutig IM. Cancer immunotherapy: The beginning of the end of cancer? BMC Medicine. 2016;**14**:73

[9] O'Brien PJ, Irwin W, Diaz D, et al. Archives of Toxicology. 2006;**80**:580-592 https://doi.org/10.1007/s00204-006-0091-3

[10] Bannan CC, Calabró G, Kyu DY, Mobley DL. Calculating partition coefficients of small molecules in octanol/water and cyclohexane/water. Journal of Chemical Theory and Computation. 2016;**12**:4015-4024

[11] Lipinski CA, Lombardo F, Dominy BW, Feeney PJ. Experimental and computational approaches to estimate solubility and permeability in drug discovery and development settings. Advanced Drug Delivery Reviews. 2001;**46**:3-26

[12] Nau R, Sörgel F, Eiffert H. Penetration of drugs through the blood-cerebrospinal fluid/blood-brain barrier for treatment of central nervous system infections. Clinical Microbiology Reviews. 2010;**23**:858-883

[13] Morgan LR. A rational for novel anti-neurooncology drugs. Chapter 15. In: Lichtor T, editor. Evolution of the Molecular Biology of Brain Tumors and the Therapeutic Implications. Croatia: InTech Publishing; 2013. pp. 435-458

[14] Salameh F, Karaman D, Mecca G, Scrano L, Bufo S, Karaman R. Prodrugs targeting the central nervous system (CNS). World Journal Pharmacy and Pharmaceutical Sciences. 2015;**4**:208-237

[15] Wood MJA, O'Loughlin AJ, Lakhal S. Exosomes and the Blood–Brain Barrier: Implications for Neurological Diseases. Published Online: 14 Sep 2011. https://doi.org/10.4155/tde.11.83

[16] Sebak S, Mirzaei M, Malhotra M, Kulamarva A, Prakash S. Human serum albumin nanoparticles as an efficient noscapine drug delivery system for potential use in breast cancer:

Preparation and *in vitro* analysis. International Journal of Nanomedicine. 2010;**5**:525-532

[17] Upadhyay RK. Drug delivery systems, CNS protection, and the blood brain barrier. BioMed Research International. 2014:869269. DOI: 10.1155/2014/869269

[18] Lajoie JM, Shusta EV. Targeting receptor-mediated transport for delivery of biologics across the blood-brain barrier. Annual Review of Pharmacology and Toxicology. 2015;**55**:613-631

[19] Fan C-H, Yeh C-K. Microbubble-enhanced focused ultrasound-induced blood–brain barrier opening for local and transient drug delivery in central nervous system disease. Journal of Medical Ultrasound. 2014;**22**:183-193

[20] Carpentier A, Canney M, Vignot A, Reina V, Beccaria K, Horodyckid C, et al. Clinical trial of blood-brain barrier disruption by pulsed ultrasound. Science Translational Medicine. 2016;**8**:343-347

Section 2

Diagnosis of CNS Tumors

Chapter 2

IDH-Mutant Gliomas

Kensuke Tateishi and Tetsuya Yamamoto

Abstract

Isocitrate dehydrogenase (*IDH*) mutation is one of the most critical genomic alterations in lower grade and secondary glioblastoma patient. More than 90% of *IDH* mutation is located at codon R132 of *IDH1* gene. *IDH* mutation produces oncometabolite "2-hydroxyglutarate" and induces epigenetic alteration, such as DNA global methylation and histone methylation. As a result, *IDH* mutation promotes early gliomagenesis. Since *IDH* mutation is the earliest genomic event and almost always retained during tumor progression, *IDH* mutation is expected as novel therapeutic target. Herein, we review the clinical characteristics of *IDH*-mutant gliomas, biological role of *IDH* mutation for gliomagenesis, and current and future therapeutic approach for *IDH* mutant tumors.

Keywords: *IDH* mutation, glioma, 2-hydroxyglutarate, tumor biology, cancer metabolism, target therapy

1. Introduction

The WHO 2016 classification integrates molecular and histological features in the diagnosis of gliomas. Among numerous genomic alterations, the *isocitrate dehydrogenase* (*IDH*) mutation is one of the most important genetic alterations found in this kind of tumor. As *IDH* mutation is a ubiquitous mutation in lower grade gliomas, the development of molecular target therapies against *IDH* mutations is expected. Here, we review *IDH*-mutant gliomas, focusing on their role in tumorigenesis and as novel therapeutic targets.

2. Discovery of *IDH* mutations in cancers

The presence of an *isocitrate dehydrogenase* (*IDH*) mutation was first discovered in colorectal cancers [1]. Parsons et al. [2] found mutations of the *IDH1* (2q.33) in 12% of the glioblastomas (GBMs). Other large scale studies validated that *IDH1* and *IDH2* (*IDH*) mutations were found in the majority of secondary GBM and lower grade (WHO grade II and III) gliomas, whereas these were rarely found in adult primary and pediatric GBMs [2–4]. Almost all of the *IDH1* mutations occur at codon 132, >90% of them exhibit a c.395G>A (R132H) substitution, followed by R132C [3, 5, 6]. Although the frequency was low, *IDH2* mutations were also identified at codon 172 in gliomas [4, 7].

Besides, *IDH* mutation was found in hematopoietic cancers, including acute myeloid leukemia (AML; 10–15%, *IDH2*) [8, 9], angioimmunoblastic T-cell lymphoma (AITL, 20%) [10], chondrosarcoma (~50%) [11–13], intrahepatic cholangiocarcinoma (15–20%, *IDH1*) [13], and at lower frequency in other hematopoietic and solid cancers, such as B-acute lymphoblastic leukemia (B-ALL), esophageal cancer, colorectal cancer, melanoma, prostate carcinoma, and breast adenocarcinoma [1, 4, 14–16].

3. Tumorigenesis of *IDH*-mutant gliomas

3.1 Genomic characteristics of *IDH*-mutant glioma

The discovery of *IDH* mutations allowed the distinction of primary GBM, which is genetically characterized by *TERT* promoter mutation, gene alteration of epidermal growth factor receptor (*EGFR*), phosphatase and tensin homolog (*PTEN*) mutation or deletion, trisomy 7, monosomy 10, and cyclin-dependent kinase inhibitor 2A (*CDKN2A*) homozygous deletion, from secondary GBM (GBM, *IDH*-mutant) [3, 5, 17, 18].

In astrocytic tumors, most of the tumor cells have co-mutations in *IDH1, TP53*, and *ATRX*. Moreover, WHO 2016 [19] defined the presence of *IDH* mutation and co-deletion of chromosome1p and 19q as necessary for the diagnosis of oligodendroglial tumors. Also, in oligodendroglial tumors, *TERT* promoter mutation is almost always present (>95%), while *CIC and FUBP1* are commonly (>40%) observed. These genetic abnormalities for astrocytic and oligodendroglial tumors are mutually exclusive [20–24]. Importantly, the *IDH* mutation is the earliest genetic alteration observed; it is commonly retained during tumor progression [25–28], but in a subset of mutants, *IDH1* was either deleted or amplified at tumor recurrence [29], indicating the critical role of *IDH* mutation for tumorigenesis. It has also been shown that *IDH* mutations do not select or create *ATRX* or *TERT* promoter mutations [30].

3.2 Developmental hierarchy in *IDH*-mutant gliomas

Two recent large scale single cell RNA-sequencing studies revealed a developmental hierarchy in *IDH1*-mutant gliomas [31, 32]. Accordingly, *IDH1*-mutant astrocytoma and oligodendroglioma shared a similar developmental hierarchy, consisting of three subpopulations of malignant cells: nonproliferative astrocytic and oligodendrocytic cells, proliferative, and undifferentiated neural stem/progenitor cells. In contrast, tumor micro environment (TME) was different in the abundance microglia/macrophage cells between astrocytic and oligodendroglial tumors. TME also differs between astrocytic tumors of different grades. Though TME and genomic alterations are distinctive, evidence indicates the existence of common progenitor cells in *IDH1*-mutant gliomas. In higher grade tumors, undifferentiated glioma stem/progenitor cells were increased [32]. In addition, almost all proliferating cancer cells were composed of subpopulations of undifferentiated cells (stem-like) in oligodendroglioma [31], suggesting a significant role for undifferentiated cells in cell proliferation and malignant progression.

3.3 *IDH*-mutant xenograft model

Although *IDH1* mutation induced proliferation *in vitro* [33], *IDH1* mutation did not promote xenograft formation [34–36]. Intriguingly, Bardella et al. [37] demonstrated that IDH1^{R132H} overexpression in the murine subventricular zone induced the formation of early gliomagenesis, where stem and transit amplifying/progenitor cell populations were expanded, indicating the pivotal role of *IDH1* mutation in glioma formation. Moreover, Wakimoto et al. demonstrated that "tertiary mutations," such as *PIK3CA* mutation, *PDGFRA* amplification, and *MYC* amplification, promote

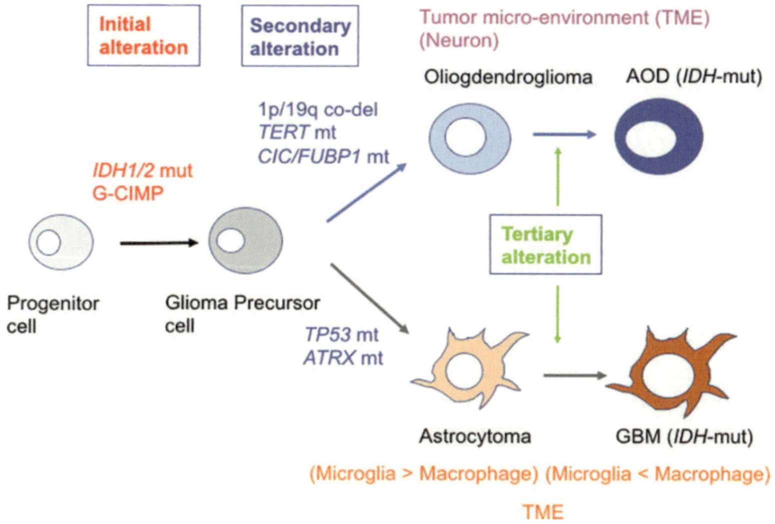

Figure 1.
Genomic alteration and tumor microenvironment in IDH-mutant astrocytic and oligodendroglial tumors.

IDH1-mutant glioma formation in xenograft models. Importantly, tumor harboring tertiary mutations were associated with unfavorable prognosis in *IDH1*-mutant glioma patients [38]. Recently, large genomic analyses demonstrated that malignant progression in *IDH1*-mutant glioma is associated with the *PI3K* pathway and *MYC* activation [39, 40]. Thus, *IDH* mutation induces gliomagenesis, whereas tertiary mutations are critical to promote tumor progression in lower grade gliomas (**Figure 1**).

4. The 2016 WHO classification

The 2016 World Health Organization (WHO) Classification of Tumors of the Central Nervous System (CNS) integrated phenotypic and genotypic parameters for CNS tumor classification. According to this classification, all diffusely infiltrating gliomas are grouped as diffuse astrocytic and oligodendroglial tumors. These tumors were histologically and genetically classified based on the presence of *IDH* mutation, co-deletion of chromosome1p and 19q, or *ATRX* and *TP53* mutations. Accordingly, gliomas are classified as follows: (1) diffuse astrocytoma (WHO grade II) or anaplastic astrocytoma (AA, WHO grade III): *IDH*-mutant, -wildtype, or not otherwise specified (NOS); (2) oligodendroglioma (WHO grade II) or anaplastic oligodendroglioma (WHO grade III): *IDH*-mutant and 1p/19q-codeleted or NOS; (3) oligoastrocytoma (grade II) and anaplastic oligoastrocytoma (WHO grade III): NOS; (4) GBM (WHO grade IV): *IDH*-mutant, -wildtype, or NOS; and (5) diffuse midline glioma (WHO grade IV): H3K27M-mutant.

IDH-wildtype GBM (about 90% of cases) is known as primary GBM, while *IDH*-mutant GBM (about 10% of cases) corresponds to secondary GBM [19].

5. Epidemiology of *IDH*-mutant gliomas

5.1 Age distribution of *IDH*-mutant gliomas

According to some statistical analyses, the *IDH*-mutant GBM or anaplastic astrocytoma patients were more than 20 years younger than those with

IDH-wildtype GBM [4]. In contrast, *IDH*-mutant GBM patients were only 4 years older than those with *IDH1*-mutant grade II and III astrocytoma [41]. This indicates that *IDH*-mutant glioma arises earlier than *IDH*-wildtype glioma (mostly GBM).

5.2 Prognosis of *IDH*-mutant gliomas

Parsons et al. [2] initially demonstrated that *IDH1*-mutant GBM patients survived about threefold longer than those with *IDH1*-wildtype GBM. Other groups verified that *IDH1* mutation is a favorable prognostic biomarker in gliomas [4, 42, 43]. In addition to GBM, large amounts of clinical studies indicated that the *IDH* mutation was an independent prognostic factor in grade II and III gliomas [4, 28, 43–47]. Notably, the prognosis of *IDH1*-mutant GBM is better than of *IDH1*-wildtype AA [48]. Also, a prospective randomized study (NOA-04) revealed that *IDH1* mutation, hypermethylation of the *O^6-methylguanine DNA-methyltransferase* (*MGMT*) promoter, age, extent of resection, and oligodendroglial histology are independent prognostic factors in anaplastic gliomas [44]. Among them, the impact of *IDH1* mutation conferred a stronger favorable prognosis than 1p/19q co-deletion, *MGMT* promoter methylation, and histology [44]. Collectively, *IDH1* mutation is a convincing prognostic factor in gliomas, irrespective of tumor grade and histology.

5.3 Prognostic classification for gliomas

Suzuki et al. [28] distinguished lower grade gliomas on the basis of the presence of *IDH1* mutation, *TP53* mutation, and 1p/19q co-deletion. Accordingly, tumors were classified into three groups: type I (*IDH1*-mutant with 1p/19q co-deletion; favorable prognostic group), type II (*IDH1*-mutant with TP53 mutation; intermediate prognostic group), and type III (*IDH1*-wildtype; poor prognostic group). Eckel-Passow et al. [47] classified gliomas into five groups based on the mutation status of *IDH1* and *TERT* promoter and on 1p/19q co-deletion. This group also demonstrated that *TERT* promoter mutations and *ATRX* alterations provided additional information for a tailored prognostic classification [49]. Besides, Arita et al. [50] proposed a classification of grade II–IV gliomas based on the mutations in *IDH* and the hotspot in *TERT* promoter.

Among *IDH*-mutant astrocytic tumors, *CDKN2A/B* homozygous deletion was demonstrated to be an unfavorable prognostic molecular marker [51]. Similarly, another group demonstrated that *PIK3R1* mutation and altered retinoblastoma pathway genes, including *RB1* and *CDKN2A*, were independent predictors of poor survival in astrocytic tumors. In oligodendrogliomas, NOTCH pathway inactivation and PI3K pathway activation were associated with poor prognosis [52, 53]. Collectively, these molecular markers could predict prognosis in glioma patients.

6. The mechanism of tumorigenesis in *IDH1*-mutant gliomas

6.1 *IDH* mutation drives production of oncometabolite D-2-hydroxyglutarate

In humans, IDH is composed of three types of isozymes (IDH1, IDH2, and IDH3). IDH1 is located in the cytoplasm and peroxisomes, whereas IDH2 and IDH3 are localized in the mitochondria and are involved in the TCA cycle. IDH1 and IDH2 are NADP+ dependent, whereas IDH3 is NAD+ dependent. IDH converts isocitrate into α-ketoglutarate (α-KG). No mutation in *IDH3* has been detected in human cancers. If *IDH* is mutated, it blocks normal enzymatic activity and instead produces D-2-hydroxyglutarate (2-HG) from α-KG in an NADPH dependent manner, irrespective of the substituted amino acid [54–56]. Compared with *IDH*-wildtype cells, the 2-HG level in *IDH*-mutant cells is 50–100-fold higher [54, 57]. *IDH* mutations are almost always heterozygous, and both mutant and wildtype *IDH1* alleles are required for 2-HG production in glioma cells [58].

6.2 *IDH*-mutation induced epigenetic alterations

6.2.1 IDH-mutation inducible DNA hypermethylator phenotype

Since the structure of 2-HG is similar to that of α-KG, 2-HG inhibits a variety of α-KG-dependent dioxygenases [59, 60]. Among them, 10–11 translocation-2 (TET2) induces global demethylation of DNA by catalyzing the conversion of 5-methylcytosine (5-mC) to 5-hydroxymethylcytosine (5-hmC). Forced mutant *IDH1* caused increased 5mC concentrations, instead of decreased 5hmC [37, 61]. *IDH* mutation also promotes methylation of DNA by TET2 inhibition, resulting in a glioma CpG island methylator phenotype (G-CIMP), a specific DNA methylation pattern in *IDH*-mutant tumor cells [61–63]. Indeed, forced overexpression of mutant *IDH* ($IDH1^{R132H}$ and $IDH2^{R172K}$) produced high concentrations of 2-HG and increased global 5-mC levels [61]. Similarly, *TET2* mutations, which are mutually exclusive to *IDH* mutations, induce a global hypermethylation signature [61]. Turcan et al. [64] demonstrated that a G-CIMP-like phenotype and G-CIMP positive proneural glioblastomas were formed after the introduction of an *IDH1* mutation into normal human astrocytes (NHA). These data indicate that mutant *IDH* induced TET2 suppression, followed by G-CIMP, in cancer cells. Consistent with *IDH*-mutant glioma patients, glioma patients with G-CIMP are younger at diagnosis and survive longer than those without G-CIMP [62]. Intriguingly, about 10% of G-CIMP tumors were relapsed as G-CIMP low tumors with poor clinical outcome [65].

The Cancer Genome Atlas (TCGA) performed comprehensive transcriptome analysis. Accordingly, GBM was classified into four groups (classic, mesenchymal, proneural, and neural groups). Aberrations and gene expression of *EGFR* and *NF1* define the classical and mesenchymal subtypes, whereas tumors with an *IDH1* mutation were classified within the proneural group. The proneural group is also accompanied by a *PDGFRA* gene abnormality and the G-CIMP feature [66]. DNA methylation induced by the *IDH1* mutation caused hypermethylation at cohesion and CCCTC-binding factor (CTCF) binding sites and compromised the binding of the insulator protein. As a result, loss of CTCF at a domain permits a constitutive enhancer to interact aberrantly with the receptor tyrosine kinase gene *PDGFRA* [67].

6.2.2 IDH mutation promotes global histone methylation

IDH mutation is also known to increase histone methylation. Lysine methylation of histone tails modifies chromatin structure and regulates gene expression. By competition with α-KG, 2-HG inhibits histone demethylases including members of the Jumonji transcription factor family (JMJD2A, JMJD2C/KDM4C, and JHDM1A/FBXL11), resulting in histone hypermethylation [68]. Indeed, hypermethylation in H3K4me1, H3K4me3, H3K9me2, H3K27me2, H3K79me2, H3K27me3, H3K9me3, and H3K36me3 was observed in cells with exogenous 2-HG or mutant *IDH1* induction [60, 63, 64, 69]. Sasaki et al. [63] also demonstrated that $IDH1^{R132H}$ knock in mice showed significantly increased early hematopoietic progenitors, histone hypermethylation, and DNA methylation. Interestingly, the elevation of H3K9me3 levels was observed earlier than the DNA methylation change in NHA upon IDH1^{R132H} induction [69], suggesting that histone methylation may be an early event in *IDH1*-mutant cancers. The hypermethylation of histones blocks cell differentiation in cancer cells [60, 63, 64, 69]. Using a histone demethylating agent or a specific mutant IDH1 inhibitor, suppressed cell differentiation can be restored [70, 71]. Besides, 2-HG impairs collagen maturation, which leads to basement membrane aberrations that play a part in glioma progression [72]. Taken together, these data show that DNA hypermethylation and histone methylation promote tumorigenesis through a wide range of gene function changes (**Figure 2**).

6.3 *IDH* mutation inducible metabolic alterations

In addition to the epigenetic changes, *IDH1* mutation is known to alter hypoxia inducible factor 1α (HIF-1α) activity. Under oxidative conditions, α-KG-dependent prolyl hydroxylases (PHDs), which form the Egl nine homolog (EglN) families, induce HIF-1α hydroxylation. Hydroxylated protein is then bound by the von Hippel-Lindau tumor suppressor protein (VHL), ubiquitylated, and degraded via proteasome. In contrast, under hypoxia, the hydroxylation reaction is inhibited and HIF-1α is upregulated. HIF-1α then activates the transcription of several genes to mediate a switch from oxidative to glycolytic metabolism and induces angiogenesis by regulating the expression of vascular endothelial growth factor (VEGF) [73, 74]. Koivunen et al. [33] demonstrated that *IDH1* mutation attenuates HIF-1α through the activation of HIF prolyl 4-hydroxylase (EGLN), enhancing the proliferation and soft agar growth of NHA.

While several studies demonstrated that the *IDH1* mutation induced aerobic glycolysis via HIF-1α activity [59, 75], other group reported that HIF-1α responsive genes, including lactate dehydrogenase (LDHA) were downregulated; silenced LDHA was associated with increased methylation of the LDHA promoter [76]. Another group showed that *IDH1* mutation reduces pyruvate flux to lactate and suppresses monocarboxylate transporters MCT1 and MCT4, which mediate lactate transmembrane transport [77]. *IDH* mutation also alters pyruvate metabolism, including pyruvate dehydrogenase and pyruvate carboxylase enzymes, resulting in anaplerosis of the TCA cycle [78, 79].

Cancer cells are known to depend on reductive carboxylation (RC) of glutamine-derived α-KG for *de novo* lipogenesis under hypoxia [80]. It is worth noticing

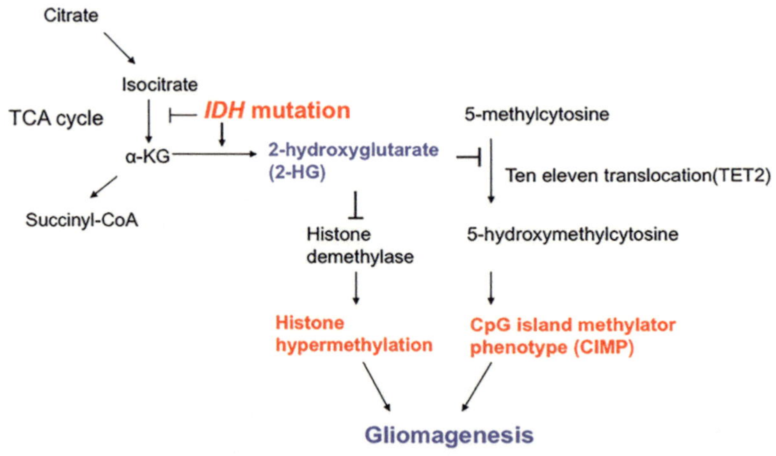

Figure 2.
Biological role of IDH mutation to induce gliomagenesis.

that the RC pathway is inhibited by *IDH* mutation [55]. Under hypoxia, *IDH1* mutation upregulated the contribution of glutamine to lipogenesis [81, 56].

Altered amino acids, glutathione, choline derivatives, and tricarboxylic acid (TCA) cycle intermediates were observed in *IDH*-mutant cells [82, 83]. Glutamate dehydrogenase (GDH)1 and GDH2 were overexpressed in *IDH1*-mutant tumors, and the orthotopic growth of an *IDH1*-mutant glioma is inhibited by a double GDH1/2 knockdown [84]. Another group demonstrated that GDH2 was critical for IDH1-mutation induced metabolic alterations and IDH1-mutant glioma growth [85]. The presence of 2-HG also inhibited ATP synthase and mTOR signaling [41].

Importantly, branched-chain amino acid transaminase (BCAT), which catalyzes the α-KG to glutamate conversion, was expressed at lower levels in *IDH1*-mutant gliomas than in *IDH1*-wildtype [86, 87]. As a result, the glutamate level was decreased, and cell proliferation and invasiveness were suppressed in *IDH*-mutant gliomas [87].

7. Role of extensive resection in *IDH1*-mutant gliomas

There is a huge amount of evidence showing that surgical resection has a pivotal role in survival benefit of glioma patients. Extensive resection is known to prolong survival in low grade glioma and also in GBM (*IDH1*-wildtype) [88–91]. In *IDH1*-mutant gliomas, an MRI study demonstrated that *IDH1*-mutant tumors were rarely located in high risk areas of the brain and show unilateral patterns of growth, sharp tumor margins, and less contrast enhancement [92, 93]. Indeed, radiographic atlas revealed *IDH1*-mutant gliomas were frequently located at frontal lobe [94]. A diffusion-tensor imaging study demonstrated that *IDH*-mutant GBM has a less invasive phenotype than *IDH*-wildtype GBM [95]. Intriguingly, patients with *IDH1*-wildtype gliomas had a reduced neurocognitive function and lower performance score than those with *IDH1*-mutant gliomas [96]. In addition, lesion volume was not associated with neurocognitive function for patients with *IDH1*-mutant tumors, but associated for those with *IDH1*-wildtype tumors [96]. Consequently, *IDH1*-mutant gliomas may be relatively less invasive to the surrounding eloquent area than *IDH*-wildtype GBM.

In addition, Beiko et al. [97] reported that extensive resection, including nonenhancing area, prolonged survival in *IDH1*-mutant anaplastic astrocytoma and glioblastoma. They also mentioned, since *IDH1*-mutant gliomas were predominantly located at frontal lobe, that maximal resection was relatively amenable. Another group independently demonstrated that gross total resection extended survival in grade III *IDH1*-mutant gliomas without 1p/19q co-deletion [98]. In contrast, survival advantage was controversial in grade II astrocytoma [99, 100]. These results suggest that for *IDH1*-mutant gliomas, especially grade III astrocytoma, maximal resection should be considered.

8. Prediction of *IDH* status

To establish *IDH* status-based treatment strategies, including surgery, advanced preoperative or intraoperative molecular analysis is important. Magnetic resonance spectroscopy (MRS) can be used to detect 2-HG and glutamate changes [101–107]. A recent MRS study demonstrated that 2-HG peaks rapidly decrease in accordance with tumor regression, whereas they increase with tumor progression in *IDH*-mutant gliomas [108], suggesting that 2-HG concentration, measured by MRS, may be a reliable approach to evaluate disease states in *IDH*-mutant gliomas.

In addition, several MR techniques, including diffusion tensor imaging and MR methods for determining relative cerebral blood volume, have been proposed to detect mutant *IDH1* noninvasively [109–111]. Moreover, T2-FLAIR mismatch sign was found as a highly specific imaging marker for *IDH*-mutant astrocytoma [112–114]. Intraoperative technologies to assess *IDH1* mutation have also been established [115–117]. These advanced technologies may allow the development of tailored surgical strategies for *IDH*-mutant gliomas. Other group demonstrated that urinary 2-HG is increased in patients with *IDH1*-mutant gliomas [118]. These findings indicate the possibility of application of indirectly assessed 2-HG as a clinical biomarker.

9. Treatment vulnerability in *IDH*-mutant gliomas

9.1 Radiotherapy for *IDH*-mutant gliomas

It has been shown that there is a higher relative sensitivity to radiotherapy and concurrent temozolomide (TMZ) in *IDH1*-mutant GBM patients than in those with *IDH1*-wildtype GBM [119], although there is no prospective clinical evidence of radiation therapy to extend survival in glioma patients with *IDH1* mutation. As described above, *IDH* mutation inhibits NADPH and glutamate production, resulting in reduced glutathione levels and increased reactive oxygen species (ROS) [120–123]. Conversely, radiosensitivity in *IDH1*-mutant tumors was diminished by IDH1 inhibitor [124]. These findings support selective vulnerability to radiation therapy in *IDH*-mutant gliomas.

9.2 Chemotherapeutic evidence for *IDH*-mutant gliomas

9.2.1 Temozolomide

Current standard management of GBM consists of surgical tumor resection, following local radiotherapy with temozolomide treatment [125]. Additionally, adjuvant TMZ prolonged survival in anaplastic astrocytoma [126]. Several studies demonstrated *IDH1*-mutation as a predictive biomarker for TMZ sensitivity in low grade gliomas and secondary GBM [127, 128].

Cytotoxicity of TMZ is provoked by the formation of O^6-methylguanine (O^6G)-DNA adducts. O^6G-DNA adducts induce DNA strand break and apoptosis through the O^6G-thymine-mediated mismatch repair pathway [129, 130]. It has also been established that the activation of DNA repairing pathways, including methylguanine methyltransferase (MGMT) repair enzyme, together with mismatch repair (MMR) system proteins deficiency, such as mutation-induced MSH2 and MSH6, result in drug resistance [131–133]. *MGMT* promoter methylation is highly methylated in *IDH1*-mutant gliomas, particularly oligodendrogliomas, compared with *IDH*-wildtype [43].

Some preclinical studies demonstrated that forced *IDH* mutation sensitized cells to chemotherapy by increased ROS [134–136]. Conversely, forced *IDH1* mutation revealed that *IDH1* mutation-induced temozolomide (TMZ) resistance and rapid G2 cell cycle arrest through increased RAD-51-mediated homologous recombination (HR) [137, 138]. Importantly, among DNA adducts, O^6G represents less than 10%, while the majority of TMZ-induced DNA lesions are N^7-methylguanine (60–80%) and N^3-methyladenine (10–20%) adducts, which are immediately repaired through poly(ADP-ribose)polymerase (PARP)-dependent base excision repair (BER) [129, 139, 140]. We have recently shown that there are lower steady state NAD+ levels in *IDH1*-mutant gliomas [141], and that TMZ immediately induces NAD+ consumption through PARP activation-mediated BER in *IDH1*-mutant gliomas [142]. Besides, Lu et al. [143] reported that the PARP associated DNA repair pathway was extensively compromised in *IDH1*-mutant cells due to decreased NAD+ availability, thus, cells were sensitive to TMZ, suggesting that deregulated NAD+ metabolism may be related with chemosensitivity. Taken together, these studies show that *IDH* mutation may increase susceptibility to chemotherapy; however, it remains unclear if *IDH* mutation itself promotes TMZ sensitivity.

In contrast, TMZ-induced hypermethylation is a critical problem. Long-term TMZ exposure induces MMR inactivation, followed by DNA hypermutation phenotype. Among numerous mutations, gene alterations in RB and AKT-mTOR pathways promoted malignant progression in *IDH1*-mutant gliomas [27].

9.2.2 Other chemotherapeutic agents

Sulkowski et al. [144] demonstrated that 2-HG inhibits KDM4A and KDM4B, histone demethylases that play a critical role in double strand repair. As a result, *IDH1* mutation suppresses HR and induces PARP inhibitor sensitivity. Additionally, *IDH1*-mutant downregulates the DNA double strand break sensor ATM by altering histone methylation, resulting in impaired DNA repair. As a result, *IDH1* mutation causes DNA damage susceptibility to radiation and daunorubicin and reduces self-renewal of hematopoietic stem cells in acute myeloid leukemia [145].

10. Novel therapeutic target in *IDH1*-mutant tumors

10.1 Specific IDH inhibitor

In 2013, specific inhibitors for *IDH1* and *IDH2* mutations were discovered [70, 146]. In *IDH2*-mutant AML cells, an $IDH2^{R140Q}$ inhibitor induced both histone and DNA demethylation [147]. These effects reversed blocked cell differentiation and resulted in cytotoxicity *in vitro* [146, 147]. It is interesting to note that histone hypermethylation is more rapidly reversed than DNA hypermethylation [147]. In *IDH1*-mutant AML cells, differentiation and DNA demethylation were also induced by a next generation IDH1 inhibitor [148]. Since the *IDH2* mutation is crucial for proliferation and maintenance of leukemia cells [149], an IDH inhibitor may be used as a novel and efficient chemotherapeutic agent against *IDH*-mutant AML cells. Indeed, clinical trials demonstrated durable response for *IDH1/2*-mutant refractory AML patients [150, 151].

In *IDH1*-mutant glioma cells, Rohle et al. [70] reported that a specific IDH1 inhibitor, AGI-5198, blocked 2-HG production, histone demethylation, cell differentiation, and inhibited cell growth in endogenous *IDH1*-mutant glioma cells. Other group demonstrated that BAY 1436032, a pan inhibitor of IDH1 mutation, promoted mild cytotoxic effects *in vivo* [152]. In contrast, we established that, even with a long-term IDH1 inhibitor treatment, 2-HG depletion does not induce demethylation of global-DNA and histones, cell differentiation, nor cytotoxicity [141]. Studies using another IDH1 inhibitor also revealed minimal cytotoxicity despite a rapid decrease in 2-HG levels in glioma cells [153, 154]. Similarly, treatment with an IDH1 inhibitor did not contribute to cytotoxicity, and the CpG island methylation status as well as histone trimethylation levels were largely retained in malignant glioma and chondrosarcoma [155, 156]. Intriguingly, in immortalized human astrocytes with an inducible $IDH1^{R132H}$ expression system, a specific IDH1 inhibitor induced demethylation and inhibited tumorigenesis when forced expression was prior or concomitant to inhibitor treatment, but these effects were not observed if the treatment was delayed [157]. These results indicate that 2-HG depletion or blocked mutant *IDH1* might be insufficient to control tumor growth and reprogramming of epigenomic alterations in progressed *IDH1*-mutant gliomas. Indeed, preliminary results indicate that the 6-month progression-free survival of *IDH1*-mutant glioma, chondrosarcoma, and cholangiocarcinoma is 25, 56, and 43%, respectively, suggesting that the potential of the IDH1 inhibitor may be weaker in *IDH1*-mutant gliomas than in other cancers [158].

10.2 Other treatment strategies

10.2.1 DNA demethylating agents

In addition to IDH1 inhibitor treatments, other strategies to control *IDH1*-mutant tumor cells have been proposed. Because the *IDH1* mutation promotes proliferation by blocking DNA demethylation, treatment with DNA demethylating agents reverses DNA methylation and inhibits proliferation in *IDH1*-mutant cells [71, 159]. Intriguingly, treatment with both the DNA demethylating agent 5-azacytidine (5-Aza) and TMZ demonstrated extensively prolonged survival in an *IDH1*-mutant orthotopic xenograft model [160].

10.2.2 Bcl-2 family inhibitors

Since 2-HG suppresses the activity of cytochrome c oxidase in mitochondrial complex IV, the mitochondrial threshold for apoptosis was decreased after BCL-2 inhibition in *IDH1* and *IDH2*-mutant AML [161]. Similarly, another Bcl-2 family member, the Bcl-xL inhibitor, induced apoptosis in *IDH*-mutant cells, including endogenous *IDH1*-mutant glioma cells [162]. Together, inhibition of Bcl-2 family members may be targetable to control growth in *IDH*-mutant cells.

10.2.3 DNA damaging agents

Because PLK1 activation provokes a rapid bypass through the G2 checkpoint after TMZ treatment in *IDH1*-mutant tumors, combination treatments with TMZ and a PLK1 inhibitor significantly suppressed tumor growth in an *IDH1*-mutant *in vivo* model [138]. In tumors with ATRX mutation-associated alternative lengthening telomeres (ALT), ATR inhibitor is highly sensitive [163], implying that such inhibition may be useful for treatments of *IDH1*-mutant astrocytic tumors with positive ALT. *IDH1* mutation blocked HR, so-called "BRCA ness" phenotype provided specific sensitivity for PARP inhibitor both *in vitro* and *in vivo* [144].

10.2.4 DLL-3 targeting therapy

Since Notch ligand DLL-3 is overexpressed in *IDH*-mutant gliomas, anti-DLL3 antibody-drug conjugate (ADC), rovalpituzumab tesirine (Rova-T), is a potent therapeutic agent for *IDH*-mutant gliomas [164].

10.2.5 Vaccination therapy

Schumacher et al. [165] reported an immunological approach to control *IDH1*-mutant cells. They showed that an epitope derived from the *IDH1*-mutant amino acid sequence is presented in HLA class II molecules of antigen-presenting cells, which elicit a strong immune response via CD4 + T cells. In addition, they showed that constitutive stimulation with synthetic peptides having the *IDH1*-mutation sequence developed an immune response that eradicated *IDH1* mutated tumors in a mouse model with human HLA molecules. Thus, vaccine therapy targeting for *IDH1*-mutation is expected to develop for future clinical trial [165, 166]. Moreover, *IDH1*-mutation caused downregulation of leukocyte chemotaxis, resulting in repression of the tumor-associated immune system including immune cells, such as macrophages [167]. Additionally, tumor infiltrating lymphocytes (TILs) and programmed death ligand 1 (PD-L1) were expressed at low levels in *IDH1*-mutant gliomas [168]. In contrast, Kohanbash et al. [153] demonstrated reduced expression of cytotoxic T lymphocyte-associated genes and IFN-gamma inducible chemokines in *IDH1*-mutant cells; these results were reversed by specific IDH1 inhibitor. Therefore, combination treatments with vaccine immunotherapy and IDH1 inhibitor result in enhanced toxicity in *IDH*-mutant tumors.

10.2.6 Target for altered metabolism

IDH1 mutation induced altered metabolism is also expected as a novel therapeutic target. Based on the fact that the main carbon source for α-KG and 2-HG synthesis in *IDH1*-mutant cells is glutamine from glutaminolysis, a suitable target therapy would be the use of glutaminase (GLS) inhibitor or anti-diabetic drug metformin via the inhibition of mitochondrial complex I in the electron transport system [83, 169–171]. Since reduced glutamate blocks glutathione synthesis, inhibition of glutaminase specifically sensitizes *IDH*-mutant glioma cells to oxidative stress and radiation [86].

Mutant *IDH1* alters steady state levels of NAD+ through inhibiting NAPRT1, one rate limiting enzyme for NAD+ biosynthesis. Therefore, inhibition of nicotinamide phosphoribosyltransferase (NAMPT), another rate limiting enzyme, induced high cytotoxicity in *IDH1*-mutant patient-derived glioma cells [141]. Since TMZ rapidly consumes NAD+ through PARP activation, combination treatments with TMZ and NAMPT inhibitor further enhanced NAD+ depletion-mediated cytotoxicity in *IDH1*-mutant cancers [142]. Similarly, Lu et al. [143] reported that the PARP-associated DNA repair pathway was extensively compromised in *IDH1*-mutant cells due to decreased NAD+ availability, thus sensitive to TMZ.

Because of the relationships between *IDH1* mutation and *MYC* activation [38, 40, 172], target therapy to regulate *MYC*, by using bromodomain and extra-terminal (BET) inhibitors, CDK7 or MYC-induced glycolysis may be used for *IDH*-mutant gliomas [40, 173–175]. Given the results of these studies, *IDH1* mutation-specific biological alterations and metabolic feature may be expected as novel therapeutic targets.

11. Conclusions

In summary, investigations on *IDH* mutations enabled distinctive tumor classification and may allow the development of specific therapeutic strategies. Further preclinical and clinical studies are warranted to overcome the outcomes of cancer development in *IDH*-mutant glioma patients.

Author details

Kensuke Tateishi* and Tetsuya Yamamoto
Department of Neurosurgery, Yokohama City University, Yokohama, Japan

*Address all correspondence to: ktate12@yokohama-cu.ac.jp

References

[1] Sjoblom T, Jones S, Wood LD, Parsons DW, Lin J, Barber TD, et al. The consensus coding sequences of human breast and colorectal cancers. Science. 2006;**314**(5797):268-274

[2] Parsons DW, Jones S, Zhang X, Lin JC, Leary RJ, Angenendt P, et al. An integrated genomic analysis of human glioblastoma multiforme. Science. 2008;**321**(5897):1807-1812

[3] Ichimura K, Pearson DM, Kocialkowski S, Backlund LM, Chan R, Jones DT, et al. IDH1 mutations are present in the majority of common adult gliomas but rare in primary glioblastomas. Neuro-Oncology. 2009;**11**(4):341-347

[4] Yan H, Parsons DW, Jin G, McLendon R, Rasheed BA, Yuan W, et al. IDH1 and IDH2 mutations in gliomas. The New England Journal of Medicine. 2009;**360**(8):765-773

[5] Balss J, Meyer J, Mueller W, Korshunov A, Hartmann C, von Deimling A. Analysis of the IDH1 codon 132 mutation in brain tumors. Acta Neuropathologica. 2008;**116**(6):597-602

[6] Pusch S, Schweizer L, Beck AC, Lehmler JM, Weissert S, Balss J, et al. D-2-hydroxyglutarate producing neo-enzymatic activity inversely correlates with frequency of the type of isocitrate dehydrogenase 1 mutations found in glioma. Acta Neuropathologica Communications. 2014;**2**:19

[7] Hartmann C, Meyer J, Balss J, Capper D, Mueller W, Christians A, et al. Type and frequency of IDH1 and IDH2 mutations are related to astrocytic and oligodendroglial differentiation and age: A study of 1,010 diffuse gliomas. Acta Neuropathologica. 2009;**118**(4):469-474

[8] Mardis ER, Ding L, Dooling DJ, Larson DE, McLellan MD, Chen K, et al. Recurring mutations found by sequencing an acute myeloid leukemia genome. The New England Journal of Medicine. 2009;**361**(11):1058-1066

[9] Marcucci G, Maharry K, Wu YZ, Radmacher MD, Mrozek K, Margeson D, et al. IDH1 and IDH2 gene mutations identify novel molecular subsets within de novo cytogenetically normal acute myeloid leukemia: A Cancer and Leukemia Group B study. Journal of Clinical Oncology. 2010;**28**(14):2348-2355

[10] Cairns RA, Iqbal J, Lemonnier F, Kucuk C, de Leval L, Jais JP, et al. IDH2 mutations are frequent in angioimmunoblastic T-cell lymphoma. Blood. 2012;**119**(8):1901-1903

[11] Amary MF, Bacsi K, Maggiani F, Damato S, Halai D, Berisha F, et al. IDH1 and IDH2 mutations are frequent events in central chondrosarcoma and central and periosteal chondromas but not in other mesenchymal tumours. The Journal of Pathology. 2011;**224**(3):334-343

[12] Kipp BR, Voss JS, Kerr SE, Barr Fritcher EG, Graham RP, Zhang L, et al. Isocitrate dehydrogenase 1 and 2 mutations in cholangiocarcinoma. Human Pathology. 2012;**43**(10):1552-1558

[13] Wang P, Dong Q, Zhang C, Kuan PF, Liu Y, Jeck WR, et al. Mutations in isocitrate dehydrogenase 1 and 2 occur frequently in intrahepatic cholangiocarcinomas and share hypermethylation targets with glioblastomas. Oncogene. 2013;**32**(25):3091-3100

[14] Kang MR, Kim MS, Oh JE, Kim YR, Song SY, Seo SI, et al. Mutational analysis of IDH1 codon 132 in glioblastomas and other common

cancers. International Journal of Cancer. 2009;**125**(2):353-355

[15] Fathi AT, Sadrzadeh H, Comander AH, Higgins MJ, Bardia A, Perry A, et al. Isocitrate dehydrogenase 1 (IDH1) mutation in breast adenocarcinoma is associated with elevated levels of serum and urine 2-hydroxyglutarate. The Oncologist. 2014;**19**(6):602-607

[16] Li-Chang HH, Kasaian K, Ng Y, Lum A, Kong E, Lim H, et al. Retrospective review using targeted deep sequencing reveals mutational differences between gastroesophageal junction and gastric carcinomas. BMC Cancer. 2015;**15**:32

[17] Nonoguchi N, Ohta T, Oh JE, Kim YH, Kleihues P, Ohgaki H. TERT promoter mutations in primary and secondary glioblastomas. Acta Neuropathologica. 2013;**126**(6):931-937

[18] Ohgaki H, Kleihues P. The definition of primary and secondary glioblastoma. Clinical Cancer Research. 2013;**19**(4):764-772

[19] Louis DN, Perry A, Reifenberger G, von Deimling A, Figarella-Branger D, Cavenee WK, et al. The 2016 world health organization classification of tumors of the central nervous system: A summary. Acta Neuropathologica. 2016;**131**(6):803-820

[20] Jiao Y, Killela PJ, Reitman ZJ, Rasheed AB, Heaphy CM, de Wilde RF, et al. Frequent ATRX, CIC, FUBP1 and IDH1 mutations refine the classification of malignant gliomas. Oncotarget. 2012;**3**(7):709-722

[21] Kannan K, Inagaki A, Silber J, Gorovets D, Zhang J, Kastenhuber ER, et al. Whole-exome sequencing identifies ATRX mutation as a key molecular determinant in lower-grade glioma. Oncotarget. 2012;**3**(10):1194-1203

[22] Liu XY, Gerges N, Korshunov A, Sabha N, Khuong-Quang DA, Fontebasso AM, et al. Frequent ATRX mutations and loss of expression in adult diffuse astrocytic tumors carrying IDH1/IDH2 and TP53 mutations. Acta Neuropathologica. 2012;**124**(5):615-625

[23] Arita H, Narita Y, Fukushima S, Tateishi K, Matsushita Y, Yoshida A, et al. Upregulating mutations in the TERT promoter commonly occur in adult malignant gliomas and are strongly associated with total 1p19q loss. Acta Neuropathologica. 2013;**126**(2):267-276

[24] Killela PJ, Reitman ZJ, Jiao Y, Bettegowda C, Agrawal N, Diaz LA Jr, et al. TERT promoter mutations occur frequently in gliomas and a subset of tumors derived from cells with low rates of self-renewal. Proceedings of the National Academy of Sciences of the United States of America. 2013;**110**(15):6021-6026

[25] Watanabe T, Nobusawa S, Kleihues P, Ohgaki H. IDH1 mutations are early events in the development of astrocytomas and oligodendrogliomas. The American Journal of Pathology. 2009;**174**(4):1149-1153

[26] Juratli TA, Kirsch M, Robel K, Soucek S, Geiger K, von Kummer R, et al. IDH mutations as an early and consistent marker in low-grade astrocytomas WHO grade II and their consecutive secondary high-grade gliomas. Journal of Neuro-Oncology. 2012;**108**(3):403-410

[27] Johnson BE, Mazor T, Hong C, Barnes M, Aihara K, McLean CY, et al. Mutational analysis reveals the origin and therapy-driven evolution of recurrent glioma. Science. 2014;**343**(6167):189-193

[28] Suzuki H, Aoki K, Chiba K, Sato Y, Shiozawa Y, Shiraishi Y, et al.

Mutational landscape and clonal architecture in grade II and III gliomas. Nature Genetics. 2015;**47**(5):458-468

[29] Mazor T, Chesnelong C, Pankov A, Jalbert LE, Hong C, Hayes J, et al. Clonal expansion and epigenetic reprogramming following deletion or amplification of mutant IDH1. Proceedings of the National Academy of Sciences of the United States of America. 2017;**114**(40):10743-10748

[30] Ohba S, Mukherjee J, Johannessen TC, Mancini A, Chow TT, Wood M, et al. Mutant IDH1 expression drives TERT promoter reactivation as part of the cellular transformation process. Cancer Research. 2016;**76**(22):6680-6689

[31] Tirosh I, Venteicher AS, Hebert C, Escalante LE, Patel AP, Yizhak K, et al. Single-cell RNA-seq supports a developmental hierarchy in human oligodendroglioma. Nature. 2016;**539**(7628):309-313

[32] Venteicher AS, Tirosh I, Hebert C, Yizhak K, Neftel C, Filbin MG, et al. Decoupling genetics, lineages, and microenvironment in IDH-mutant gliomas by single-cell RNA-seq. Science. 2017;**355**(6332)

[33] Koivunen P, Lee S, Duncan CG, Lopez G, Lu G, Ramkissoon S, et al. Transformation by the (R)-enantiomer of 2-hydroxyglutarate linked to EGLN activation. Nature. 2012;**483**(7390):484-488

[34] Piaskowski S, Bienkowski M, Stoczynska-Fidelus E, Stawski R, Sieruta M, Szybka M, et al. Glioma cells showing IDH1 mutation cannot be propagated in standard cell culture conditions. British Journal of Cancer. 2011;**104**(6):968-970

[35] Luchman HA, Stechishin OD, Dang NH, Blough MD, Chesnelong C, Kelly JJ, et al. An in vivo patient-derived model of endogenous IDH1-mutant glioma. Neuro-Oncology. 2012;**14**(2):184-191

[36] Balvers RK, Kleijn A, Kloezeman JJ, French PJ, Kremer A, van den Bent MJ, et al. Serum-free culture success of glial tumors is related to specific molecular profiles and expression of extracellular matrix-associated gene modules. Neuro-Oncology. 2013;**15**(12):1684-1695

[37] Bardella C, Al-Dalahmah O, Krell D, Brazauskas P, Al-Qahtani K, Tomkova M, et al. Expression of Idh1R132H in the murine subventricular zone stem cell niche recapitulates features of early gliomagenesis. Cancer Cell. 2016;**30**(4):578-594

[38] Wakimoto H, Tanaka S, Curry WT, Loebel F, Zhao D, Tateishi K, et al. Targetable signaling pathway mutations are associated with malignant phenotype in IDH-mutant gliomas. Clinical Cancer Research. 2014;**20**(11):2898-2909

[39] Kamoun A, Idbaih A, Dehais C, Elarouci N, Carpentier C, Letouze E, et al. Integrated multi-omics analysis of oligodendroglial tumours identifies three subgroups of 1p/19q co-deleted gliomas. Nature Communications. 2016;**7**:11263

[40] Bai H, Harmanci AS, Erson-Omay EZ, Li J, Coskun S, Simon M, et al. Integrated genomic characterization of IDH1-mutant glioma malignant progression. Nature Genetics. 2016;**48**(1):59-66

[41] Reuss DE, Mamatjan Y, Schrimpf D, Capper D, Hovestadt V, Kratz A, et al. IDH mutant diffuse and anaplastic astrocytomas have similar age at presentation and little difference in survival: A grading problem for WHO. Acta Neuropathologica. 2015;**129**(6):867-873

[42] Nobusawa S, Watanabe T, Kleihues P, Ohgaki H. IDH1 mutations as molecular signature and predictive factor of secondary glioblastomas. Clinical Cancer Research. 2009;**15**(19):6002-6007

[43] Sanson M, Marie Y, Paris S, Idbaih A, Laffaire J, Ducray F, et al. Isocitrate dehydrogenase 1 codon 132 mutation is an important prognostic biomarker in gliomas. Journal of Clinical Oncology. 2009;**27**(25):4150-4154

[44] Wick W, Hartmann C, Engel C, Stoffels M, Felsberg J, Stockhammer F, et al. NOA-04 randomized phase III trial of sequential radiochemotherapy of anaplastic glioma with procarbazine, lomustine, and vincristine or temozolomide. Journal of Clinical Oncology. 2009;**27**(35):5874-5880

[45] Killela PJ, Pirozzi CJ, Healy P, Reitman ZJ, Lipp E, Rasheed BA, et al. Mutations in IDH1, IDH2, and in the TERT promoter define clinically distinct subgroups of adult malignant gliomas. Oncotarget. 2014;**5**(6):1515-1525

[46] Minniti G, Scaringi C, Arcella A, Lanzetta G, Di Stefano D, Scarpino S, et al. IDH1 mutation and MGMT methylation status predict survival in patients with anaplastic astrocytoma treated with temozolomide-based chemoradiotherapy. Journal of Neuro-Oncology. 2014;**118**(2):377-383

[47] Eckel-Passow JE, Lachance DH, Molinaro AM, Walsh KM, Decker PA, Sicotte H, et al. Glioma groups based on 1p/19q, IDH, and TERT promoter mutations in tumors. The New England Journal of Medicine. 2015;**372**(26):2499-2508

[48] Hartmann C, Hentschel B, Wick W, Capper D, Felsberg J, Simon M, et al. Patients with IDH1 wild type anaplastic astrocytomas exhibit worse prognosis than IDH1-mutated glioblastomas, and IDH1 mutation status accounts for the unfavorable prognostic effect of higher age: Implications for classification of gliomas. Acta Neuropathologica. 2010;**120**(6):707-718

[49] Pekmezci M, Rice T, Molinaro AM, Walsh KM, Decker PA, Hansen H, et al. Adult infiltrating gliomas with WHO 2016 integrated diagnosis: Additional prognostic roles of ATRX and TERT. Acta Neuropathologica. 2017;**133**(6):1001-1016

[50] Arita H, Yamasaki K, Matsushita Y, Nakamura T, Shimokawa A, Takami H, et al. A combination of TERT promoter mutation and MGMT methylation status predicts clinically relevant subgroups of newly diagnosed glioblastomas. Acta Neuropathologica Communications. 2016;**4**(1):79

[51] Shirahata M, Ono T, Stichel D, Schrimpf D, Reuss DE, Sahm F, et al. Novel, improved grading system(s) for IDH-mutant astrocytic gliomas. Acta Neuropathologica. 2018;**136**(1):153-166

[52] Halani SH, Yousefi S, Vega JV, Rossi MR, Zhao Z, Amrollahi F, et al. Multi-faceted computational assessment of risk and progression in oligodendroglioma implicates NOTCH and PI3K pathways. NPJ Precision Oncology. 2018;**2**:24

[53] Aoki K, Nakamura H, Suzuki H, Matsuo K, Kataoka K, Shimamura T, et al. Prognostic relevance of genetic alterations in diffuse lower-grade gliomas. Neuro-Oncology. 2018;**20**(1):66-77

[54] Dang L, White DW, Gross S, Bennett BD, Bittinger MA, Driggers EM, et al. Cancer-associated IDH1 mutations produce 2-hydroxyglutarate. Nature. 2009;**462**(7274):739-744

[55] Leonardi R, Subramanian C, Jackowski S, Rock CO. Cancer-associated isocitrate dehydrogenase mutations inactivate

NADPH-dependent reductive carboxylation. The Journal of Biological Chemistry. 2012;**287**(18):14615-14620

[56] Grassian AR, Parker SJ, Davidson SM, Divakaruni AS, Green CR, Zhang X, et al. IDH1 mutations alter citric acid cycle metabolism and increase dependence on oxidative mitochondrial metabolism. Cancer Research. 2014;**74**(12):3317-3331

[57] Ward PS, Patel J, Wise DR, Abdel-Wahab O, Bennett BD, Coller HA, et al. The common feature of leukemia-associated IDH1 and IDH2 mutations is a neomorphic enzyme activity converting alpha-ketoglutarate to 2-hydroxyglutarate. Cancer Cell. 2010;**17**(3):225-234

[58] Jin G, Reitman ZJ, Duncan CG, Spasojevic I, Gooden DM, Rasheed BA, et al. Disruption of wild-type IDH1 suppresses D-2-hydroxyglutarate production in IDH1-mutated gliomas. Cancer Research. 2013;**73**(2):496-501

[59] Zhao S, Lin Y, Xu W, Jiang W, Zha Z, Wang P, et al. Glioma-derived mutations in IDH1 dominantly inhibit IDH1 catalytic activity and induce HIF-1alpha. Science. 2009;**324**(5924): 261-265

[60] Xu W, Yang H, Liu Y, Yang Y, Wang P, Kim SH, et al. Oncometabolite 2-hydroxyglutarate is a competitive inhibitor of alpha-ketoglutarate-dependent dioxygenases. Cancer Cell. 2011;**19**(1):17-30

[61] Figueroa ME, Abdel-Wahab O, Lu C, Ward PS, Patel J, Shih A, et al. Leukemic IDH1 and IDH2 mutations result in a hypermethylation phenotype, disrupt TET2 function, and impair hematopoietic differentiation. Cancer Cell. 2010;**18**(6):553-567

[62] Noushmehr H, Weisenberger DJ, Diefes K, Phillips HS, Pujara K, Berman BP, et al. Identification of a CpG island methylator phenotype that defines a distinct subgroup of glioma. Cancer Cell. 2010;**17**(5):510-522

[63] Sasaki M, Knobbe CB, Munger JC, Lind EF, Brenner D, Brustle A, et al. IDH1(R132H) mutation increases murine haematopoietic progenitors and alters epigenetics. Nature. 2012;**488**(7413):656-659

[64] Turcan S, Rohle D, Goenka A, Walsh LA, Fang F, Yilmaz E, et al. IDH1 mutation is sufficient to establish the glioma hypermethylator phenotype. Nature. 2012;**483**(7390):479-483

[65] de Souza CF, Sabedot TS, Malta TM, Stetson L, Morozova O, Sokolov A, et al. A distinct DNA methylation shift in a subset of glioma CpG island methylator phenotypes during tumor recurrence. Cell Reports. 2018;**23**(2):637-651

[66] Verhaak RG, Hoadley KA, Purdom E, Wang V, Qi Y, Wilkerson MD, et al. Integrated genomic analysis identifies clinically relevant subtypes of glioblastoma characterized by abnormalities in PDGFRA, IDH1, EGFR, and NF1. Cancer Cell. 2010;**17**(1):98-110

[67] Flavahan WA, Drier Y, Liau BB, Gillespie SM, Venteicher AS, Stemmer-Rachamimov AO, et al. Insulator dysfunction and oncogene activation in IDH mutant gliomas. Nature. 2016;**529**(7584):110-114

[68] Chowdhury R, Yeoh KK, Tian YM, Hillringhaus L, Bagg EA, Rose NR, et al. The oncometabolite 2-hydroxyglutarate inhibits histone lysine demethylases. EMBO Reports. 2011;**12**(5):463-469

[69] Lu C, Ward PS, Kapoor GS, Rohle D, Turcan S, Abdel-Wahab O, et al. IDH mutation impairs histone demethylation and results in a block to cell differentiation. Nature. 2012;**483**(7390):474-478

[70] Rohle D, Popovici-Muller J, Palaskas N, Turcan S, Grommes C, Campos C, et al. An inhibitor of mutant IDH1 delays growth and promotes differentiation of glioma cells. Science. 2013;**340**(6132):626-630

[71] Turcan S, Fabius AW, Borodovsky A, Pedraza A, Brennan C, Huse J, et al. Efficient induction of differentiation and growth inhibition in IDH1 mutant glioma cells by the DNMT inhibitor decitabine. Oncotarget. 2013;**4**(10):1729-1736

[72] Sasaki M, Knobbe CB, Itsumi M, Elia AJ, Harris IS, Chio II, et al. D-2-hydroxyglutarate produced by mutant IDH1 perturbs collagen maturation and basement membrane function. Genes & Development. 2012;**26**(18):2038-2049

[73] Semenza GL. HIF-1 mediates metabolic responses to intratumoral hypoxia and oncogenic mutations. The Journal of Clinical Investigation. 2013;**123**(9):3664-3671

[74] Semenza GL. Regulation of metabolism by hypoxia-inducible factor 1. Cold Spring Harbor Symposia on Quantitative Biology. 2011;**76**:347-353

[75] Nie Q, Guo P, Guo L, Lan J, Lin Y, Guo F, et al. Overexpression of isocitrate dehydrogenase-1R(1)(3)(2)H enhances the proliferation of A172 glioma cells via aerobic glycolysis. Molecular Medicine Reports. 2015;**11**(5):3715-3721

[76] Chesnelong C, Chaumeil MM, Blough MD, Al-Najjar M, Stechishin OD, Chan JA, et al. Lactate dehydrogenase A silencing in IDH mutant gliomas. Neuro-Oncology. 2014;**16**(5):686-695

[77] Viswanath P, Najac C, Izquierdo-Garcia JL, Pankov A, Hong C, Eriksson P, et al. Mutant IDH1 expression is associated with down-regulation of monocarboxylate transporters. Oncotarget. 2016;**7**(23):34942-34955

[78] Izquierdo-Garcia JL, Cai LM, Chaumeil MM, Eriksson P, Robinson AE, Pieper RO, et al. Glioma cells with the IDH1 mutation modulate metabolic fractional flux through pyruvate carboxylase. PLoS ONE. 2014;**9**(9):e108289

[79] Izquierdo-Garcia JL, Viswanath P, Eriksson P, Cai L, Radoul M, Chaumeil MM, et al. IDH1 mutation induces reprogramming of pyruvate metabolism. Cancer Research. 2015;**75**(15):2999-3009

[80] Metallo CM, Gameiro PA, Bell EL, Mattaini KR, Yang J, Hiller K, et al. Reductive glutamine metabolism by IDH1 mediates lipogenesis under hypoxia. Nature. 2012;**481**(7381):380-384

[81] Reitman ZJ, Duncan CG, Poteet E, Winters A, Yan LJ, Gooden DM, et al. Cancer-associated isocitrate dehydrogenase 1 (IDH1) R132H mutation and d-2-hydroxyglutarate stimulate glutamine metabolism under hypoxia. The Journal of Biological Chemistry. 2014;**289**(34):23318-23328

[82] Reitman ZJ, Jin G, Karoly ED, Spasojevic I, Yang J, Kinzler KW, et al. Profiling the effects of isocitrate dehydrogenase 1 and 2 mutations on the cellular metabolome. Proceedings of the National Academy of Sciences of the United States of America. 2011;**108**(8):3270-3275

[83] Ohka F, Ito M, Ranjit M, Senga T, Motomura A, Motomura K, et al. Quantitative metabolome analysis profiles activation of glutaminolysis in glioma with IDH1 mutation. Tumour Biology. 2014;**35**(6):5911-5920

[84] Chen R, Nishimura MC, Kharbanda S, Peale F, Deng Y, Daemen A, et al. Hominoid-specific enzyme GLUD2 promotes growth of IDH1R132H glioma. Proceedings of

the National Academy of Sciences of the United States of America. 2014;**111**(39):14217-14222

[85] Waitkus MS, Pirozzi CJ, Moure CJ, Diplas BH, Hansen LJ, Carpenter AB, et al. Adaptive evolution of the GDH2 allosteric domain promotes gliomagenesis by resolving IDH1(R132H)-induced metabolic liabilities. Cancer Research. 2018;**78**(1):36-50

[86] McBrayer SK, Mayers JR, DiNatale GJ, Shi DD, Khanal J, Chakraborty AA, et al. Transaminase inhibition by 2-hydroxyglutarate impairs glutamate biosynthesis and redox homeostasis in glioma. Cell. 2018;**175**(1):101-116 e25

[87] Tonjes M, Barbus S, Park YJ, Wang W, Schlotter M, Lindroth AM, et al. BCAT1 promotes cell proliferation through amino acid catabolism in gliomas carrying wild-type IDH1. Nature Medicine. 2013;**19**(7):901-908

[88] Lacroix M, Abi-Said D, Fourney DR, Gokaslan ZL, Shi W, DeMonte F, et al. A multivariate analysis of 416 patients with glioblastoma multiforme: Prognosis, extent of resection, and survival. Journal of Neurosurgery. 2001;**95**(2):190-198

[89] Smith JS, Chang EF, Lamborn KR, Chang SM, Prados MD, Cha S, et al. Role of extent of resection in the long-term outcome of low-grade hemispheric gliomas. Journal of Clinical Oncology. 2008;**26**(8):1338-1345

[90] Sanai N, Polley MY, McDermott MW, Parsa AT, Berger MS. An extent of resection threshold for newly diagnosed glioblastomas. Journal of Neurosurgery. 2011;**115**(1):3-8

[91] Marko NF, Weil RJ, Schroeder JL, Lang FF, Suki D, Sawaya RE. Extent of resection of glioblastoma revisited: Personalized survival modeling facilitates more accurate survival prediction and supports a maximum-safe-resection approach to surgery. Journal of Clinical Oncology. 2014;**32**(8):774-782

[92] Qi S, Yu L, Li H, Ou Y, Qiu X, Ding Y, et al. Isocitrate dehydrogenase mutation is associated with tumor location and magnetic resonance imaging characteristics in astrocytic neoplasms. Oncology Letters. 2014;**7**(6):1895-1902

[93] Darlix A, Deverdun J, Menjot de Champfleur N, Castan F, Zouaoui S, Rigau V, et al. IDH mutation and 1p19q codeletion distinguish two radiological patterns of diffuse low-grade gliomas. Journal of Neuro-Oncology. 2017;**133**(1):37-45

[94] Ellingson BM, Lai A, Harris RJ, Selfridge JM, Yong WH, Das K, et al. Probabilistic radiographic atlas of glioblastoma phenotypes. AJNR. American Journal of Neuroradiology. 2013;**34**(3):533-540

[95] Price SJ, Allinson K, Liu H, Boonzaier NR, Yan JL, Lupson VC, et al. Less invasive phenotype found in isocitrate dehydrogenase-mutated glioblastomas than in isocitrate dehydrogenase wild-type glioblastomas: A diffusion-tensor imaging study. Radiology. 2017;**283**(1):215-221

[96] Wefel JS, Noll KR, Rao G, Cahill DP. Neurocognitive function varies by IDH1 genetic mutation status in patients with malignant glioma prior to surgical resection. Neuro-Oncology. 2016;**18**(12):1656-1663

[97] Beiko J, Suki D, Hess KR, Fox BD, Cheung V, Cabral M, et al. IDH1 mutant malignant astrocytomas are more amenable to surgical resection and have a survival benefit associated with

maximal surgical resection. Neuro-Oncology. 2014;**16**(1):81-91

[98] Kawaguchi T, Sonoda Y, Shibahara I, Saito R, Kanamori M, Kumabe T, et al. Impact of gross total resection in patients with WHO grade III glioma harboring the IDH 1/2 mutation without the 1p/19q co-deletion. Journal of Neuro-Oncology. 2016;**129**(3):505-514

[99] Wijnenga MMJ, French PJ, Dubbink HJ, Dinjens WNM, Atmodimedjo PN, Kros JM, et al. The impact of surgery in molecularly defined low-grade glioma: An integrated clinical, radiological, and molecular analysis. Neuro-Oncology. 2018;**20**(1):103-112

[100] Patel T, Bander ED, Venn RA, Powell T, Cederquist GY, Schaefer PM, et al. The role of extent of resection in IDH1 wild-type or mutant low-grade gliomas. Neurosurgery. 2018;**82**(6):808-814

[101] Andronesi OC, Kim GS, Gerstner E, Batchelor T, Tzika AA, Fantin VR, et al. Detection of 2-hydroxyglutarate in IDH-mutated glioma patients by in vivo spectral-editing and 2D correlation magnetic resonance spectroscopy. Science Translational Medicine. 2012;**4**(116):116ra4

[102] Choi C, Ganji SK, DeBerardinis RJ, Hatanpaa KJ, Rakheja D, Kovacs Z, et al. 2-hydroxyglutarate detection by magnetic resonance spectroscopy in IDH-mutated patients with gliomas. Nature Medicine. 2012;**18**(4):624-629

[103] Lazovic J, Soto H, Piccioni D, Lou JR, Li S, Mirsadraei L, et al. Detection of 2-hydroxyglutaric acid in vivo by proton magnetic resonance spectroscopy in U87 glioma cells overexpressing isocitrate dehydrogenase-1 mutation. Neuro-Oncology. 2012;**14**(12):1465-1472

[104] Andronesi OC, Rapalino O, Gerstner E, Chi A, Batchelor TT, Cahill DP, et al. Detection of oncogenic IDH1 mutations using magnetic resonance spectroscopy of 2-hydroxyglutarate. The Journal of Clinical Investigation. 2013;**123**(9):3659-3663

[105] de la Fuente MI, Young RJ, Rubel J, Rosenblum M, Tisnado J, Briggs S, et al. Integration of 2-hydroxyglutarate-proton magnetic resonance spectroscopy into clinical practice for disease monitoring in isocitrate dehydrogenase-mutant glioma. Neuro-Oncology. 2016;**18**(2):283-290

[106] Emir UE, Larkin SJ, de Pennington N, Voets N, Plaha P, Stacey R, et al. Noninvasive quantification of 2-hydroxyglutarate in human gliomas with IDH1 and IDH2 mutations. Cancer Research. 2016;**76**(1):43-49

[107] Nagashima H, Tanaka K, Sasayama T, Irino Y, Sato N, Takeuchi Y, et al. Diagnostic value of glutamate with 2-hydroxyglutarate in magnetic resonance spectroscopy for IDH1 mutant glioma. Neuro-Oncology. 2016;**18**(11):1559-1568

[108] Choi C, Raisanen JM, Ganji SK, Zhang S, McNeil SS, An Z, et al. Prospective longitudinal analysis of 2-hydroxyglutarate magnetic resonance spectroscopy identifies broad clinical utility for the management of patients with IDH-mutant glioma. Journal of Clinical Oncology. 2016;**34**(33):4030-4039

[109] Tan WL, Huang WY, Yin B, Xiong J, Wu JS, Geng DY. Can diffusion tensor imaging noninvasively detect IDH1 gene mutations in astrogliomas? A retrospective study of 112 cases. AJNR. American Journal of Neuroradiology. 2014;**35**(5):920-927

[110] Kickingereder P, Sahm F, Radbruch A, Wick W, Heiland S, Deimling A, et al. IDH mutation status is associated with a distinct hypoxia/angiogenesis transcriptome

signature which is non-invasively predictable with rCBV imaging in human glioma. Scientific Reports. 2015;**5**:16238

[111] Yamashita K, Hiwatashi A, Togao O, Kikuchi K, Hatae R, Yoshimoto K, et al. MR imaging-based analysis of glioblastoma multiforme: Estimation of IDH1 mutation status. AJNR. American Journal of Neuroradiology. 2016;**37**(1):58-65

[112] Juratli TA, Tummala SS, Riedl A, Daubner D, Hennig S, Penson T, et al. Radiographic assessment of contrast enhancement and T2/FLAIR mismatch sign in lower grade gliomas: Correlation with molecular groups. Journal of Neuro-Oncology. 2019;**141**(2):327-335

[113] Broen MPG, Smits M, Wijnenga MMJ, Dubbink HJ, Anten M, Schijns O, et al. The T2-FLAIR mismatch sign as an imaging marker for non-enhancing IDH-mutant, 1p/19q-intact lower-grade glioma: A validation study. Neuro-Oncology. 2018;**20**(10):1393-1399

[114] Patel SH, Poisson LM, Brat DJ, Zhou Y, Cooper L, Snuderl M, et al. T2-FLAIR mismatch, an imaging biomarker for IDH and 1p/19q status in lower-grade gliomas: A TCGA/TCIA project. Clinical Cancer Research. 2017;**23**(20):6078-6085

[115] Kanamori M, Kikuchi A, Watanabe M, Shibahara I, Saito R, Yamashita Y, et al. Rapid and sensitive intraoperative detection of mutations in the isocitrate dehydrogenase 1 and 2 genes during surgery for glioma. Journal of Neurosurgery. 2014;**120**(6):1288-1297

[116] Santagata S, Eberlin LS, Norton I, Calligaris D, Feldman DR, Ide JL, et al. Intraoperative mass spectrometry mapping of an onco-metabolite to guide brain tumor surgery. Proceedings of the National Academy of Sciences of the United States of America. 2014;**111**(30):11121-11126

[117] Shankar GM, Francis JM, Rinne ML, Ramkissoon SH, Huang FW, Venteicher AS, et al. Rapid intraoperative molecular characterization of glioma. JAMA Oncology. 2015;**1**(5):662-667

[118] Fathi AT, Nahed BV, Wander SA, Iafrate AJ, Borger DR, Hu R, et al. Elevation of urinary 2-hydroxyglutarate in IDH-mutant glioma. The Oncologist. 2016;**21**(2):214-219

[119] Tran AN, Lai A, Li S, Pope WB, Teixeira S, Harris RJ, et al. Increased sensitivity to radiochemotherapy in IDH1 mutant glioblastoma as demonstrated by serial quantitative MR volumetry. Neuro-Oncology. 2014;**16**(3):414-420

[120] Li S, Chou AP, Chen W, Chen R, Deng Y, Phillips HS, et al. Overexpression of isocitrate dehydrogenase mutant proteins renders glioma cells more sensitive to radiation. Neuro-Oncology. 2013;**15**(1):57-68

[121] Wang XW, Labussiere M, Valable S, Peres EA, Guillamo JS, Bernaudin M, et al. IDH1(R132H) mutation increases U87 glioma cell sensitivity to radiation therapy in hypoxia. BioMed Research International. 2014;**2014**:198697

[122] Kessler J, Guttler A, Wichmann H, Rot S, Kappler M, Bache M, et al. IDH1(R132H) mutation causes a less aggressive phenotype and radiosensitizes human malignant glioma cells independent of the oxygenation status. Radiotherapy and Oncology. 2015;**116**(3):381-387

[123] Bleeker FE, Atai NA, Lamba S, Jonker A, Rijkeboer D, Bosch KS, et al. The prognostic IDH1(R132) mutation is associated with reduced NADP+-dependent IDH activity in

glioblastoma. Acta Neuropathologica. 2010;**119**(4):487-494

[124] Molenaar RJ, Botman D, Smits MA, Hira VV, van Lith SA, Stap J, et al. Radioprotection of IDH1-mutated cancer cells by the IDH1-mutant inhibitor AGI-5198. Cancer Research. 2015;**75**(22):4790-4802

[125] Stupp R, Mason WP, van den Bent MJ, Weller M, Fisher B, Taphoorn MJ, et al. Radiotherapy plus concomitant and adjuvant temozolomide for glioblastoma. The New England Journal of Medicine. 2005;**352**(10):987-996

[126] van den Bent MJ, Baumert B, Erridge SC, Vogelbaum MA, Nowak AK, Sanson M, et al. Interim results from the CATNON trial (EORTC study 26053-22054) of treatment with concurrent and adjuvant temozolomide for 1p/19q non-co-deleted anaplastic glioma: A phase 3, randomised, open-label intergroup study. Lancet. 2017;**390**(10103):1645-1653

[127] Houillier C, Wang X, Kaloshi G, Mokhtari K, Guillevin R, Laffaire J, et al. IDH1 or IDH2 mutations predict longer survival and response to temozolomide in low-grade gliomas. Neurology. 2010;**75**(17):1560-1566

[128] SongTao Q, Lei Y, Si G, YanQing D, HuiXia H, XueLin Z, et al. IDH mutations predict longer survival and response to temozolomide in secondary glioblastoma. Cancer Science. 2012;**103**(2):269-273

[129] Fu D, Calvo JA, Samson LD. Balancing repair and tolerance of DNA damage caused by alkylating agents. Nature Reviews. Cancer. 2012;**12**(2):104-120

[130] Fan CH, Liu WL, Cao H, Wen C, Chen L, Jiang G. O6-methylguanine DNA methyltransferase as a promising target for the treatment of temozolomide-resistant gliomas. Cell Death & Disease. 2013;**4**:e876

[131] Hegi ME, Diserens AC, Gorlia T, Hamou MF, de Tribolet N, Weller M, et al. MGMT gene silencing and benefit from temozolomide in glioblastoma. The New England Journal of Medicine. 2005;**352**(10):997-1003

[132] Hunter C, Smith R, Cahill DP, Stephens P, Stevens C, Teague J, et al. A hypermutation phenotype and somatic MSH6 mutations in recurrent human malignant gliomas after alkylator chemotherapy. Cancer Research. 2006;**66**(8):3987-3991

[133] Cahill DP, Levine KK, Betensky RA, Codd PJ, Romany CA, Reavie LB, et al. Loss of the mismatch repair protein MSH6 in human glioblastomas is associated with tumor progression during temozolomide treatment. Clinical Cancer Research. 2007;**13**(7):2038-2045

[134] Fu Y, Huang R, Zheng Y, Zhang Z, Liang A. Glioma-derived mutations in isocitrate dehydrogenase 2 beneficial to traditional chemotherapy. Biochemical and Biophysical Research Communications. 2011;**410**(2):218-223

[135] Mohrenz IV, Antonietti P, Pusch S, Capper D, Balss J, Voigt S, et al. Isocitrate dehydrogenase 1 mutant R132H sensitizes glioma cells to BCNU-induced oxidative stress and cell death. Apoptosis. 2013;**18**(11):1416-1425

[136] Shi J, Sun B, Shi W, Zuo H, Cui D, Ni L, et al. Decreasing GSH and increasing ROS in chemosensitivity gliomas with IDH1 mutation. Tumour Biology. 2015;**36**(2):655-662

[137] Ohba S, Mukherjee J, See WL, Pieper RO. Mutant IDH1-driven cellular transformation increases RAD51-mediated homologous recombination

and temozolomide resistance. Cancer Research. 2014;**74**(17):4836-4844

[138] Koncar RF, Chu Z, Romick-Rosendale LE, Wells SI, Chan TA, Qi X, et al. PLK1 inhibition enhances temozolomide efficacy in IDH1 mutant gliomas. Oncotarget. 2017;**8**(9):15827-15837

[139] Trivedi RN, Almeida KH, Fornsaglio JL, Schamus S, Sobol RW. The role of base excision repair in the sensitivity and resistance to temozolomide-mediated cell death. Cancer Research. 2005;**65**(14):6394-6400

[140] Yoshimoto K, Mizoguchi M, Hata N, Murata H, Hatae R, Amano T, et al. Complex DNA repair pathways as possible therapeutic targets to overcome temozolomide resistance in glioblastoma. Frontiers in Oncology. 2012;**2**:186

[141] Tateishi K, Wakimoto H, Iafrate AJ, Tanaka S, Loebel F, Lelic N, et al. Extreme Vulnerability of IDH1 Mutant Cancers to NAD+ Depletion. Cancer Cell. 2015;**28**(6):773-784

[142] Tateishi K, Higuchi F, Miller J, Koerner MVA, Lelic N, Shankar GM, et al. The alkylating chemotherapeutic temozolomide induces metabolic stress in IDH1-mutant cancers and potentiates NAD+ depletion-mediated cytotoxicity. Cancer Research. 2017;**77**(15):4102-4115

[143] Lu Y, Kwintkiewicz J, Liu Y, Tech K, Frady LN, Su YT, et al. Chemosensitivity of IDH1 mutant gliomas due to an impairment in PARP1-mediated DNA repair. Cancer Research. 2017;**77**(7):1709-1718

[144] Sulkowski PL, Corso CD, Robinson ND, Scanlon SE, Purshouse KR, Bai H, et al. 2-Hydroxyglutarate produced by neomorphic IDH mutations suppresses homologous recombination and induces PARP inhibitor sensitivity. Science Translational Medicine. 2017;**9**(375)

[145] Inoue S, Li WY, Tseng A, Beerman I, Elia AJ, Bendall SC, et al. Mutant IDH1 downregulates ATM and alters DNA repair and sensitivity to DNA damage independent of TET2. Cancer Cell. 2016;**30**(2):337-348

[146] Wang F, Travins J, DeLaBarre B, Penard-Lacronique V, Schalm S, Hansen E, et al. Targeted inhibition of mutant IDH2 in leukemia cells induces cellular differentiation. Science. 2013;**340**(6132):622-626

[147] Kernytsky A, Wang F, Hansen E, Schalm S, Straley K, Gliser C, et al. IDH2 mutation-induced histone and DNA hypermethylation is progressively reversed by small-molecule inhibition. Blood. 2015;**125**(2):296-303

[148] Okoye-Okafor UC, Bartholdy B, Cartier J, Gao EN, Pietrak B, Rendina AR, et al. New IDH1 mutant inhibitors for treatment of acute myeloid leukemia. Nature Chemical Biology. 2015;**11**(11):878-886

[149] Kats LM, Reschke M, Taulli R, Pozdnyakova O, Burgess K, Bhargava P, et al. Proto-oncogenic role of mutant IDH2 in leukemia initiation and maintenance. Cell Stem Cell. 2014;**14**(3):329-341

[150] DiNardo CD, Stein EM, de Botton S, Roboz GJ, Altman JK, Mims AS, et al. Durable remissions with ivosidenib in IDH1-mutated relapsed or refractory AML. The New England Journal of Medicine. 2018;**378**(25):2386-2398

[151] Stein EM, DiNardo CD, Pollyea DA, Fathi AT, Roboz GJ, Altman JK, et al. Enasidenib in mutant IDH2 relapsed or refractory acute myeloid leukemia. Blood. 2017;**130**(6):722-731

[152] Pusch S, Krausert S, Fischer V, Balss J, Ott M, Schrimpf D, et al.

Pan-mutant IDH1 inhibitor BAY 1436032 for effective treatment of IDH1 mutant astrocytoma in vivo. Acta Neuropathologica. 2017;**133**(4):629-644

[153] Kohanbash G, Carrera DA, Shrivastav S, Ahn BJ, Jahan N, Mazor T, et al. Isocitrate dehydrogenase mutations suppress STAT1 and CD8+ T cell accumulation in gliomas. The Journal of Clinical Investigation. 2017;**127**(4):1425-1437

[154] Davis MI, Gross S, Shen M, Straley KS, Pragani R, Lea WA, et al. Biochemical, cellular, and biophysical characterization of a potent inhibitor of mutant isocitrate dehydrogenase IDH1. The Journal of Biological Chemistry. 2014;**289**(20):13717-13725

[155] Suijker J, Oosting J, Koornneef A, Struys EA, Salomons GS, Schaap FG, et al. Inhibition of mutant IDH1 decreases D-2-HG levels without affecting tumorigenic properties of chondrosarcoma cell lines. Oncotarget. 2015;**6**(14):12505-12519

[156] Turcan S, Makarov V, Taranda J, Wang Y, Fabius AWM, Wu W, et al. Mutant-IDH1-dependent chromatin state reprogramming, reversibility, and persistence. Nature Genetics. 2018;**50**(1):62-72

[157] Johannessen TA, Mukherjee J, Viswanath P, Ohba S, Ronen SM, Bjerkvig R, et al. Rapid conversion of mutant IDH1 from driver to passenger in a model of human gliomagenesis. Molecular Cancer Research. 2016;**14**(10):976-983

[158] Fujii T, Khawaja MR, DiNardo CD, Atkins JT, Janku F. Targeting isocitrate dehydrogenase (IDH) in cancer. Discovery Medicine. 2016;**21**(117):373-380

[159] Borodovsky A, Salmasi V, Turcan S, Fabius AW, Baia GS, Eberhart CG, et al. 5-azacytidine reduces methylation, promotes differentiation and induces tumor regression in a patient-derived IDH1 mutant glioma xenograft. Oncotarget. 2013;**4**(10):1737-1747

[160] Yamashita AS, da Costa Rosa M, Borodovsky A, Festuccia WT, Chan T, Riggins GJ. Demethylation and epigenetic modification with 5-azacytidine reduces IDH1 mutant glioma growth in combination with temozolomide. Neuro-Oncology. 2018

[161] Chan SM, Thomas D, Corces-Zimmerman MR, Xavy S, Rastogi S, Hong WJ, et al. Isocitrate dehydrogenase 1 and 2 mutations induce BCL-2 dependence in acute myeloid leukemia. Nature Medicine. 2015;**21**(2):178-184

[162] Karpel-Massler G, Ishida CT, Bianchetti E, Zhang Y, Shu C, Tsujiuchi T, et al. Induction of synthetic lethality in IDH1-mutated gliomas through inhibition of Bcl-xL. Nature Communications. 2017;**8**(1):1067

[163] Flynn RL, Cox KE, Jeitany M, Wakimoto H, Bryll AR, Ganem NJ, et al. Alternative lengthening of telomeres renders cancer cells hypersensitive to ATR inhibitors. Science. 2015;**347**(6219):273-277

[164] Spino M, Kurz SC, Chiriboga L, Serrano J, Zeck B, Sen N, et al. Cell surface Notch ligand DLL3 is a therapeutic target in isocitrate dehydrogenase mutant glioma. Clinical Cancer Research. 2019;**25**(4):1261-1271

[165] Schumacher T, Bunse L, Pusch S, Sahm F, Wiestler B, Quandt J, et al. A vaccine targeting mutant IDH1 induces antitumour immunity. Nature. 2014;**512**(7514):324-327

[166] Pellegatta S, Valletta L, Corbetta C, Patane M, Zucca I, Riccardi Sirtori F, et al. Effective immuno-targeting of the IDH1 mutation R132H in a murine

model of intracranial glioma. Acta Neuropathologica Communications. 2015;**3**:4

[167] Amankulor NM, Kim Y, Arora S, Kargl J, Szulzewsky F, Hanke M, et al. Mutant IDH1 regulates the tumor-associated immune system in gliomas. Genes & Development. 2017;**31**(8):774-786

[168] Berghoff AS, Kiesel B, Widhalm G, Wilhelm D, Rajky O, Kurscheid S, et al. Correlation of immune phenotype with IDH mutation in diffuse glioma. Neuro-Oncology. 2017;**19**(11):1460-1468

[169] Seltzer MJ, Bennett BD, Joshi AD, Gao P, Thomas AG, Ferraris DV, et al. Inhibition of glutaminase preferentially slows growth of glioma cells with mutant IDH1. Cancer Research. 2010;**70**(22):8981-8987

[170] Emadi A, Jun SA, Tsukamoto T, Fathi AT, Minden MD, Dang CV. Inhibition of glutaminase selectively suppresses the growth of primary acute myeloid leukemia cells with IDH mutations. Experimental Hematology. 2014;**42**(4):247-251

[171] Cuyas E, Fernandez-Arroyo S, Corominas-Faja B, Rodriguez-Gallego E, Bosch-Barrera J, Martin-Castillo B, et al. Oncometabolic mutation IDH1 R132H confers a metformin-hypersensitive phenotype. Oncotarget. 2015;**6**(14):12279-12296

[172] Odia Y, Orr BA, Bell WR, Eberhart CG, Rodriguez FJ. cMYC expression in infiltrating gliomas: Associations with IDH1 mutations, clinicopathologic features and outcome. Journal of Neuro-Oncology. 2013;**115**(2):249-259

[173] Chipumuro E, Marco E, Christensen CL, Kwiatkowski N, Zhang T, Hatheway CM, et al. CDK7 inhibition suppresses super-enhancer-linked oncogenic transcription in MYCN-driven cancer. Cell. 2014;**159**(5):1126-1139

[174] Christensen CL, Kwiatkowski N, Abraham BJ, Carretero J, Al-Shahrour F, Zhang T, et al. Targeting transcriptional addictions in small cell lung cancer with a covalent CDK7 inhibitor. Cancer Cell. 2014;**26**(6):909-922

[175] Tateishi K, Iafrate AJ, Ho Q, Curry WT, Batchelor TT, Flaherty KT, et al. Myc-driven glycolysis is a therapeutic target in glioblastoma. Clinical Cancer Research. 2016;**22**(17):4452-4465

Section 3

Spinal Tumors

Chapter 3

Intradural Extramedullary Spinal Tumors

Saleh Rasras and Arash Kiani

Abstract

Intradural extramedullary (IDEM) spinal tumors are common pathologies, and despite their name, they can extend beyond dural confinements. IDEMs can have both sporadic and syndromic patterns, and various genetic abnormalities are believed to be responsible for these mainly benign pathologies. Meningiomas, nerve sheath tumors (NST), and ependymomas are the three most common subtypes, and due to their pathologically benign nature, surgical total resection plays the most important role in their management. These tumors have always been challenging entities to neurosurgeons, and many surgical techniques have been described in order to achieve gross total resection, and these techniques have continued to evolve over time. Adjuvant therapies such as radiotherapy or radiosurgery are usually considered when total resection is not possible or sometimes in syndromic patients in order to avoid multiple surgical procedures in a short period of time.

Keywords: intradural extramedullary (IDEM), spinal cord, tumor, nerve sheath tumors (NST), meningioma, ependymoma

1. Introduction

A wide variety of tumors can affect spinal column and cord causing functional or neurological impairment. Axial skeleton tumors can be either primary or secondary with metastatic lesions being the most common and are classified as secondary malignant tumors. On the other hand, primary tumors of the axial skeletons are the ones arising from vertebral bony structures and can also be benign or malignant.

The skeletal system is one the most common sites for metastasis with spinal part being the most frequent site [1] due to its cancellous structure and extensive arterial and venous supplies [2]. Cancers with tendency to affect the spinal column are in descending order: prostate, breast, kidney, lung, and thyroid [3] (**Figure 1**).

Benign tumors of the spinal column can be diagnosed in both children and adults; in children they could be similar to the tumors of other skeletal areas like giant cell tumors (GCT) or osteoblastomas. Regarding the autopsy studies, vertebral hemangiomas are the most common benign primary lesions of the spinal column in adults and could be seen in up to 20% of the population. Other common benign primary tumors are aneurysmal bone cyst, osteoblastoma, osteoid osteoma, GCT, osteochondroma, and enchondroma (**Figure 1**) [4].

Malignant primary spinal column tumors tend to occur in older patients than primary ones, and the most commonly occurring tumors are multiple myeloma and plasmacytoma, chordoma, and osteosarcoma in order of frequency (**Figure 1**).

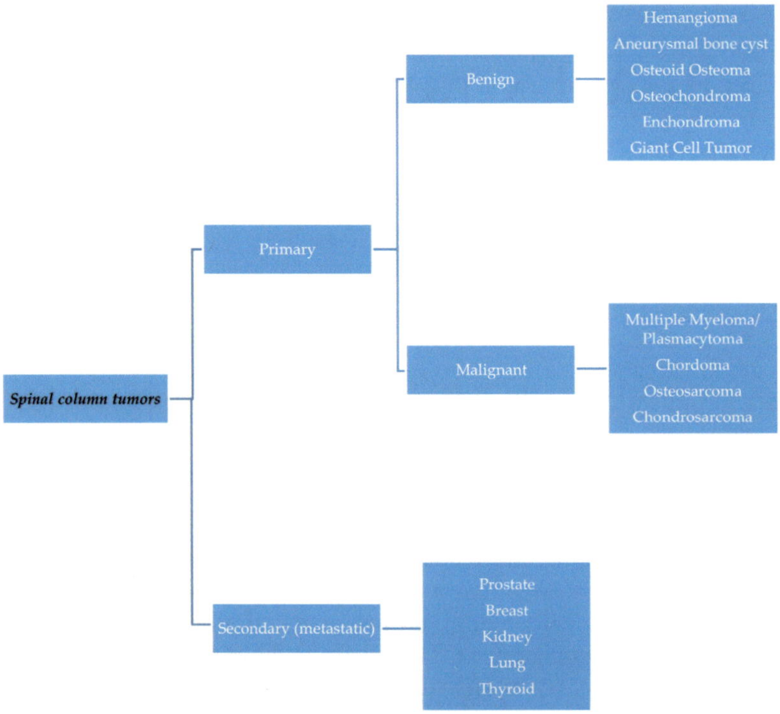

Figure 1.
Spinal column tumors.

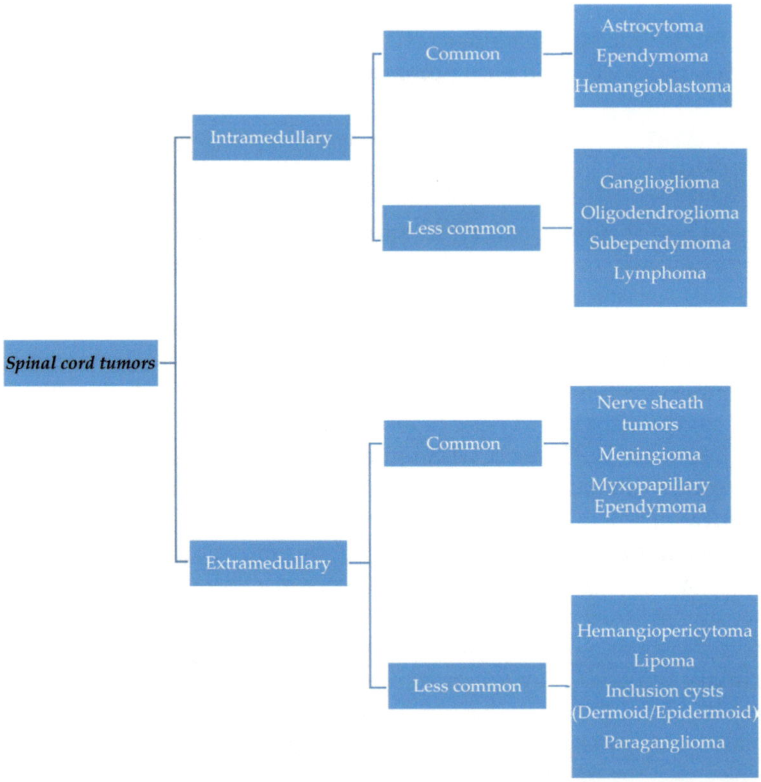
Spinal cord tumors
Intramedullary
Common
Astrocytoma
Ependymoma
Hemangioblastoma
Less common
Ganglioglioma
Oligodendroglioma
Subependymoma
Lymphoma
Extramedullary
Common
Nerve sheath tumors
Meningioma
Myxopapillary Ependymoma
Less common
Hemangiopericytoma
Lipoma
Inclusion cysts (Dermoid/Epidermoid)
Paraganglioma

Figure 2.
Intradural spinal cord tumors.

Tumors that arise within the dural sac are termed as intradural tumors and can be within the substance of the spinal cord (intramedullary) or outside of it (extramedullary); however, a small portion of tumors can be both intra- and extramedullary and usually are seen at the conus medullaris transition site to filum terminale or at the nerve root entry zone areas.

Intramedullary tumors are usually benign but can also be malignant, and the most common pathologies are astrocytoma, ependymoma, and hemangioblastoma (**Figure 2**); other less common tumors are gangliogliomas, oligodendrogliomas, subependymomas, and in very rare cases lymphomas.

Intradural extramedullary (IDEM) tumors consist almost 70% of all intradural lesions [5], and the most frequent types are nerve sheath tumors, meningiomas, and myxopapillary ependymomas. Other less common tumors include hemangiopericytomas, lipomas, paragangliomas, and inclusion cysts such as dermoid and epidermoid cysts (**Figure 2**).

In this chapter we focus on fundamentals of assessment, diagnosis, and treatment of intradural extramedullary tumors.

2. Epidemiology and histology

IDEM tumors are mostly consisted of meningiomas, nerve sheath tumors (schwannomas and neurofibromas), and at the filum terminale myxopapillary ependymomas.

Meningiomas are the most frequent intradural tumors and usually happen at the thoracic region. Psammomatous subtype is the most common histologic subtype, and they resemble the intracranial ones in which numerous psammoma bodies can be observed [6, 7]. Meningiomas have female preponderance with female to male ratio of 3–4:1 and tend to affect the elder population of 50–70 years of age [8].

Nerve sheath tumors affect both sexes equally with the peak incidence in the fourth and fifth decade of life. Schwannomas are the far more common subtype in this category and usually happen sporadically but also can be seen in neurofibromatosis type 2 [9]. Spinal NSTs arise from ventral or dorsal nerve rootlets with the dorsal nerve rootlet being more common. These tumors can be purely extradural especially at the cervical regions or purely intradural; they also can have both intra- and extradural components and present in dumbbell shape pattern.

The transition zone of the myelin-producing cells from oligodendrocytes to Schwann cell is believed to be where schwannomas arise from a nonfunctional nerve fascicle, and as they grow, these well-capsulated lesions can cause compression on adjacent functional fascicles [10]. Schwannomas can be seen in a compact cellular pattern with palisading verocay bodies (Antoni A) or in a less cellular pattern (Antoni B) [11].

Neurofibromas primarily are seen in patients with neurofibromatosis type 2 but can also happen sporadically. Unlike schwannomas these tumors can involve multiple nerve fascicles and expand the whole nerve which makes it sometimes impossible to totally resect the tumor without sacrificing the nerve of origin. The presence of axons in gross pathology can help in distinguishing these lesions from schwannomas.

Filum terminale ependymomas are well-capsulated tumors with slight male preponderance with peak incidence at 36 years of age [12]. Histologic smears reveal well-differentiated radially arranged cuboidal or columnar cells around vascularized myxoid cores with a myxopapillary appearance.

3. Genetic considerations

Genetic syndromes such as neurofibromatosis can be associated with IDEMs. Spinal neurofibromas can be associated with NF1 and NF2 in which NF1 is far more common than NF2.

Neurofibromatosis type 1 (NF1) caused by a mutation in the NF1 gene on chromosome 17 that codes neurofibromin is an autosomal dominant inherited syndrome that can be associated with multiple spinal neurofibromas.

Schwannomas, neurofibromas, and meningiomas are associated with NF2 which is inherited as an autosomal dominant syndrome and caused by mutation at chromosome 22 (NF2 gene) that codes merlin protein which is the responsible etiology [13]. Schwannomatosis a syndrome which is characterized by multiple schwannomas without defining other features of NF1 or NF2 is also another syndrome that may cause spinal schwannomas.

Spinal irradiation and NF2 are two main predisposing factors that cause spinal meningiomas. Intramedullary ependymomas are associated with NF2, but myxopapillary ependymoma is believed to be a distinct entity and is not related to NF2.

4. Sign and symptoms

IDEM tumors are usually benign slow-growing tumors, and there can be a long period of time between the initiation of symptoms and the diagnosis. Axial back pain can be present for a long time before diagnosis and can be the only symptom. Radicular pain is another symptom especially in patients with NSTs. Spinal cord compression can cause myelopathy or cauda equina syndrome.

Syndromic patients may reveal symptoms at younger age with more rapid progression of functional or neural impairment.

5. Imaging

Plain X-ray is not usually indicated in evaluation of patients with IDEM tumors, but due to the slow-growing nature of these tumors, reactive bony responses such as foraminal widening, vertebral body scalloping, laminar thinning, and increased inter-pedicular space can be seen.

Computed tomographic studies are quite helpful regarding the evaluation of bony structures, spinal stability, and tumoral calcification and are also helpful in surgical planning.

Magnetic resonance imaging is the modality of choice for the diagnosis of these lesions and delineating their relative anatomy regarding the spinal cord and nerve rootlets.

Schwannomas and neurofibromas have decreased or equal signals in T1W imaging and increased signal in T2W imaging, and they show avid heterogeneous or homogeneous enhancement in contrast studies (**Figure 3**).

Meningiomas have more homogeneous imaging patterns than NSTs and show equal to decreased signals in T1WI and equal to slightly increased signals in T2WI; they show more homogeneous contrast enhancement, and dural enhancement (dural tail) can also be observed (**Figure 4**).

Myxopapillary ependymomas usually represent themselves as isointense lesions in T1W imaging, but the mucinous component can show hypersignality in T1WI. Ependymomas are usually hypersignal in T2W imaging studies and

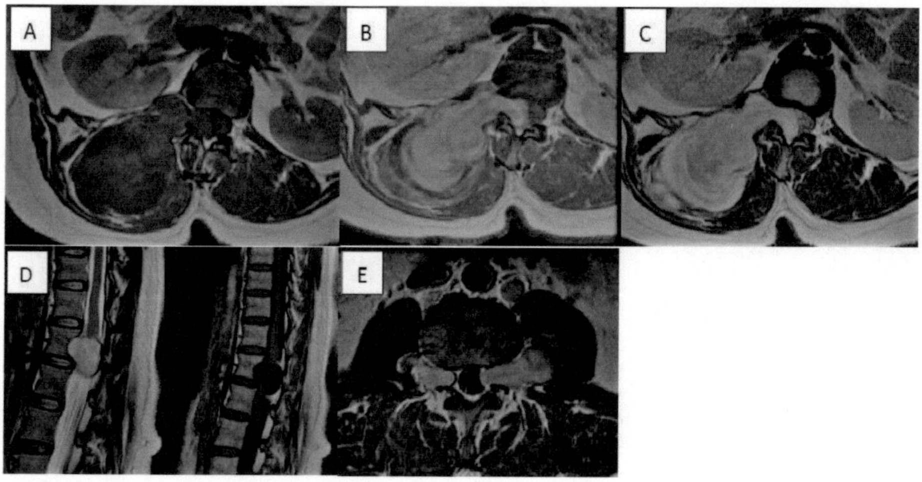

Figure 3.
T1W non-contrast-enhanced (A), T1W contrast-enhanced (B), and T2W (C) axial images of a thoracic schwannoma showing cord compression and massive retroperitoneal and paraspinal component. Midsagittal T1W and T2W MR images of a patient with thoracic schwannoma (D). Axial T2W MR image of a syndromic patient with NF1 showing bilateral spinal neurofibroma (E).

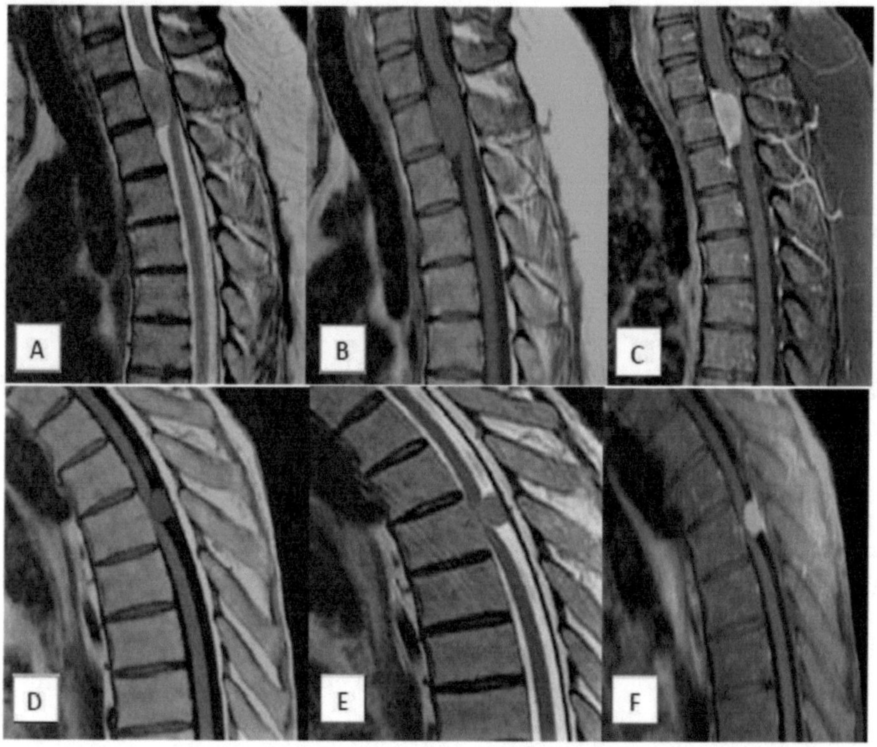

Figure 4.
Sagittal T2W (A), T1 non-contrast, (B) and contrast-enhanced (C) images of a patient with ventral thoracic meningioma. Sagittal T1W (D), T2W (E), and (F) T1 contrast-enhanced images of a patient with dorsal thoracic meningioma.

are enhanced in contrast studies. Myxopapillary ependymomas are most prone to hemorrhage, and when present, MR images show heterogeneous signals and heterogeneous enhancement pattern (**Figure 5**).

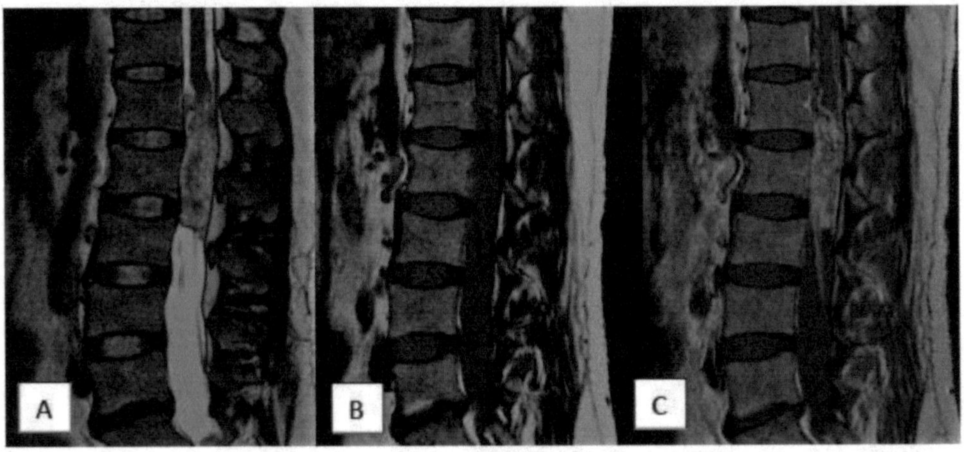

Figure 5.
Sagittal T2W (A), T1 non-contrast, (B) and contrast-enhanced (C) images of a patient with filum terminale ependymoma.

6. Indications for surgery and surgical routes

Surgical intervention is required in almost all symptomatic patients, but in syndromic patients with mild symptoms, due to higher chance of regrowth and multiple lesions, surgery might not be performed in order to avoid multiple surgeries in a short period of time.

All patients with progressive neural or functional impairment and those with rapid tumor growth in serial MR studies should undergo surgery.

Asymptomatic patients can be followed by serial clinical and radiological examinations, and surgery is not advised for diagnostic purposes only; the only exception would be myxopapillary ependymoma in which asymptomatic patients may be advised to undergo surgical evacuation for CSF seeding prevention [14, 15].

Most of IDEM tumors can be approached via simple posterior standard laminectomy, though the tumor location in the spinal axis and its relation to the spinal cord are the major factors determining the surgical route.

Cervical lesions can be addressed via both anterior and posterior approaches. Tumors located posteriorly, laterally, and ventrolaterally can be approached by posterior laminectomy procedure.

For the lesions above C2 when located ventrally, an extensive lateral approach to the foramen magnum can be used which needs vertebral artery transposition and sigmoid sinus skeletonization; on the other hand, ventral subaxial lesions can be addressed via standard anterior cervical procedure.

Thoracic IDEM tumors are generally operated via posterior approaches due to complications and difficulties of the transthoracic technique described by Bohlman which needs significant lung retraction and may cause serious vascular injuries [16]. Various posterior techniques have been described for ventral thoracic lesion removal including the traditional extracavitary technique described by Larson which is suitable for both ventrally located tumors and tumors with large extra-foraminal component and costotransversectomy technique which is also suitable for lateral and ventrolateral lesions but not for tumors located ventrally due to limited surgical view of the contralateral side passing the midline [17].

Most of lumbar and sacral IDEM tumors are operated via posterior approach or its modifications; anterior trans- or retroperitoneal approaches are barely used now.

The key to a successful surgery is minimal cord or nerve root retraction, and for this purpose extensive resection of bony structures may be necessary, and this might lead to spinal instability. There are multiple reports of successful spinal instrumented fusion surgeries in treated patients with IDEM [18].

Bilateral laminectomy and medial facetectomies usually do not cause spinal instability, while total unilateral facetectomy especially at cervical or lumbar area makes spinal column unstable [19].

7. Surgical treatment of nerve sheath tumors

Patients undergoing standard posterior approach are placed in prone position with head fixed in Mayfield head holder for cervical tumors or placed at the headrest frame. Arms are placed along side of the trunk in upper thoracic lesions or are abducted by 90° in lower thoracic or lumbosacral lesions.

Motor and sensory evoked potential monitoring system is applied, and for cervical and lumbosacral lesions, continuous nerve root EMG monitoring should also be performed.

Midline skin and fascia incisions are made, and classic subperiosteal dissection of the paravertebral muscles is performed. Small laterally located lesions can be reached by a simple hemilaminectomy, but bilateral laminectomy widens the surgical view and may be preferred in most surgeries. Laminectomy length should exceed the whole length of the tumor, and regarding the tumor size and location, unilateral facetectomy may also be performed; intraoperative ultrasonography is helpful in determining the adequacy of the laminectomy extension.

Dura is usually opened posteriorly in a linear fashion which makes duraplasty much easier but also can be opened in a T-shaped fashion or at the paramedian site. Dural opening length should exceed the tumors' length, and when opened, it is sutured to the paraspinal musculature, and then the arachnoid layer is opened. Surgical microscope is mandatory in intradural tumor resection surgeries, and under microscopic view careful dissection of the arachnoid layer, cord, and nerve roots from the tumor is carried out. NSTs are usually originated from dorsal nerve rootlets, but the normal anatomy might be distorted; careful identification of the afferent and efferent origin nerve roots should be performed before tumor resection. Large tumors obstructing the surgical view should be entered and debulked by an ultrasonic aspirator, and then careful identification of the origin roots is carried out. Sensory origin nerve roots are usually bulge and vascular, but motor ones can appear totally normal, and motor evoked potential monitoring can be helpful in distinguishing the motor nerve of origin.

NSTs might extend into the pial surface of the spinal cord, and so, no obvious sensory afferent root might be distinguishable; in these cases, careful dissection of the tumor from the cord substance should be performed. At the cervical and lumbar spine, preservation of the functional motor roots is important, and only those confirmed to be nonfunctional by motor evoked potential studies can be sacrificed. After identification and ligation of the origin afferent and efferent roots with preservation of all functional ones, the tumor is carefully dissected and resected. Subarachnoid space is irrigated vigorously until the blood is cleared. Dural closure is performed with running sutures in a watertight fashion, and then multilayer suturing of the paraspinal muscles, fascia, subcutaneous layer, and skin is carried out. Some surgeons advocate the use of lumbar drain post-op for 48–72 hours to avoid CSF leakage from the incision site.

NSTs can grow extradurally and into neural foramina and even beyond that and get to a significant size at the paraspinal regions; in these cases, we prefer to operate the intradural part first and decompress the spinal canal; the extradural part can be evacuated at the same procedure or may be addressed to in a staged surgery via the same route or in another surgical route depending on the size of the extra-foraminal part.

8. Surgical treatment of spinal meningiomas

In order to approach a spinal meningioma, a surgeon must consider the site and the location of the tumor regarding the cord and boney structures. Meningiomas barely have extradural components and are commonly ventral to the cord.

Cervical meningiomas are addressed by a posterior standard technique if located dorsally or by an anterior approach if located ventrally. Thoracic meningiomas are usually reached via posterior routes, and if located ventrally, extracavitary or costotransversectomy techniques might be used; sectioning and suture rotating the dentate ligament may be helpful for a better and wider surgical view. Lumbar meningiomas are usually operated via posterior approaches because the surgeon is able to safely retract the nerve roots.

Patients are positioned in the same way as patients with NSTs, and motor and sensory evoked potentials are monitored before and during the surgery.

Meningiomas are dural-based lesions, and the extent of dural involvement may be greater than the amount shown in MR studies so the laminectomy length should exceed the cephalad and caudal poles of the tumor, and intraoperative sonography is very helpful in this regard. Durotomy should be performed in an ellipsoid fashion in dorsally located tumors so that the tumor and the involved dura matter could be resected totally.

Ventrally located meningiomas are more challenging both in surgical resection and dural reconstitution which the latter might even be impossible; hence, many prefer dural coagulation instead of resection. Dural coagulation at the tumor base reduces intraoperative bleeding.

When the tumor poles are exposed, the dentate ligament can be sectioned and rotated by a suture for surgical view improvement. Large tumors compressing the cord should be debulked by an ultrasonic aspirator before resection so that spinal cord gets decompressed and a better view of the tumor margins could be achieved.

9. Surgical treatment of filum terminale ependymomas

Myxopapillary ependymomas are solid fleshy lesions originating from filum terminale and can have a large size at the time of diagnosis. These lesions are exclusively approached via posterior surgical procedure, and care must be taken to resect these tumors in an en bloc fashion so that CSF seeding and metastasis would not occur [20, 21].

Standard posterior approach in a prone position is performed under electrophysiologic monitoring evaluation, and when laminectomy is completed, dura is opened dorsally in a linear fashion and then sutured to paraspinal musculature. Arachnoid layer is opened, and careful microdissection of the neural roots from tumor is performed, and filum is identified proximal and distal to the tumor and tested by a neurostimulator.

Filum is cauterized and sectioned at both ends of the tumor, and then en bloc tumor resection is achieved with caution not to retract adjacent nerve roots excessively.

In some cases, en bloc resection of the tumor cannot be obtained especially when the tumor is too fragile and falls apart even with most careful microdissection or when it's too large, and safe en bloc resection is impossible. The presence of functional nerve roots in the tumor substance also makes en bloc resection impossible, and subtotal resection would be the only option.

Dura is approximated by running sutures in a watertight fashion, and multilayer closure of the overlying compartments is carried out.

10. Adjuvant therapies

Adjuvant therapies do not play a major role in treatment of IDEM tumors, and microsurgical gross total resection still is the gold standard modality of treatment.

Radiotherapy has a defined role in patients with myxopapillary ependymoma and improves their progression-free survival when administered postsurgery [21].

Radiotherapy is administered in multiple recurrent meningiomas or the ones with atypical or malignant histology [22]. Stereotactic radiosurgery has been shown to be beneficial in patients with NSTs or meningiomas as the primary modality of treatment or as an adjuvant therapy in patients with post-operation radiologic tumor growth [23, 24].

Stereotactic radiosurgery is of more importance in syndromic patients who might have multiple lesions and also a higher tumor progression rate and helps them to face less surgical procedures in their lifetime.

Author details

Saleh Rasras* and Arash Kiani
Ahvaz Jundishapour University of Medical Sciences, Ahvaz, Iran

*Address all correspondence to: dr.rasras@gmail.com

References

[1] Jaffe HL. Tumors and Tumorous Conditions of Bones and Joints. Philadelphia: Lea & Febiger; 1958

[2] Akram H, Allibone J. Spinal surgery for palliation in malignant spinal cord compression. Clinical Oncology (Royal College of Radiologists). 2010;**22**:792-800

[3] Maccauro G, Spinelli MS, Mauro S, et al. Physiopathology of spine metastasis. International Journal of Surgical Oncology. 2011;**2011**:107969

[4] Fox MW, Onofrio BM. The natural history and management of symptomatic and asymptomatic vertebral hemangiomas. Journal of Neurosurgery. 1993;**78**:36-45

[5] Traul DE, Shaffrey ME, Schiff D. Part I: Spinal-cord neoplasms–intradural neoplasms. The Lancet Oncology. 2007;**8**:35-45

[6] Gottfried ON, Gluf W, Quinones-Hinojosa A, et al. Spinal meningiomas: Surgical management and outcome. Neurosurgical Focus. 2003;**14**(6):e2

[7] Schaller B. Spinal meningioma: Relationship between histological subtypes and surgical outcome? Journal of Neuro-Oncology. 2005;**75**:157-161

[8] Preston-Martin S. Descriptive epidemiology of primary tumors of the spinal cord and spinal meninges in Los Angeles County, 1972-1985. Neuroepidemiology. 1990;**9**:106-111

[9] Seppälä MT, Haltia MJ, Sankila RJ, et al. Long-term outcome after removal of spinal schwannoma: A clinicopathological study of 187 cases. Journal of Neurosurgery. 1995;**83**:621-626

[10] Kim P, Ebersold MJ, Onofrio BM, et al. Surgery of spinal nerve schwannoma. Risk of neurological deficit after resection of involved root. Journal of Neurosurgery. 1989;**71**:810-814

[11] Requena L, Sangüeza OP. Benign neoplasms with neural differentiation: A review. The American Journal of Dermatopathology. 1995;**17**:75-96

[12] Sonneland PR, Scheithauer BW, Onofrio BM. Myxopapillary ependymoma. A clinicopathologic and immunocytochemical study of 77 cases. Cancer. 1985;**56**:883-893

[13] National Institutes of Health Consensus Development Conference Statement: Neurofibromatosis. Bethesda, Md., USA, July 13-15, 1987. Neurofibromatosis. 1988;**1**:172-178

[14] Mridha AR, Sharma MC, Sarkar C, et al. Myxopapillary ependymoma of lumbosacral region with metastasis to both cerebellopontine angles: Report of a rare case. Child's Nervous System. 2007;**24**:1209-1213

[15] Fassett DR, Pingree J, Kestle JRW, et al. The high incidence of tumor dissemination in myxopapillary ependymoma in pediatric patients. Report of five cases and review of the literature. Journal of Neurosurgery. 2005;**102**(1 suppl):59-64

[16] Bohlman HH, Zdeblick TA. Anterior excision of herniated thoracic discs. The Journal of Bone and Joint Surgery. American Volume. 1988;**20**:1038-1047

[17] McCormick PC. Surgical management of dumbbell and paraspinal tumors of the thoracic and lumbar spine. Neurosurgery. 1996;**38**:67-74

[18] Ando K, Imagama S, Ito Z, et al. Unilateral instrumented fixation for cervical dumbbell tumors. Journal of

Orthopaedic Surgery and Research. 2014;**9**:2

[19] Abumi K, Panjabi M, Kramer K, et al. Biomechanical evaluation of lumbar spinal stability after graded facetectomies. Spine. 1990;**15**:1142-1147

[20] Wen BC, Hussey DH, Hitchon PW, et al. The role of radiation therapy in the management of ependymomas of the spinal cord. International Journal of Radiation Oncology, Biology, Physics. 1991;**20**:781-786

[21] Akyurek S, Chang EL, Yu TK, et al. Spinal myxopapillary ependymoma outcomes in patients treated with surgery and radiotherapy at M.D. Anderson Cancer Center. Neuro-Oncology. 2006;**80**:177-183

[22] Schiebe ME, Hoffmann W, Kortmann RD, et al. Radiotherapy in recurrent malignant meningiomas with multiple spinal manifestations. Acta Oncologica. 1997;**36**:88-90

[23] Dodd RL, Ryu MR, Kamnerdsupaphon P, et al. CyberKnife radiosurgery for benign intradural extramedullary spinal tumors. Neurosurgery. 2006;**58**:674-685

[24] Gerszten PC, Burton SA, Ozhasoglu C, et al. Radiosurgery for benign intradural spinal tumors. Neurosurgery. 2008;**62**:887-896

Chapter 4

Jugular Foramen Paragangliomas

Breno Nery, Rodrigo Antônio Fernandes Costa, Eduardo Quaggio, Ricardo Lopes Araújo, Bernardo Alves Barbosa, Diogo Fabricio Coelho de Melo, Carolina Salviano de Abreu Nery, Fred Bernardes Filho and George Peter Stevens

Abstract

Jugular foramen paragangliomas are rare neoplasms occurring with a myriad of symptoms originating from paraganglionic tissue derived from the neural crest, comprising about 0.03% of all human tumors. Patients usually present with symptoms of dysfunction of VI, VII, VIII, IX, X, XI, XII nerves and sympathetic trunk. Depending on the tumor's topography, various approaches might be used to obtain its gross total resection. Jugular Foramen's paraganglioma classification, nuances of the approaches, pathology, postoperative complications, and outcomes are revised as follows. In conclusion, anatomical knowledge and the disease's comprehension are essential when dealing with such tumors, and despite their rarity, we must be obstinately committed to the surgical technique and devoted to the patient's functional postoperative outcome.

Keywords: paraganglioma, brain neoplasms

1. Introduction

Tumors located in the jugular foramen are rare, being one of the significant challenges in the surgical practice for cranial base neurosurgeons. Several tumors can affect this region, among them schwannomas, paragangliomas, and meningiomas representing the most common. Head and neck paragangliomas are rare neoplasms comprising about 0.03% of all human tumors. The yearly incidence is estimated to be at around 0.001% [1, 2]. Rarely, tumors located in the jugular foramen show intracranial and extracranial extension and, thus, present a myriad of symptoms, with several clinical syndromes described in the literature (see clinical presentation). The term "glomus tumor" has been used to describe the most common tumor related to this region, representing a tumor originating from paraganglionic tissue derived from the neural crest whose cells have the capacity to reserve and release catecholamines and may have clinical implications (see preoperative preparation) [3, 4].

Malignant tumors can also affect the jugular foramen, including metastatic tumors (carcinomas), chondrosarcomas and chordomas, as part of the differential diagnosis of these lesions [3]. The detailed discussion of the differential diagnosis of these lesions is not part of the scope of this chapter and can be seen in other references [3-5].

Advances in diagnostic imaging and surgical technique have allowed the understanding of these tumors and their exeresis with lower morbidity and mortality. A brief review of the clinical, diagnostic, imaging, histopathological and surgical aspects related to the glomus tumors of the jugular foramen is given below.

2. Clinical presentation

Glomus tumors of the jugular foramen present with slow growth and with early signs and clinical symptoms, being diagnosed on average after 5 years of onset of symptoms. These tumors have an average growth rate of approximately 1 mm per year [6]. The symptoms are directly related to the site of involvement and infiltration. Tumors of glomus jugulare represent neoplastic lesions that originate in the adventitia of the jugular vein and most commonly present with symptoms related to the involvement of lower cranial nerves, such as vagus (X), accessory (XI) and hypoglossus (XII). In the variant of glomus tympanicum, which are tumors related to the Jacobson's nerve, the most common initial clinical presentation is the presence of tinnitus, followed by conductive deafness and vertigo. Jacobson's nerve represents a tympanic branch of the glossopharyngeal nerve, which conveys the sensitivity of the tympanic membrane, auditory tube, and mastoid region. In the third anatomotopographic variety of this tumor we have the glomus vagale, originating from Arnold's nerve. Arnold's nerve emerges between the superior and inferior ganglia of the vagus nerve (auricular branch of the vagus nerve) and

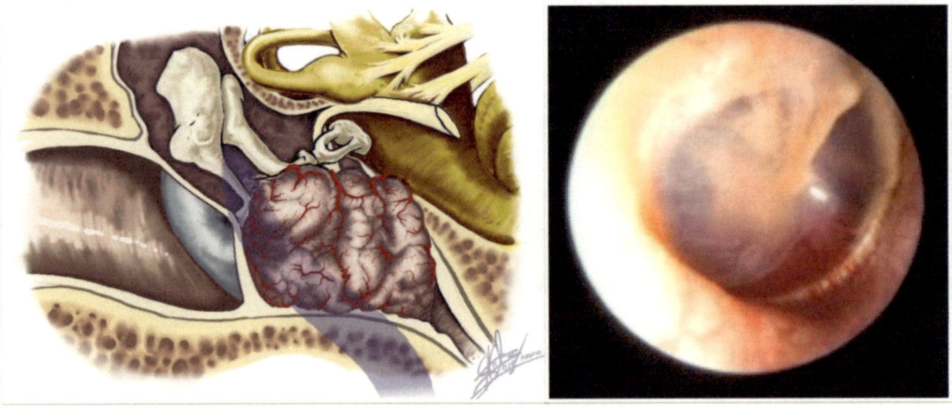

Figure 1.
On the left, anatomical relationships of the glomus tumor of the jugular foramen; on the right, otoscopy revealing the presence of a tumor in the lower right field.

Jugular foramen syndromes and respective affected nerves	Vernet	Collet-Sicard	Vilaret	Tapia	Jackson	Schmidt
IX	+	+	+			
X	+	+	+	+	+	+
XI	+	+	+	+/—	+	+
XII	—	+	+	+	+	—
Sympathetic fibers	—	—	+	+/—	—	+

Table 1.
Syndromes related to the jugular foramen.

is responsible for the sensitive innervation of the skin over the outer ear's shell. Detailed examination through otoscopy may reveal the presence of tympanic membrane invasion, and otorhinolaryngology may be evidenced in some cases (**Figure 1**). Classical syndromes related to this type of tumor and their respective locations are described in **Table 1**.

3. Pre-operative diagnosis and image classification

Detailed clinical examination is essential for accurate lesion location and scheduling of resection of the intra- and extracranial portions of the tumor. Detailed examinations of the functions of VI, VII, VIII, IX, X, XI, XII and sympathetic trunk should be performed, seeking to predict the intraoperative relations of the tumor with the cranial nerves. Prior to the decision to resect the lesion, evaluation of lesion growth pattern through serial imaging is not considered bad practice. Computed tomography (CT) scans and fine sections (1.0 mm) with reconstruction in the coronal and sagittal planes are essential to delineate the bone relations of the tumor during the chosen surgical approach, as well as the study by the magnetic resonance imaging (MRI) with gadolinium is essential for the evaluation of the neurovascular relationships of the lesion. Tomography can show a smoother surface and have associated bone erosion in cases of schwannoma of the jugular foramen, in contrast to paragangliomas of this region, which demonstrate a more irregular

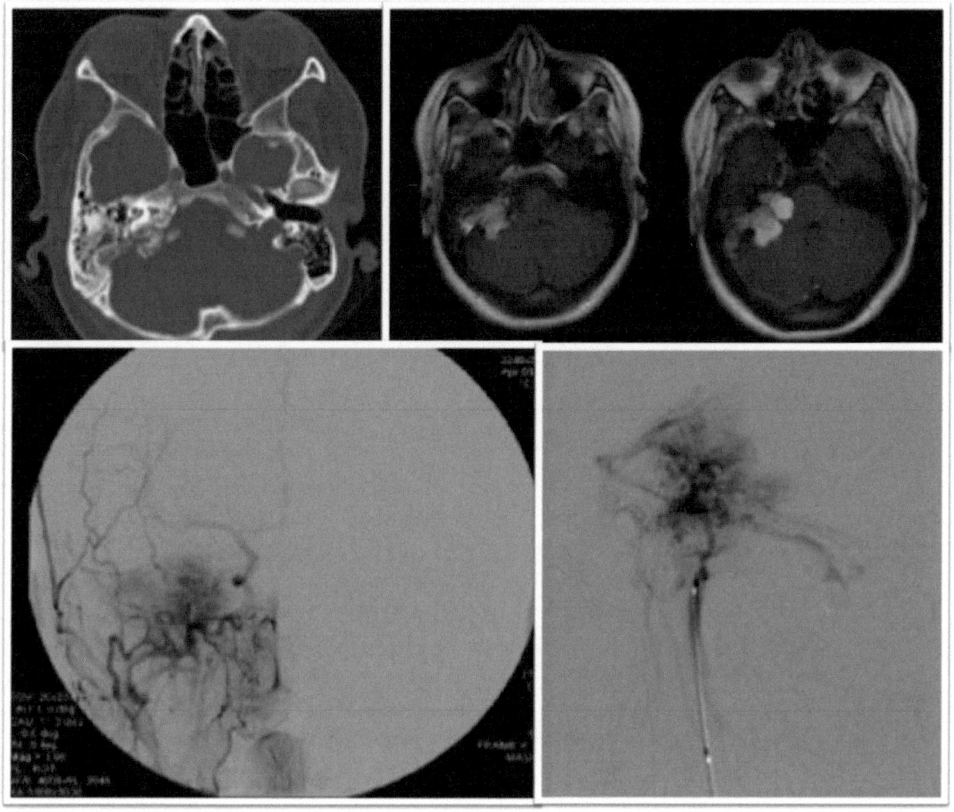

Figure 2.
On the superior left, glomus tumor of the right jugular foramen seen on the tomography (moth-eaten pattern); on the superior right, magnetic nuclear resonance with "salt and pepper" appearance; below, angiography evidencing irrigation of a glomus tumor of the head predominantly by the right ascending pharyngeal artery.

tumoral surface with adjacent bone destruction (**Figure 1**). Neurovascular relationships with the internal carotid artery, cephalic trunk, as well as its intra and extracranial extension are better visualized through the MRI. In T1 weighted images, the glomus tumor is hypo/isointense to the brainstem, and gadolinium injection presents the classic salt and pepper enhancement pattern (**Figure 1**).

Pepper's image represents the hypointense void sign, and the "salt" image represents the hyperintense signal caused by low vascular flow or intratumoral subacute hemorrhage. These tumors typically have a distinct pattern of infiltration, generally following pathways of lower resistance, such as air mastoid cells, vascular channels, Eustachian tube and neural foramina [7, 8].

Angioresonance, angiotomography, or venography may help to demonstrate the type of vascularization of the tumor and its local venous circulation (**Figure 2**). Digital angiography is a prerequisite in patients with extremely vascular lesions, for whom preoperative embolization is necessary to reduce bleeding during surgery. **Table 2** shows the imaging modalities and the peculiar characteristics of the tumors of this region during the preoperative study, aiming to differentiate the three most common lesions of this region. A balloon occlusion test should be performed in case of involvement of the internal carotid artery.

The most relevant laboratory exams prior to surgery are serum and urinary catecholamines, as well as urinary levels of vanilmandelic acid and urinary metanephrines, to determine the possibility of neuroendocrine secretion of the tumor. Five percent of glomus tumors of the jugular foramen (JF) are secretory, and in

Tumor type and radiological features by imaging studies	**Computed tomography**	**Nuclear magnetic resonance**	**Digital angiography**
Glomus tumors	• "Moth-eaten" pattern of temporal bone • Dehiscence of the floor of the tympanic cavity • Erosion of the ossicular chain	• T1 weighted images heterogeneously enhanced with gadolinium "salt and pepper" pattern	• Irrigation of the inferomedial portion of the tumor by the ascending pharyngeal artery • Posterior auricular, stylomastoid and • occipital arteries irrigate the posterolateral portion of the tumor • Internal maxillary artery and ACI may contribute to larger tumors
Schwannoma	• Isodense tumors • Enlargement of the jugular foramen without destruction	• T1 hypointense, T2 hyperintense and moderate enhancement with gadolinium	• Absence of significant irrigation or compression of the jugular vein
Meningioma	• Isodense with intense and homogeneous contrast enhancement • Hyperostosis, intralesional calcifications	• Characteristic and homogeneous enhancement • Presence of dural tail	• Early enhancement with slow emptying

Table 2.
Differential diagnoses by imaging of the main lesions affecting the jugular foramen.

A	Tumors limited to the space of the middle ear
B	Tumors limited to the middle ear or mastoid, without involvement of the infralabirintic space of the temporal bone
C	Tumor involving the infralabirintic space and apical spaces of the temporal bone, with extension to the petrous apex
C1	Tumor with little involvement of the vertical portion of the carotid canal
C2	Tumor invading the vertical portion of the carotid canal
C3	Tumor invading the horizontal portion of the carotid canal
D1	Tumor invading the horizontal portion of the carotid canal
D2	Tumor with intracranial extension >2 cm in diameter

Table 3.
Fisch classification for glomus tumors of temporal region.

I	Tumor involving jugular bulb, middle ear and mastoid
II	Tumor extending below the internal acoustic meatus; may present intracranial extension
III	Tumor extending to the petrous apex; may present intracranial extension
IV	Tumor extending beyond the petrous apex to the infratemporal clivus or infratemporal fossa; may present intracranial extension

Table 4.
Glasscock-Jackson classification for glomus tumors of jugular foramen.

these cases, the preoperative use of alpha and beta-blockers are essential to avoid complications. The most commonly used radiological classification in the preoperative evaluation of patients with glomus tumors of the jugular foramen are Fisch [9] (**Table 3**) and Glasscock-Jackson [10] (**Table 4**). The most used classification of schwannomas of the jugular foramen is Samii's classification, who divided the schwannomas of the jugular foramen into four groups: type A which represents the primary tumors of the cerebellar angle with minimal enlargement of the JF; type B that are the primary tumors of the JF with intracranial extension; type C which have extracranial tumors with extension to the jugular foramen (with clinical signs of involvement of the XII nerve); and type D being the "hourglass" tumors with intra and extracranial involvement [11].

4. Histopathological characteristics

Glomus tumors of the jugular foramen present polygonal epithelioid cells with clear and abundant cytoplasm arranged in small lobes (alveolar arrangement). These cellular clusters were given the name Zellballen, which means "cellular balls" in German. Numerous capillaries can also be observed in the proximity of tumor cells that perform tumor irrigation (**Figure 3**).

5. Surgical approaches

Patients should be routinely monitored, and preoperative antibiotic (30 min before incision) should be administered. The ideal approach for each patient should be chosen after a meticulous preoperative study of lesion's location. Tumors that

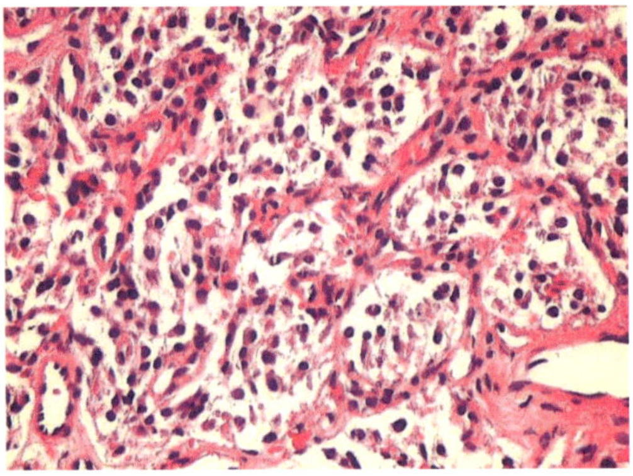

Figure 3.
Typical alveolar pattern with presence of Zellballen, which are classic epithelioid clusters of these tumors.

are primarily intracranial located (Samii type A schwannomas) or tumors with a more significant intracranial extension may be approached by the classic lateral suboccipital retrosigmoid approach. The patient should be ideally positioned in a semi-sited position, since the presence of tumor bleeding gravitates downward, maintaining the surgical field with better visibility throughout the resection. Ideally, central venous access and pre-cordial Doppler should be used to prevent and treat air embolism. Pneumatic compression boots should be used to facilitate venous return. The head should be rotated about 30° to the same side of the lesion, aiming a straight direction in relation to the jugular foramen, as well as a smaller cerebellar retraction, and be fixed in a Mayfield head holder. Discrete flexion helps to expose the suboccipital region, facilitating the positioning of the surgeon during the approach. Vigorous rotation and flexion should be avoided as they may compromise jugular venous return; so a space of two fingers should separate the chin from the ipsilateral clavicle for this purpose. A cutaneous incision should be made with an upper limit on the pinna to the posterior musculature of the neck, maintaining a distance of about 3 cm from the mastoid. After incision of the muscular plane, suboccipital craniectomy is performed, ideally exposing the inferior portion of the transverse sinus and medial portion of the sigmoid sinus. The most crucial step of the craniectomy is its inferior extension to the posterior border of the magnum foramen. The dura mater should be cut in a "C" fashion with its convex portion of the cut close to the transverse and sigmoid sinuses. The dura mater, when cut in this way, not only protects the cerebellar hemisphere from contusions but also prevents dural redundancy in the visual field of the surgeon, also allowing more adequate closure at the end of the procedure.

Next, the arachnoid trabeculae of the Magna cistern of the pontocerebellar angle (PCA) should be cut, and careful aspiration of cerebrospinal fluid should follow, allowing relaxation of the neurovascular structures. Then, the anterior and medial portion of the cerebellum must be carefully covered with cottonoids and retracted medially and superiorly with a spatula, and then fixed in a static position. Dialogue with neurophysiologists is essential during this time of surgery, and repositioning of the spatula may be necessary in case of disturbed auditory brainstem evoked potential. It is essential to determine the exact position of the tumor in relation to the sigmoid sinus and bulb of the jugular vein, because in larger tumors of this region the wall of these vessels may be compromised, with catastrophic bleeding that is difficult to control. Extradural drilling of the jugular foramen helps to define the margins of the tumor, and after this maneuver follows the careful debulking of the tumor.

We carefully proceed with the dissection between the tumor and the lower cranial nerves, as well as its separation of the sigmoid sinus and bulb of the jugular vein when they are involved. The use of ultrasonic aspiration helps significantly during the resection of these tumors. As the tumor resection is performed, we maintain an incessant dialogue with the neurophysiologist observing the changes during the monitoring of the lower cranial nerves (IX, X, XI, XII). At the end of resection, hemostasis is followed, and defects in the skull base and mastoid should be covered with autologous fat and fibrin glue. The closure in subsequent layers is done, and extubation is monitored by an anesthesiologist in the operating room when there is no cranial nerve injury. Larger tumors (schwannomas B, C, and D of Samii) or glomus tumors involving the infralabirintic space, auditory meatus, jugular bulb, and mastoid need an exposition that allows a more adequate vascular control and more significant bone resection to allow complete or near-total resection of the lesions.

The patient should be ideally placed in the supine position, and his/her head should be rotated about 60–70 degrees contralaterally and fixed with the Mayfield head holder. Due to the need for a more considerable amount of autologous fat graft to later wound closure, we suggest the abdominal preparation for its eventual use. The incision follows from the anterior sternocleidomastoid (ECM) muscle to the retroauricular region, taking care to preserve the larger auricular nerve, since it may be a neural graft donor source for an eventual injury of intracranial nerves. Dissection of the neck allows adequate identification of the lower cranial nerves after their emergence of the skull, as well as carotid artery and internal jugular vein. Suboccipital craniectomy prior to mastoidectomy greatly facilitates control over the sigmoid sinus and jugular bulb, since the dura of the posterior fossa is less adhered to the sigmoid sinus and craniectomy facilitates its identification, reducing the possibility of injury to the sigmoid sinus even during mastoid air cells drilling. The cortical portion of the mastoid can be removed and used for the reconstruction of that region at the end of the procedure, and the mastoid air cells are drilled until a thin layer of bone remains over the sigmoid sinus/jugular vein's bulb. The venous structures are carefully separated, and the retrolabyrinthine bony portion resected until exposure of the posterior fossa dura. Care should be taken when drilling the anterior portion of this approach, avoiding entering the labyrinth and injuring the facial nerve. By drilling the intralabyrinthine portion, the extracranial portion of the tumor can be adequately resected. If there is an intracranial lesion, the opening of the dura mater in the presigmoid retrolabyrinthine region is followed, and the intradural resection is completed. In the case of preoperative anacusis (diagnosed by audiometry), presigmoid translabyrinthine approach, transcochlear approach and even posterior or total petrosectomy can be performed to maximize resection (**Figures 4–9**).

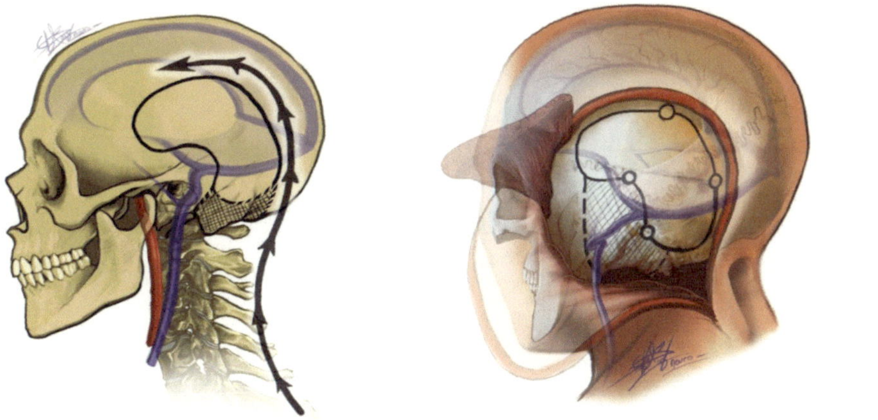

Figure 4.
Skin incision (arrows on the left), muscle dissection and bur hole demarcations (on the right) for a posterior petrosal approach.

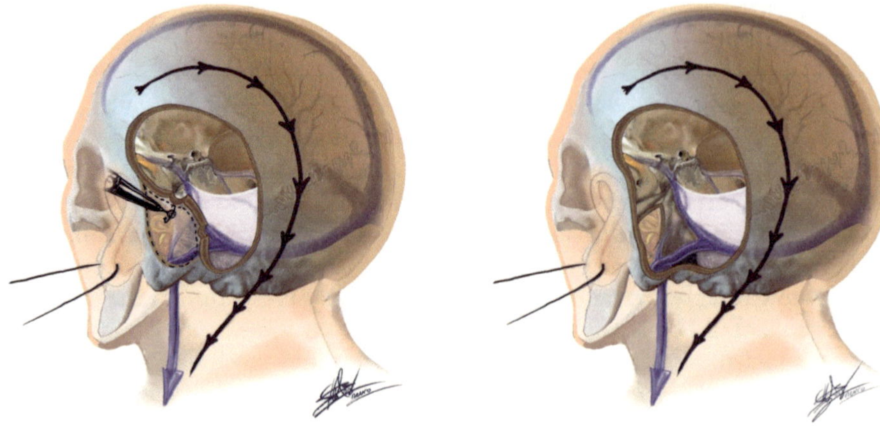

Figure 5.
Skin incision and bur hole demarcations for a posterior petrosal approach after the craniotomy (left side) and after mastoid drilling (right side).

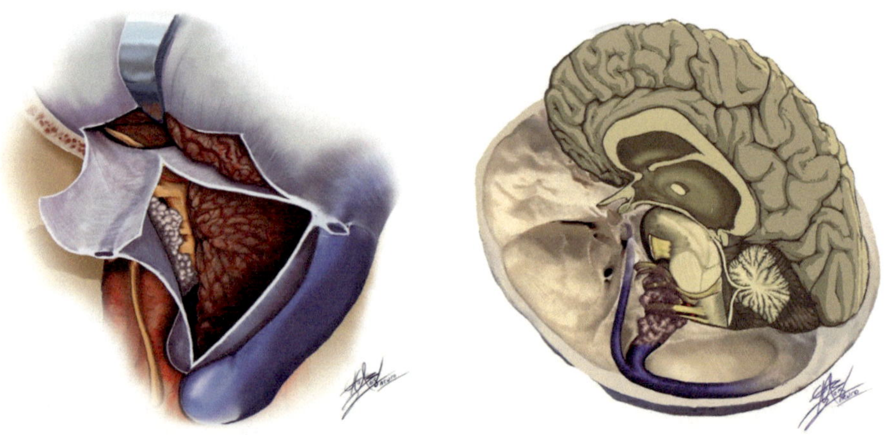

Figure 6.
Presigmoid approach and tentorial incision (on the left). Three-dimensional perspective of the tumor and its relationship with neural, vascular and skull base structures (right side).

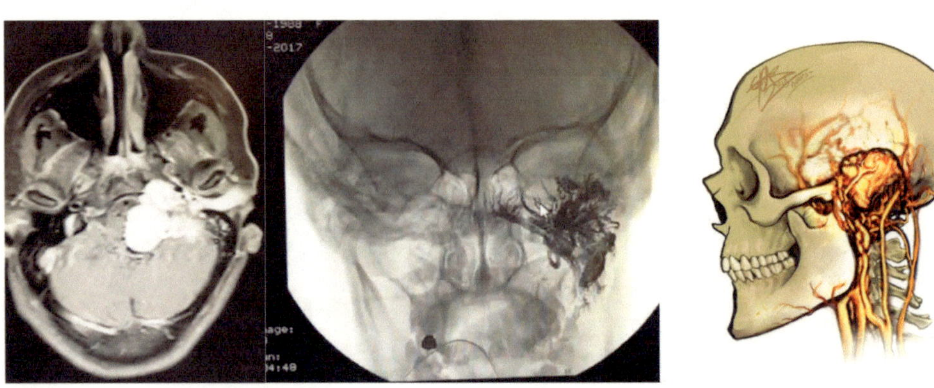

Figure 7.
On the left side, preoperative T1 weighted MRI with gadolinium from a patient operated in our institution; in the middle, preoperative embolization, 1 day before surgery. On the right side, artist's depiction of the tumor and its vascularity.

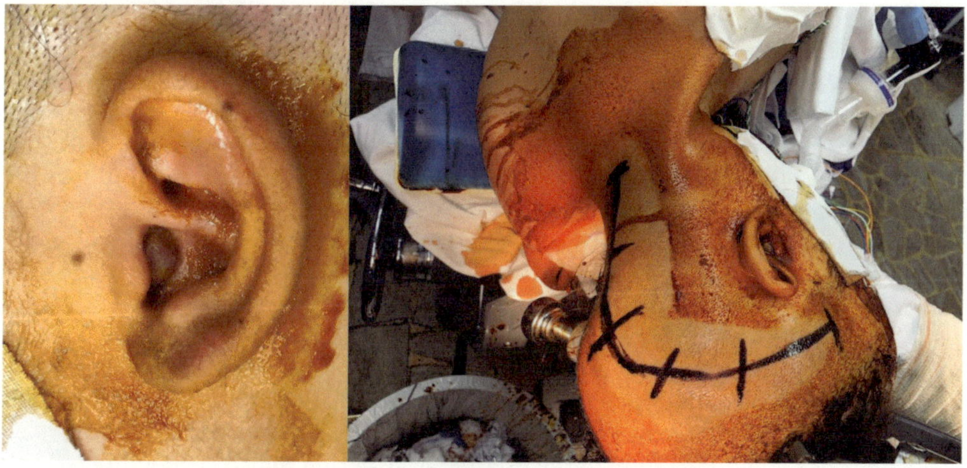

Figure 8.
External auditory meatus invasion by the tumor on the left side and skin incision on the right side.

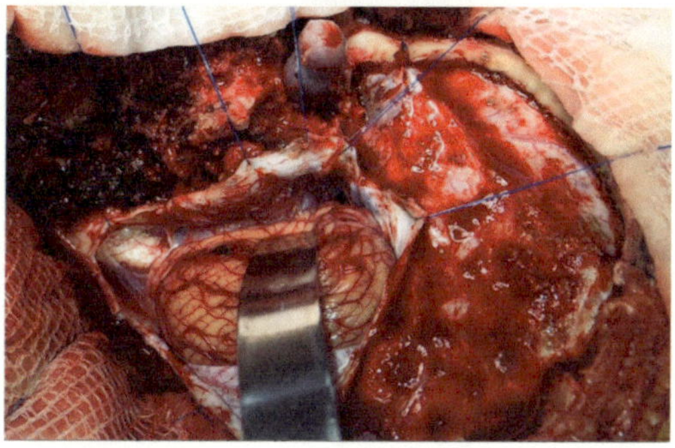

Figure 9.
Approaches' visualization after craniotomy, partial incision of the tentorium.

In cases of infiltration or occlusion of the sigmoid sinus by the tumor, its proximal and distal ligation can be performed, generally without the addition of deficits since the collateral venous drainage is developed by slow tumor growth. After hemostasis and verification of cranial nerve function by neurophysiologists, hemostasis follows. The retroauricular space with the mastoid should be filled with autologous fat graft and fibrin glue. Closure should than be performed.

6. Treatment with radiotherapy

Increasing evidence demonstrates that stereotactic radiosurgery, particularly Gamma-Knife (GK) surgery may play a relevant role in the treatment of these tumors. Results show no change in neurological signs and symptoms in up to 65% of patients [12]. Due to the best results with microsurgery, we prefer microsurgical resection with the use of radiosurgery in residual or recurrent tumor.

7. Postoperative complications and results

Possible complications include facial nerve damage, injury to the lower cranial nerves, injury to the internal carotid artery, excessive bleeding due to lesions of the venous structures (sigmoid sinus and internal jugular vein), and other complications such as cerebrospinal fluid fistula and infection. Larger tumors (C and D of Fisch) represent a greater surgical challenge, and cranial nerve deficits can be seen postoperatively and in around 6% of cases [13]. Facial paralysis can be seen in around 6% of cases, and cerebrospinal fluid fistula occurs in about 5% of cases [13]. Giant tumors with invasion of multiple structures have a more difficult but feasible resection, and malignant tumors have a reserved prognosis [14].

8. Conclusion

Resection of paragangliomas is possible as long as accurate clinical evaluation and preoperative examinations are rigorously performed. Complications can occur during and after the surgery, and we must be adequately prepared for its treatment. The use of embolization in the preoperative period may considerably reduce bleeding during surgery, but it is not considered an innocuous procedure and may present cranial nerve paralysis due to vasa nervorum obstruction culminating with nerve ischemia. Once again we consider that experience is essential for its effective treatment.

Conflict of interest

Authors declare no conflict of interest.

Author details

Breno Nery[1*], Rodrigo Antônio Fernandes Costa[1], Eduardo Quaggio[1], Ricardo Lopes Araújo[2], Bernardo Alves Barbosa[2], Diogo Fabricio Coelho de Melo[2], Carolina Salviano de Abreu Nery[3], Fred Bernardes Filho[4] and George Peter Stevens[5]

1 Department of Neurosurgery, São Francisco Hospital, Ribeirão Preto, SP, Brazil

2 Department of Neurosurgery, Heliopolis Hospital, São Paulo, São Paulo, Brazil

3 Department of Radiology and Medical Imaging, Diagnóstico por Imagem de Alta Performance (DIAP), Ribeirão Preto, SP, Brazil

4 Department of Internal Medicine, São Francisco Hospital, Ribeirão Preto, SP, Brazil

5 College of Osteopathic Medicine, William Carey University, Hattiesburg, MS, USA

*Address all correspondence to: brenonery84@gmail.com

References

[1] Persky MS, Setton A, Niimi Y, Hartman J, Frank D, Berenstein A. Combined endovascular and surgical treatment of head and neck paragangliomas—A team approach. Head & Neck. 2002;**24**:423-431. DOI: 10.1002/hed.10068

[2] Lee JH, Barich F, Karnell LH, Robinson RA, Zhen WK, Gantz BJ, et al. National cancer data base report on malignant paragangliomas of the head and neck. Cancer. 2002;**94**:730-737. DOI: 10.1002/cncr.10252

[3] Guinto G, Kageyama M, Trujillo-Luarca VH, Abdo M, Ruiz-Than A, Romero-Rangel A. Nonglomic tumors of the jugular foramen: Differential diagnosis and prognostic implications. World Neurosurgery. 2014;**82**:1283-1290. DOI: 10.1016/j.wneu.2014.1207.1013

[4] Nowak A, Dziedzic T, Czernicki T, Kunert P, Marchel A. Surgical treatment of jugular foramen meningiomas. Neurologia i neurochirurgia polska. 2014;**48**:391-396. DOI: 10.1016/j.pjnns.2014.1009.1008

[5] Thomas AJ, Wiggins RH 3rd, Gurgel RK. Nonparaganglioma jugular foramen tumors. Otolaryngologic Clinics of North America. 2015;**48**:343-359. DOI: 10.1016/j.otc.2014.1012.1008

[6] Jansen JC, van den Berg R, Kuiper A, van der Mey AG, Zwinderman AH, Cornelisse CJ. Estimation of growth rate in patients with head and neck paragangliomas influences the treatment proposal. Cancer. 2000;**88**:2811-2816. DOI: 10.1002/1097-0142(20000615)88:12<2811

[7] Dickens WJ, Million RR, Cassisi NJ, Singleton GT. Chemodectomas arising in temporal bone structures. The Laryngoscope. 1982;**92**:188-191. DOI: 10.1002/lary.1982.92.2.188

[8] Gulya AJ. The glomus tumor and its biology. The Laryngoscope. 1993;**103**:7-15

[9] Oldring D, Fisch U. Glomus tumors of the temporal region: Surgical therapy. The American Journal of Otology. 1979;**1**:7-18

[10] Jackson CG, Glasscock ME 3rd, Harris PF. Glomus tumors. Diagnosis, classification, and management of large lesions. Archives of Otolaryngology. 1982;**108**:401-410

[11] Samii M, Babu RP, Tatagiba M, Sepehrnia A. Surgical treatment of jugular foramen schwannomas. Journal of Neurosurgery. 1995;**82**:924-932. DOI: 10.3171/jns.1995.82.6.0924

[12] Gerosa M, Visca A, Rizzo P, Foroni R, Nicolato A, Bricolo A. Glomus jugulare tumors: The option of gamma knife radiosurgery. Neurosurgery. 2006;**59**:561-569. DOI: 10.1227/01.NEU.0000228682.92552.CA

[13] Makiese O, Chibbaro S, Marsella M, Tran Ba Huy P, George B. Jugular foramen paragangliomas: Management, outcome and avoidance of complications in a series of 75 cases. Neurosurgical Review. 2012;**35**: 185-194; discussion 194. DOI: 10.1007/s10143-10011-10346-10141

[14] Al-Mefty O, Teixeira A. Complex tumors of the glomus jugulare: Criteria, treatment, and outcome. Journal of Neurosurgery. 2002;**97**:1356-1366. DOI: 10.3171/jns.2002.97.6.1356

Section 4

Surgical Approaches to CNS Tumors

Chapter 5

Surgery for Recurrent Glioblastoma

Vamsi Krishna Yerramneni, Ramanadha Reddy Kanala, Vasundhara S. Rangan and Thirumal Yerragunta

Abstract

Recurrence of glioblastoma (GB) is inevitable. As the optimal management for recurrent glioblastoma continues to evolve, clear treatment guidelines for are lacking. Existing literature does not clarify the role that second surgery plays in the treatment of these patients. Although few studies report that second surgery is beneficial in select patients and leads to longer overall survival (OS), other studies have demonstrated the limited impact that repeat surgery has on the eventual patient outcome. Maximal safe resection (high extent of resection—EOR) has been proven to improve the OS at reoperation, even when undertaken for cases where the first surgery achieved only a limited EOR. Karnofsky Performance Score (KPS) and age at presentation are valuable prognostic factors that predict better OS and aid in better patient selection for surgical management. The true value of reoperation versus systemic treatment, their effects the patient's QoL and the added increase in overall survival is better judged after detailed investigation by means of a prospective, randomized trial.

Keywords: EOR—extent of resection, KPS—Karnofsky Performance Score, rGB—recurrent glioblastoma

1. Introduction

Glioblastoma (GB) is not only the most common primary intrinsic brain tumor of adulthood, but also the most frequently encountered malignant subtype. The standard treatment for newly diagnosed GB remains maximal surgical resection followed by concomitant or adjuvant chemotherapy [1]. The culmination of all the developments in diagnostics, imaging, surgical refinements and adjuvant therapies has not translated into any significant boost to the median overall survival (OS) of these patients. Prognosis continues to be dismal and OS has risen by just about 3.3 months (from 11.3 to 14.6 months) [2]. In select cohorts (consisting of a very favorable subset of patients), a median OS of 20.5 months has been observed. Recurrence is inevitable in GB despite every kind of known therapy. The standard care of the recurrent GB (rGB) is incompletely defined. Considering the ineffectiveness of therapy for first time disease, patients with recurrent disease are left with even more limited truly useful treatment options. With no clear standard of care, available options include reexcision of the lesion, angiogenesis inhibitor agents, and other targeted therapies, some of which have been the subject of clinical trials. In current practice, second surgery is performed in less than one half of the patients who present with rGB. This might be either due to a seemingly inoperability of the lesion or poor surgical fitness of the patient [3, 4]. Several studies and reviews are published, but undertaking extensive surgery in the recurrence of a disease defined by poor prognosis continues to remain controversial.

2. Criteria for diagnosis of recurrent GB

Criteria for diagnosis have undergone many modifications over past decade. Magnetic resonance imaging every 2–3 months remains the gold standard for assessment of response and progression of the GB. The Macdonald criteria have served as the standard tool in follow up and evaluation of this disease until 2010 and their widespread use has led to the observation of several shortcomings [5, 6]. These include the problem of measuring tumor deposits shaped irregularly (including tumor forming the lining of cystic or excision cavities), observer to observer variability, lack of guidance for the evaluation of multifocal tumors as well as non-enhancing portion(s) of the tumor [5, 6]. Wen et al. published updated criteria in 2010 with restricted parameters for diagnosis of progressive disease within 3 months after completion of adjuvant therapy and integration of the evaluation of T2/FLAIR sequences as well of corticosteroid use [6].

According to the Macdonald et al. [5] criteria, progression of the tumor is defined as development of one or more of the following features:

"25% increase in sum of the products of perpendicular diameters of enhancing lesions, development of any new lesion on imaging and/or clinical deterioration."

The lack of specificity of enhancement in GB patients treated with surgery, radiation or chemotherapy as well as other difficulties in standardization of assessment by the above criteria led to the need for updated Response Assessment in Neurooncology group (RANO) criteria. These criteria define progression as presence of any one of the following:

"≥25% increase in sum of the products of perpendicular diameters of enhancing lesions compared with the smallest tumor measurement obtained either at baseline (if no decrease) or best response, on stable or increasing doses of corticosteroids; significant increase in T2/FLAIR nonenhancing lesion on stable or increasing doses of corticosteroids compared with baseline scan or best response after initiation of therapy not caused by comorbid events (e.g., radiation therapy, demyelination, ischemic injury, infection, seizures, postoperative changes, or other treatment effects); any new lesion; clear clinical deterioration not attributable to other causes apart from the tumor (e.g., seizures, medication adverse effects, complications of therapy, cerebrovascular events, infection, and so on) or changes in corticosteroid dose; failure to return for evaluation as a result of death or deteriorating condition; or clear progression of nonmeasurable disease."

Figure 1 is an example of recurrent GBM managed by surgery followed by Bevacizumab chemotherapy.

3. Indications of surgery

Surgery is indicated in patients who show both:

1. Progression of disease according to MacDonald or RANO radiological criteria.

2. Deterioration in clinical status (as manifested by development of new deficits, change in neurological status due to mass effect of the lesion, seizures, or, features of raised intracranial pressure).

The decision to undertake repeat surgery is especially valid in young patients, patients with good functional status and a conveniently resectable tumor.

In rGB, surgery is undertaken with the main aim of cytoreduction. The reduced tumor burden is thought to cause an improvement in OS [7, 8]. Lu et al. in their meta-analysis concluded that repeat surgery has an overall positive role in managing recurrent GBM. It was observed that surgery resulted in a prognostic benefit that was observed to be independent of demographic as well as clinical parameters [8]. Various factors which are found to affect prognosis are age, extent of resection at repeat surgery, adjuvant chemoradiation, tumor location, methylation status, in addition to

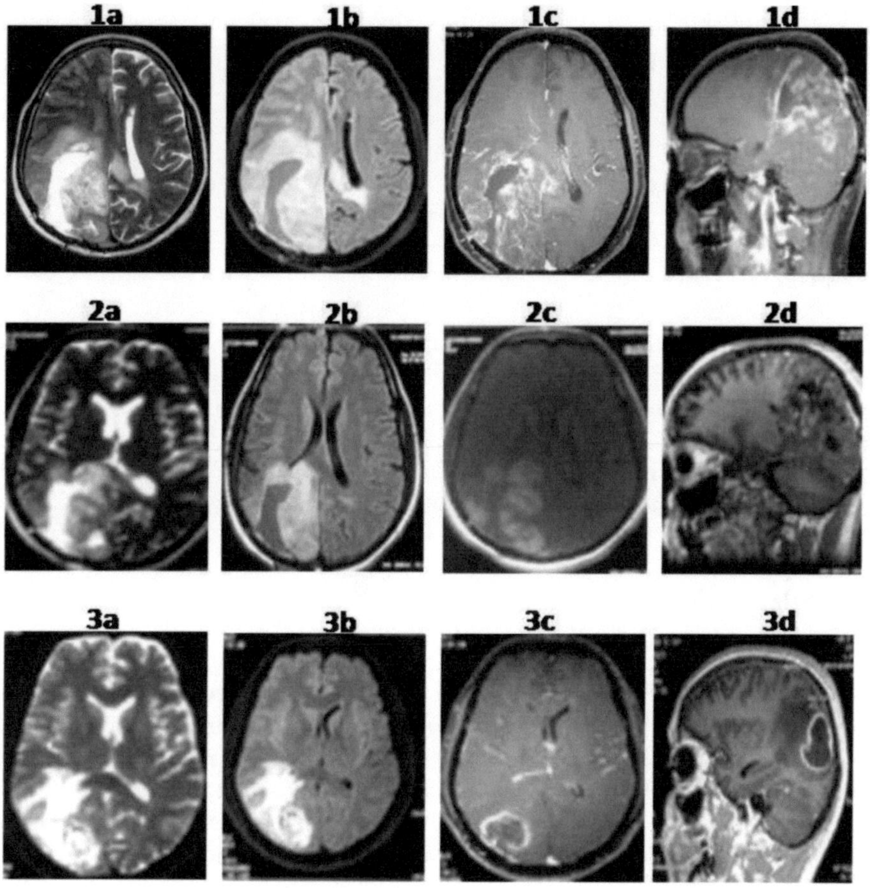

Figure 1.
(1a–1d) MRI brain T2 Axial, Axial FLAIR, Axial contrast and sagittal contrast images showing Right ParietoOcciptial mass with surrounding edema with corresponding enhancement on the contrast. Surgical excision of the tumor was done with around 60% excision followed by chemoradiotherapy as per Stupp Protocol. (2a–2d) One year after the initial treatment patient follow up MRI (2a–d) shows Tumor regrowth. Patient was taken up for Redo surgical excision and around 70% of the tumor excision was achieved. After second surgery patient was treated in another center with bevacizumab and he came back to us in 3 months with regrowth of the tumor. (3a–3d) Patient had low platelet count as a result of the bevacizumab therapy and was in poor general condition. Surgery excision was not considered as the outcome in patients with poor performance score in recurrent tumor is bad though the MRI does not show an extensive tumor. Poor performance scores with a not so extensive gross tumor on MRI indicate microscopic infiltration.

functional assessment of the patient using scores like Karnofsky Performance Status (KPS) and Eastern Cooperative Oncology Group (ECOG) score. Nonetheless, studies conducted that have analyzed patient groups after matching for many of these factors have still observed the prognostic advantage conferred by surgery undertaken for recurrent disease. The potential benefit is not limited to the first recurrence only. Superior OS in patients with GB experiencing more repeat surgeries for continuously recurring GB independent of other features has been previously shown [9, 10].

Various factors have been analyzed with respect to surgery in recurrent GB:

3.1 Age

Recent literature proves that age is an important prognostic factor with OS being longer in patients who are younger at the time of diagnosis, in contradiction to older studies which failed to show any meaningful correlation between age and prognosis [9, 11–14]. Although gender has not been commonly thought to be a factor affecting prognosis, a study by Tugcu et al. has interestingly noted that male gender was a factor according better prognosis.

3.2 Timing of second surgery

Studies have shown that survival is not affected by the time interval between initial diagnosis/surgery and repeat surgery [15, 16].

3.3 Performance score

Studies have reported that better performance score at the time of presentation (KPS $\geq$ 70) correlates strongly with a longer OS [14, 16–18]. Chang et al. [16, 18, 19] documented that the most important factor affecting OS is KPS at the time of recurrence. Quick et al., on the same lines, have demonstrated that good statistical parallel exists between KPS score and OS in their series [20]. Moreover, Michaelsen et al. have reported that the ECOG Performance Status significantly affects the OS following therapy [13].

3.4 Molecular markers

The role of molecular markers in predicting/affecting survival in recurrent GB has been controversial. Studies have shown an association between loss of MGMT expression and survival in patients with GB. Although this correlation was confirmed to have a prognostic significance at the time of first surgery, Brandes et al. reported that MGMT methylation status has no particular place in the prediction of outcome following repeat surgery. Similarly, multiple authors have noted that MGMT status at the time of redo surgery in GB patients has no effect on OS or on SFR [21, 22]. Mutations of IDH1 and IDH2 are known to be suggestive of secondary GB and to confer favorable prognosis [23, 24]. This was confirmed by Hartmann et al. who reported longer OS in patients with IDH mutant tumors as compared to the IDH wild-type ones. On the contrary, Amelot et al. have reported comparable long term survival in patients with and without IDH1/2 mutation [25, 26].

3.5 Extent of resection

That a greater extent of resection (EOR) confers an obvious advantage in patients being treated for GB has been demonstrated by multiple studies. This has been more widely evaluated and concluded at the time of first surgery [27–32].

It suffices to say that surgical resection of the tumor is still the most effective therapy in GB, leading to instant decompression and improvement in the efficacy of adjuvant radiation by reducing tumor bulk. An increase in survival by an average of 5.5 months was noted by Quick et al. in patients in whom atleast 95% of tumor was excised. This benefit was noted irrespective of tumor size. However, it is not as clear if such an advantage is conferred again during operation for recurrence [20]. On inquiry into whether this same benefit holds true in cases of recurrent GB, Robin et al., in their review article found 16 studies reinforcing the role of EOR in patient survival.

According to Stupp et al. surgery (5ALA fluorescence guided complete tumor resection) [35] done at the time of noting disease progression, along with additional chemotherapy (Temozolamide) and radiotherapy improved the average patient survival to more than 14 months. It was thereby suggested that, in patients where surgery for tumor recurrence is deemed prudent, Maximal Safe Resection of the GB should be aimed for [33].

The next logical question that arises would be the role of such ambitious surgery in further recurrences after the second operation. In a series of 578 primary GB patients were studied with reference to the number of repeat surgeries undertaken, Chaichana et al. concluded that patients who underwent multiple resections had better median survival than those who had single time surgery. The 15 patients in this study who underwent resection four times had a median survival of 26.6 months compared to those who were operated once (354 patients), twice (168 patients) and thrice (41 cases). These patients were found to have a median survival of 6.8, 15.5, 22.4 respectively [9].

Bloch et al. also conducted a valuable study on results of multiple resections in 107 patients by four-way subgroup analysis after noting EORs during both first and second surgery. Whether the initial as well as subsequent surgery achieved Gross Total Resection (GTR) or Sub Total Resection (STR) of the tumor was made note of. Patients were then categorized into four resection groups: GTR/GTR, GTR/STR, STR/GTR, and, STR/STR. On follow up, the study established that a survival advantage was conferred by performing complete tumor resection during both initial surgery as well as second surgery for recurrence of GB [31].

A series by Oppenlander and colleagues also confirms the advantage conferred by increased EOR in patients operated for rGB. A survival advantage was observed with even 80% resection of tumor volume. The OS for the entire cohort studied was 19.0 months while median survival on Kaplan-Meier curves showed survival upto 20 months and even 30 months when EOR was greater than 81 and 97%, respectively. Multivariate analysis identified EOR, age, and KPS as independent predictors of survival [30].

Of particular interest is a study by Sanai et al. where in cases when a more complete resection was deemed imprudent due to the tumor being located in eloquent brain, more limited resection (78% EOR) of the contrast enhancing lesion did correspond to a survival benefit that was of significance statistically [4]. Despite being largely based on class II to III evidence, surgically reducing the amount of residual tumor does translate to longer PFS and better OS.

4. Survival following reoperation for recurrent or progressive glioblastoma

With the advancement of refinement in surgical techniques and in nonsurgical adjunctive therapies, our understanding of the impact of surgery on survival in both newly diagnosed and recurrent GB increases. As elaborated so far, varied studies have come to the common conclusion that a survival benefit is accorded by surgery, especially by the maximization of EOR, not only in newly diagnosed GB, but also in recurrent cases [9, 11, 16, 20, 34].

A detailed review of relevant literature by Ryken et al. suggests that reoperation adds about 8 or 9 months to the OS in select patients, without the added burden of significant morbidity. This positive outcome is especially observed in patients with age less than or equal to 50, KPS scores equal to or greater than 60 or 70 as well as favorable tumor location [36].

It can now be safely said that the most effective therapy in recurrent GB is surgical resection as it improves the efficacy of radiotherapy. Patient selection should take into consideration the so far observed positive prognostic factors and maximal safe tumor volume resection should be the surgical goal [33] in those patients who are candidates to second surgery.

5. Complications

Although surgery logically aims at maximal cytoreduction, the safety of this goal is compromised by factors such as highly infiltrative nature of tumor, eloquent, deep seated/periventricular location, advanced age and/or coexistence of comorbidities. A multicenter retrospective study documented a 2–4% increase in the rate of neurological and non-neurological complications in repeat surgery when compared with initial surgery [37].

Following surgery for rGB, mortality rate has been shown to lie in the range of 0–11% with morbidity rate varying from 13 to 69%, leaving a significant number of rGB patients in a condition that precludes administration of adjuvant therapy [19]. This risk, therefore, appeared to nullify the survival benefit of reoperation at recurrence when compared with patients of recurrence who received no treatment at all. Hence, the importance of safer surgery avoiding morbidity as well as judiciousness in decision making cannot be overstated.

6. Conclusions

The available literature suggests a higher OS in selected patients who were managed with repeat excision of tumor at the time of recurrence of Glioblastoma. Although a debate remains open regarding the benefit of such excision, a clear trend in its favor has become more evident. The decision of undertaking surgery for rGB should be individualized and should surely be considered in patients with a favorable functional score at the time of presentation with recurrent disease as well as favorable preoperative neurological and radiological characteristics. The goal of such repeat surgery should be the resolution of symptoms, stabilization or improvement in QoL, increase in the time to further progression and reduction in requirement of steroid therapy. There is also the additional advantage of the possibility to offer intracavitary adjunctive therapy as well as an improved response to other adjunctive therapies [36]. As is customary to state, the actual value of such repeat surgery in comparison with systemic treatments and the effect of each on patient QoL and survical remains a topic for further prospective, randomized trials.

Author details

Vamsi Krishna Yerramneni*, Ramanadha Reddy Kanala, Vasundhara S. Rangan and Thirumal Yerragunta
Department of Neurosurgery, Nizam's Institute of Medical Sciences, Hyderabad, India

*Address all correspondence to: vamsiky.ns@gmail.com

References

[1] Central Brain Tumor Registry of the United States. Central Brain Tumor Registry of the United States Statistical Report: Primary Brain and Central Nervous System Tumors Diagnosed in the United States in 2004-2006. Hinsdale, IL: Central Brain Tumor Registry of the United States; 2010

[2] Despite advances in diagnostic technology, surgical techniques and adjuvant treatments, the prognosis remains poor and the median overall survival (OS) of patients has increased only 3.3 months (from 11.3 months to 14.6 months) over the past 25 years

[3] Robin AM, Lee I, Kalkanis SN. Reoperation for recurrent glioblastoma multiforme. Neurosurgery Clinics. 2017;**28**(3):407-428

[4] Sanai N, Polley M-Y, McDermott MW, et al. An extent of resection threshold for newly diagnosed glioblastomas. Journal of Neurosurgery. 2011;**115**(1):3

[5] Macdonald D, Cascino T, Schold SJ, et al. Response criteria for phase II studies of supratentorial malignant glioma. Journal of Clinical Oncology. 1990;**8**:1277-1280

[6] Wen PY, Macdonald DR, Reardon DA, Cloughesy TF, Sorensen AG, Galanis E, et al. Updated response assessment criteria for high-grade gliomas: Response assessment in neuro-oncology working group. Journal of Clinical Oncology. 2010;**28**(11):1963-1972

[7] Vogelbaum MA. The benefit of surgical resection in recurrent glioblastoma. Neuro-Oncology. 2016;**18**:462-463

[8] Lu VM, Jue TR, McDonald KL, Rovin RA. The survival effect of repeat surgery at glioblastoma recurrence and its trend: A systematic review and meta-analysis. World Neurosurgery. 2018;**115**:453-459

[9] Chaichana KL, Zadnik P, Weingart JD, Olivi A, Gallia GL, Blakeley J, et al. Multiple resections for patients with glioblastoma: Prolonging survival. Journal of Neurosurgery. 2013;**118**(4):812-820

[10] Chen YR, Sole J, Ugiliweneza B, Johnson E, Burton E, Woo SY, et al. National trends for reoperation in older patients with glioblastoma. World Neurosurgery. 2018;**113**:179-189

[11] Sughrue ME, Sheean T, Bonney PA, Maurer AJ, Teo C. Aggressive repeat surgery for focally recurrent primary glioblastoma: Outcomes and theoretical framework. Neurosurgical Focus. 2015;**38**(3):E11

[12] Franceschi E, Bartolotti M, Tosoni A, Bartolini S, Sturiale C, Fioravanti A, et al. The effect of re-operation on survival in patients with recurrent glioblastoma. Anticancer Research. 2015;**35**(3):1743-1748

[13] Michaelsen SR, Christensen IJ, Grunnet K, Stockhausen MT, Broholm H, Kosteljanetz M, et al. Clinical variables serve as prognostic factors in a model for survival from glioblastoma multiforme: An observational study of a cohort of consecutive non-selected patients from a single institution. BMC Cancer. 2013;**3**(13):402

[14] Stark AM, Hedderich J, Held-Feindt J, Mehdorn HM. Glioblastoma—The consequences of advanced patient age on treatment and survival. Neurosurgical Review. 2007;**30**(1):56-61

[15] Filippini G, Falcone C, Boiardi A, Broggi G, Bruzzone MG, Caldiroli D,

et al. Prognostic factors for survival in 676 consecutive patients with newly diagnosed primary glioblastoma. Neuro-Oncology. 2008;**10**(1):79-87

[16] Park JK, Hodges T, Arko L, Shen M, DelloIacono D, McNabb A, et al. Scale to predict survival after surgery for recurrent glioblastoma multiforme. Journal of Clinical Oncology. 2010;**28**(24):3838-3843

[17] Tugcu B, Postalci LS, Gunaldi O, Tanriverdi O, Akdemir H. Efficacy of clinical prognostic factors on survival in patients with glioblastoma. Turkish Neurosurgery. 2010;**20**(2):117-125

[18] Hervey-Jumper SL, Berger MS. Reoperation for recurrent high-grade glioma: A current perspective of the literature. Neurosurgery. 2014;**75**(5):491-499

[19] De Bonis P, Fiorentino A, Anile C, Balducci M, Pompucci A, Chiesa S, et al. The impact of repeated surgery and adjuvant therapy on survival for patients with recurrent glioblastoma. Clinical Neurology and Neurosurgery. 2013;**115**(7):883-886

[20] Quick J, Gessler F, Dützmann S, Hattingen E, Harter PN, Weise LM, et al. Benefit of tumor resection for recurrent glioblastoma. Journal of Neuro-Oncology. 2014;**117**(2):365-372

[21] Brandes AA, Franceschi E, Tosoni A, Bartolini S, Bacci A, Agati R, et al. O(6)-methylguanine DNA-methyltransferase methylation status can change between first surgery for newly diagnosed glioblastoma and second surgery for recurrence: Clinical implications. Neuro-Oncology. 2010;**12**(3):283-288

[22] Brandes AA, Tosoni A, Cavallo G, Bertorelle R, Gioia V, Franceschi E, et al. Temozolomide 3 weeks on and 1 week off as first-line therapy for recurrent glioblastoma: Phase II study from gruppo italiano cooperativo di neuro-oncologia (GICNO). British Journal of Cancer. 2006;**95**(9):1155-1160

[23] Weller M, Stupp R, Hegi ME, van den Bent M, Tonn JC, Sanson M, et al. Personalized care in neuro-oncology coming of age: Why we need MGMT and 1p/19q testing for malignant glioma patients in clinical practice. Neuro-Oncology. 2012;**14**(Suppl. 4):iv100-iv108

[24] Weller M, Stupp R, Reifenberger G, Brandes AA, van den Bent MJ, Wick W, et al. MGMT promoter methylation in malignant gliomas: Ready for personalized medicine? Nature Reviews. Neurology. 2010;**6**(1):39-51

[25] Hartmann C, Hentschel B, Simon M, Westphal M, Schackert G, Tonn JC, et al. Germanglioma network long-term survival in primary glioblastoma with versus without isocitrate dehydrogenase mutations. Clinical Cancer Research. 2013;**19**(18):5146-5157

[26] Amelot A, De Cremoux P, Quillien V, Polivka M, Adle-Biassette H, Lehmann-Che J, et al. IDH-mutation is a weak predictor of long-term survival in glioblastoma patients. PLoS One. 2015;**10**(7):e0130596

[27] Lacroix M, Abi-Said D, Fourney DR, et al. A multivariate analysis of 416 patients with glioblastoma multiforme: Prognosis, extent of resection, and survival. Journal of Neurosurgery. 2001;**95**(2):190-198

[28] Chaichana KL, Jusue-Torres I, Navarro-Ramirez R, et al. Establishing percent resection and residual volume thresholds affecting survival and recurrence for patients with newly diagnosed intracranial glioblastoma. Neuro-Oncology. 2014;**16**(1):113-122

[29] Orringer D, Lau D, Khatri S, et al. Extent of resection in patients with glioblastoma: Limiting factors,

perception of resectability, and effect on survival. Journal of Neurosurgery. 2012;**117**(5):851-859

[30] Oppenlander ME, Wolf AB, Snyder LA, et al. An extent of resection threshold for recurrent glioblastoma and its risk for neurological morbidity. Journal of Neurosurgery. 2014;**120**(4):846-853

[31] Bloch O, Han SJ, Cha S, et al. Impact of extent of resection for recurrent glioblastoma on overall survival: Clinical article. Journal of Neurosurgery. 2012;**117**(6):1032-1038

[32] McGirt MJ, Chaichana KL, Gathinji M, Attenello FJ, Than K, Olivi A, et al. Independent association of extent of resection with survival in patients with malignant brain astrocytoma. Journal of Neurosurgery. 2009;**110**(1):156-162

[33] Stupp R, Mason WP, van den Bent MJ, Weller M, Fisher B, Taphoorn MJ, et al. Radiotherapy plus concomitant and adjuvant temozolomide for glioblastoma. The New England Journal of Medicine. 2005;**352**(10):987-996

[34] Gorlia T, van den Bent MJ, Hegi ME, Mirimanoff RO, Weller M, Cairncross JG, et al. Nomograms for predicting survival of patients with newly diagnosed glioblastoma: Prognostic factor analysis of EORTC and NCIC trial 26981-22981/CE.3. The Lancet Oncology. 2008;**9**(1):29-38

[35] Stummer W, Reulen HJ, Meinel T, Pichlmeier U, Schumacher W, Tonn JC, et al. ALA-Glioma study group: Extent of resection and survival in glioblastoma multiforme: Identification of and adjustment for bias. Neurosurgery. 2008;**62**(3):564-576

[36] Ryken TC, Kalkanis SN, Buatti JM, Olson JJ, AANS/CNS Joint Guidelines Committee. The role of cytoreductive surgery in the management of progressive glioblastoma: A systematic review and evidence-based clinical practice guideline. Journal of Neuro-Oncology. 2014;**118**(3):479-488

[37] Ringel F, Pape H, Sabel M, et al. Clinical benefit from resection of recurrent glioblastomas: Results of a multicenter study including 503 patients with recurrent glioblastomas undergoing surgical resection. Neuro-Oncology. 2016;**18**(1):96-104

Chapter 6

Surgical Principles for Spinal and Paraspinal Neurofibromas

Feyzi Birol Sarica

Abstract

Neurofibromas are the most prevalent seen tumor in the neurofibromatosis type 1 (NF1) disease. Spinal neurofibromas, which are the major diagnostic criteria of disease, are seen in approximately 60% of the patients with NF1. They constitute 23% of all of the spinal tumors. While the spinal neurofibromas most frequently show a location in thoracic region, it is followed by their predilection in cervical and lumbar regions, respectively. The spinal neurofibromas located in the sacral region are quite rarely observed and show an asymptomatic course until reaching to the big sizes. Of these spinal neurofibromas, 72% were with intradural extramedullary, 14% with extradural, and 13% with intradural and extradural "dumbbell formation." Only 1% of the spinal neurofibromas are intramedullary located. The total taking of the single solitary neurofibroma surgically is relatively easier. But, the difficulties can be encountered in taking these tumors surgically since they are characterized by the multiple tumors in the plexiform neurofibromas, especially accompanying to the NF1. In this chapter, the surgical difficulties encountered in the region in which the tumor is localized and different surgical approaches are developed in the course of time in order to exceed these difficulties are described.

Keywords: dumbbell neurofibroma, dumbbell tumor, neurofibromatosis type 1, NF1, paraspinal neurofibroma, spinal nerve sheath tumor, spinal neurofibroma, surgery, surgical approach, surgical treatment, von Recklinghausen disease

1. Introduction

The close follow-up is clinically and radiologically suggested in the asymptomatic spinal neurofibroma cases that do not make pressure on the spinal cord and important nerve roots. But, surgical tumor resection is preferred in the tumors showing rapid growth and/or causing the progressive neurodeficits. The total taking of the single solitary neurofibroma surgically is relatively easier. But, the difficulties can be encountered in taking these tumors surgically since they are characterized by the multiple tumors in the plexiform neurofibromas, especially accompanying to the NF1. Different surgical approaches had been described for the tumor's total resection in the spinal neurofibroma cases, in which the surgical difficulty is observed at most and which show a *dumbbell formation*. While a single-stage posterior approach was used for dumbbell tumors having a small extraspinal component, the single-stage combined posteroanterior approach had been preferred in those having a big extraspinal component. In time, the two-stage combined posteroanterior approach had been started to be used instead of the single-stage combined posteroanterior approach in order to eliminate the excessive hemorrhage risk arising from the length of surgery duration. In this approach, the dumbbell tumor is firstly taken by the intraspinal component's posterior approach, and then, by giving a certain period, the tumors' extraspinal component is taken by the anterior approach. In time, the lateral approaches applied by using the extensive posterolateral exposure had been described instead of the single-stage or two-stage combined posteroanterior approaches in order to totally take the dumbbell tumors, in which especially huge extraforaminal component is found. A wider visual angle can be provided by the lateral approaches to the spinal channel lateral, intervertebral foramen, and extraforaminal regions, and the tumor can be totally taken in a single session.

2. Neurofibromatosis type 1

2.1 Epidemiology of the NF1

The neurofibromatosis expressing a tumor-predisposing syndrome group is characterized especially by the tumors found in the CNS and peripheral nervous system. NF1 constituting 96% of the neurofibromatosis patients is the most frequently seen form. It is followed by the neurofibromatosis type 2 with the rate of 3% and Schwannomatosis recently defined. The NF1, of which its most extensive definition had been made by Friedrich von Recklinghausen in 1882 for the first time, is named with "von Recklinghausen disease." Moreover, since it is described by the multiple neurofibromas that are one of the peripheral nerve sheath tumors with benign character, they are also named as the "peripheral neurofibromatosis." The NF1, the most frequently seen phakomatosis, shows an autosomal dominant hereditary transmission, and its prevalence incidence is approximately 1 per 2500–3000 births [1, 2].

2.2 Natural history and genetic alterations of the NF1

The gene that is responsible for the NF1 formation is found in the 17q11.2 chromosome and contains 280 kbp DNAs. The tumor is a suppressor gene. The *NF1 gene* provides the synthesizing protein named as the "neurofibromin" that is found in Schwann cell at a high level and acts as a tumor suppressor [3]. Neurofibromin, which has an activating effect of the GTPaz, also regulates the cellular proliferation and differentiation by inactivating the RAS that is a cytosolic signal transduction proto-oncogene [4]. Neurofibromin level decreases in varying degrees in the "NF1 gene"mutations, and as a result, it leads to a formation of the various ectodermal and mesodermal tumors that are seen in the NF1 together with the different penetration types of NFs. In conclusion, the peripheral nerve sheath tumors frequently occur in particular to the neurofibroma. Moreover, prevalence incidence of the CNS tumors such as glioma, ganglioglioma, and neuroblastoma as well as the other malignancies such as leukemia, pheochromocytoma, Wilms tumor, and sarcoma increases [4, 5]. Fifty percent of the mutations in NF1 gene are in the form of spontaneous mutations of which family history is not found, and the remaining is in the form of hereditary mutations of which family history is found. Even though there are high penetration values in those having a hereditary mutation, the different phenotypic presentations can be observed between the family members due to the probable epigenetic modification [4–6]. One thousand and five hundred different *NF1 gene* mutations have been notified until today, while a slight phenotypic represented by the NF1 table had been observed in the presence of mosaicism;

a serious phenotypic represented by the NF1 table had been observed when the 17q11.2 microdeletion was detected [7].

2.3 Clinical presentations of NF1

Diagnosis in the NF1 bases upon the clinical criteria despite the progressions in the molecular genetics. The criteria listed for the NF1 clinical diagnosis had been determined in the "NIH Consensus Development Conference" in 1987 [8] (**Table 1**).

2.3.1 Pigmentation abnormalities

Although these criteria observed in the NF1 show a variation between the patients according to the penetration type, at least two of the NIH criteria are found in 30% of the cases to the age of 1 and in 97% of the cases to the age of 8. The café au lait macules seen in 95% of the adult cases with NF1 are the skin macules that are found in an oval shape and are hyperpigmented and light brown colored. They can be observed during birth. But, its number and size increase in the first decade. Being found of the café au lait macule in number of 6 and more with the dimension of 5 mm or larger in the prepubertal period and 15 mm or larger in the postpubertal period according to the NIH criteria is in the common features of NF1. The café au lait macules, which are not only intrinsic to NF1, can be seen by the other genetic syndromes such as McCune Albright syndrome, Legius syndrome, and Silver-Russell dwarfism. The malign transformation potential is not found in these macules since they can be only seen in 10% of population [1, 2, 9]. Another pigmentation anomaly seen in the NF1 is axillary and inguinal freckling. These hyperpigmented spots that can also exist at birth come to existence afterward and are observed in 90% of the cases with NF1 under the age of 7 years [2]. The most frequently encountered eye finding in the adult patients with NF1 is Lisch nodules with the rate of 95%. Lisch nodules are asymptomatic, small, and superficial melanocytic hamartomatous nodules generally observed as multiple in the iris. They are observed in the shape of a dome and in the form of yellow-brown lesions in the slit-lamp examination [1, 10].

2.3.2 Tumors of the optic pathway

The eye finding determined in patients with NF1 in the second frequently observed finding with the rate of 15% is an optic pathway glioma and takes part

1	The presence of six or more café au lait macules 5 mm or more in size during prepuberty or 15 mm or more in size during postpuberty
2	The presence of two or more neurofibromas of any type or the presence of one plexiform neurofibroma
3	The presence of freckling in the axillary and inguinal regions
4	The presence of optic glioma
5	The presence of two or more Lisch nodules (iris hamartoma)
6	The presence of bone anomalies, such as long bones with thin cortex without arthrosis, together with sphenoid aplasia or arthrosis
7	The presence of NF1 diagnosis in first-degree relatives according to the diagnosis criteria written above

**Two or more of the above points should be present in the cases diagnosed with NF1.*

Table 1.
Neurofibromatosis type-1 diagnosis criteria of the National Institutes of Health [8].*

between the important diagnosis criteria. The optic pathway glioma is the most frequently observed glioma type in patients with NF1. They are found in the low-grade glial tumors (WHO grades I and II). The region, in which the optic pathway glioma is frequently localized, is prechiasmatic region. They are frequently presented in the form of an optic nerve pilocytic astrocytoma (WHO grade I). The visual field defects give the clinical finding such as a decrease in the visual acuity, proptosis, and diplopia in the optic pathway gliomas that are generally presented to the age of 7 [1, 6, 11, 12]. The brainstem glioma (pilocytic astrocytoma, WHO grade I), glioblastoma multiforme (GBM, WHO grade IV), and ganglioglioma (WHO grade I) can be enumerated between the other gliomas that are less frequently observed in the cases with NF1. The development risk of GBM having a quite aggressive course among them had increased approximately five times in the cases with NF1. The schwannomas and meningiomas originating from any cranial nerve sheath can be enumerated among the other intracranial tumors accompanying to the NF1.

2.3.3 Cognitive function disorders and NF1 bright object

One of the non-tumoral CNS lesions observed in patients with NF1 is the lesions named as "NF1 bright object," and they are observed at the rate of 43–93%. The hyperintense lesions, of which borders are significant in the magnetic resonance imaging (MRI) T2 sequences, are frequently localized in the subcortical white matter fields, basal ganglions, and capsula interna in the brain. These lesions named as the *NF1 bright object* are held responsible for cognitive malfunctions such as the mental retardation, learning disorder, and speech disorder observed in patients with NF1 [13, 14].

2.3.4 Skeletal manifestations

The deformities observed in the various bones accompany to the cases with NF1. The most frequently observed skeletal deformity is kyphoscoliosis, which develops depending on the vertebral bone deformities, especially in the cervicothoracic region. The neurodeficits at various levels can be observed in the cases with NF1 depending on the rapid increase in the degree of kyphosis and scoliosis. Another vertebral bone anomaly observed at the rate of 10% is the dorsal scalloping in the vertebral bones. These tables develop independently from the spinal neurofibromas observed in the NF1 [15]. Moreover, the tumor's intraspinal part can cause the destruction on the intervertebral foramen walls when extending to the extraspinal cavities by passing through the intervertebral foramen in the spinal neurofibroma cases constituting the *dumbbell formation*, and in this case, the intervertebral foramen enlargement and thinning can be radiologically observed in the adjacent vertebra pedicles.

A thinning had been also observed in cortexes of the long bones such as the radius and tibia and between the other skeletal deformities observed in patients with NF1. The ptosis is accompanied by vitamin D levels in the bone densitometer, osteopenia, and laboratory tests made for patients with NF1 [12]. It had been determined that fracture development risk secondarily increased three to five times in the cases with NF1 according to the normal population in these tables [16]. Although the body rates were normal in many cases with NF1, the growth hormone insufficiency and pubertas praecox had been held responsible as the reason of short stature developed [12].

Moreover, the anomalies also accompany to the cranial bones in the cases with NF1. The parieto-occipital bone defects, sphenoid wing dysplasia or aplasia, and pulsatile exophthalmia developed depending on the unilateral defect on the orbital superior wall are observed between them. Moreover, the head asymmetry, macrocephaly, and mandibular bone deformities can be also accompanied [1, 10].

2.3.5 Tumors of the gastrointestinal system

The tumoral formations are also observed in the gastrointestinal system in patients with NF1. The most frequently accompanying tumor to the NF1 is gastrointestinal stromal tumors with the rate of 25% between them [17], and they occur as a result of the KIT and PDGFRA mutations. These tumors, of which sizes are small, do not generally give the clinical finding. Moreover, endocrine tumors of the gastrointestinal system such as somatostatinoma, gastrinoma, and insulinoma can be also observed in the cases with NF1. These tumors are most frequently in the tendency to localize in the periampullary region. However, the gastrointestinal system can be held by the focal or prevalent neurofibromas and present the clinical findings characterized by the internal organ dysfunction.

2.3.6 Nodular (intraneural), cutaneous (diffuse), and plexiform neurofibromas

The nodular neurofibromas (*intraneural form*), which are also named as solitary, are the most frequently seen form as sporadic independent from the NF1. The localization predilection is not found in the neurofibroma, which is most frequently seen in the third and fourth decades. Their borders are relatively significant and characterized by slow-growing tumors in an oval and elastic shape since they show an intraneural growth pattern in a single nerve. The nodular neurofibromas, which frequently originate from the dorsal nerve roots, are frequently presented by ache, hearing disorders, and power loss in the clinic [18, 19].

The cutaneous neurofibromas (*diffuse form*) are seen in approximately 10% of the patients with NF1, located in the skin and subcutaneous tissue. They can be seen in the pedunculated and nodular forms or similar forms like the plaque. They are frequently observed in the neonatal and adolescent periods, and an increase is observed in their numbers together with the age [1, 11, 12, 18].

The plexiform neurofibroma is the most frequently seen one with the rate of 30% in patients with NF1. They had taken this name since they presented a plexiform growth pattern in such a way that it would contain more than one fascicule, nerve, or plexus branches. The characteristic "worm bag" term had been also used for these tumors due to their surgical macroscopic appearances. They are characterized by fusiform-formed multiple neurofibromas observed throughout peripheral nerves. They frequently hold the main nerve body including the brachial and lumbar plexuses. If a big nerve is held in the extremities, they can also lead to a local giantism table in the extremity, which is named as the "elephantiasis neuromatosa." They frequently develop in the childhood period, and the plexiform neurofibromas, which make pressure to the adjacent tissues with the mass effect by showing a rapid growth tendency, are pathognomonic [1, 11]. Moreover, the plexiform neurofibromas contain the malign transformation potential differently from the cutaneous neurofibromas, and the transformation risk into the malign peripheral nerve sheath tumor (MPNST) varies between 5 and 10% [20]. Therefore, scanning should be made by the FDG-PET in order to make early malign transformation diagnosis in the cases, in which the growth or sudden change was determined in the plexiform neurofibroma size.

3. Spinal neurofibromas and dumbbell formation

3.1 Epidemiology of the spinal neurofibroma

The neurofibromas are the most prevalent seen tumor in the NF1 disease. The schwannoma, MPNST, meningioma, and astrocytoma from the other spinal tumors less often accompany the NF1 [6]. The spinal neurofibromas, which are the major diagnostic criteria of disease, are seen in approximately 60% of the patients with NF1 [2, 6]. They constitute 23% of all of the spinal tumors [18]. While the spinal neurofibromas most frequently show a location in the thoracic region, it is followed by their predilection in cervical and lumbar regions, respectively. The neurofibromas located in the sacral region are quite rarely observed and show an asymptomatic course until reaching to the big sizes [21]. Of these spinal neurofibromas, 72% were with the intradural extramedullary, 14% with the extradural, and 13% with the intradural and extradural "dumbbell formation." Only 1% of the spinal neurofibromas are intramedullary located [22].

3.2 Dumbbell formation of the spinal neurofibroma

The tumor's intraspinal component extends throughout the peripheral segment in the extraspinal distance of the nerve through the intervertebral foramen in the dumbbell spinal neurofibroma, of which total resections have difficulty with the neurosurgical techniques required for the multidisciplinary-combined approaches. The extraspinal tumor part is usually larger than the intraspinal tumor part and can reach the giant sizes. The huge dumbbell tumors are generally in a lobule shape and show a cystic degeneration [1, 11].

The extraspinal tumor component can adhere to the adjacent tissue and organs in the body cavities and also gives the clinical finding through the pressure effect. The extraspinal tumor component's serious respiratory problems are more frequently observed as a result of the pressure of lung parenchyma to the bronchus and bronchioles in the chest cavity due to especially thoracic region predilection of dumbbell neurofibroma. Therefore, nowadays, the surgical treatment in the thoracic dumbbell neurofibromas is frequently carried out by the combined approaches planned together with the thoracic surgeons. Moreover, the progression of cervical neurofibroma in the adjacency of vertebral artery of extraspinal tumor component showing an extension to the subsurface skin is a condition constituting another difficulty in terms of the surgery. Similarly, the intraabdominal and retroperitoneal organ dysfunctions can be also observed in the lumbar *dumbbell neurofibroma* cases, and they make the multidisciplinary-combined approaches a current issue in the surgical treatments of these cases [1, 6, 23].

3.3 Pathology of the spinal neurofibroma

The neurofibromas are macroscopically in gray-white color, gelatinized, and in a soft form. Dissecting the nerve macroscopically from the neurofibroma is quite difficult due to the close relationship between the nerve and neurofibroma [24]. The solitary and plexiform neurofibromas showing the similar microscopic features consist of the thin and long fusiform cells dispersed between the collagen fibers within a mucopolysaccharide-rich matrix. In addition, these cells are in a uniform form and contain the hyperchromatic nucleus. While the cell density is less in the neurofibromas, they contain Schwann cells, neural fibroblasts, cells like the perineural cell, and mast cells [6]. Sometimes, some difficulties can be encountered in separating the neurofibroma from the schwannomas due to their common cell contents. The nuclear atypia and hyalinizing vascular component observed in the neurofibromas are less often determined as significant according to the schwannoma [20]. It immunohistochemically shows a positive staining feature with S100. But, the stained neurofibromas are more subtle since their immunoreactivity is less often in comparison with the schwannoma [24]. The neurofibromas show a positive staining feature in the different levels together with the epithelial membrane antigen (EMA), which is specific for the perineural cell [20]. Similarly, they have the strong staining features with the vimentin and fibronectin [25]. There is a CD34 positiveness showing immunoreactivity in the cutaneous (*intraneural*) neurofibromas [26]. The myelinated nerve fibers in the neurofibromas can be shown by the silvering paint and myelin paint.

3.4 Clinical presentations of the spinal neurofibroma

The spinal neurofibromas are generally asymptomatic when they are small. The unilateral radicular ache is the most frequently observed symptom with the rate of 80% in early phases of the disease since most of them are originated from the spinal dorsal nerve roots. The paradoxical ache is characterized as increasing during rest and nights. This condition depends on the venous return difficulty developed while sleeping. The other paresthesia symptoms can accompany to this table. Moreover, the deep sensory losses can be also observed as a result of affecting the posterior column. The tumor growing in the intradural extramedullary distance leads to the long-tract findings by making the spinal cord pressure in advanced stages of the disease. The muscle strength losses—motor deficits—observed at the rate of 30% in the spinal neurofibroma cases mostly occur as a result of affecting the lateral and anterior columns by the tumor. The sphincter disorders developed depending on the involvement of autonomous ways are observed at the rate of 25%. The other neurologic deficits can generally develop approximately 3–5 years later following the radicular ache in the spinal neurofibromas like in the other intradural tumors [1, 6, 27].

The tumor's extraspinal component can wrap the peripheral tissues by growing and cause the additional symptoms by making pressure in the dumbbell neurofibroma cases. The neck ache and suboccipital headache can be observed in the cervical localized tumors [28]. The tumors showing an extension to the chest cavity can lead to the respiratory distress by making pressure to the air conduction ways. The patients are asymptomatic for a long time in the dumbbell tumors showing an intraabdominal growth. However, the intraabdominal tumor leads to the related organ dysfunction symptoms by making the displacement and pressure in the abdominal organs when it reaches the big or huge sizes. The ache spreading from the abdomen toward the lumbar region can be seen in the big tumors showing an extension to the retroperitoneal region [29, 30].

3.5 Neurodiagnostic techniques of the spinal neurofibroma

There are variations that will have made a diagnosis in 50% of the cases in the direct graphies. The most frequently seen vertebra radiographies findings are pedicle erosion and scalloping in the vertebral corpus. The enlargement of the interpedicular distance and foramen can regularly and indirectly show a dumbbell tumor existence [27, 31]. It had been notified that the whole block was observed in 50% of the cases and 83% of the myelographic defects were intradural in the myelographic examination [27]. The most used important radiologic imaging method is MRI in order to detect the prevalence of disease, reveal the intraspinal and extraspinal components of spinal neurofibromas in details, evaluate the complications to be developed in the postoperative period, and detect the tumor recurrence in the cases with NF1. The spinal neurofibromas give an isointense or hypointense appearance in the spinal T1-MRIs and give a hyperintense appearance in the spinal T2-MRIs [27, 31]. The extraspinal tumor component's extensions to the lateral together with the dumbbell neurofibroma's specific appearances can be shown better by the spinal MRI. Moreover, imaging the dumbbell neurofibroma's paravertebral extension and pressure by showing an extension to the adjacent organs by the MRI is quite important in planning the surgical approaches. The MR images of our one NF1 case with multiple dumbbell neurofibromas (cervical, thoracic, and lumbar regions) are presented in **Figure 1** [22].

3.5.1 Radiological alterations of the tumors' growth

The spinal neurofibroma holds the contrast in a significant and homogenous way when its size is small [27, 31]. Especially, the cystic degeneration and

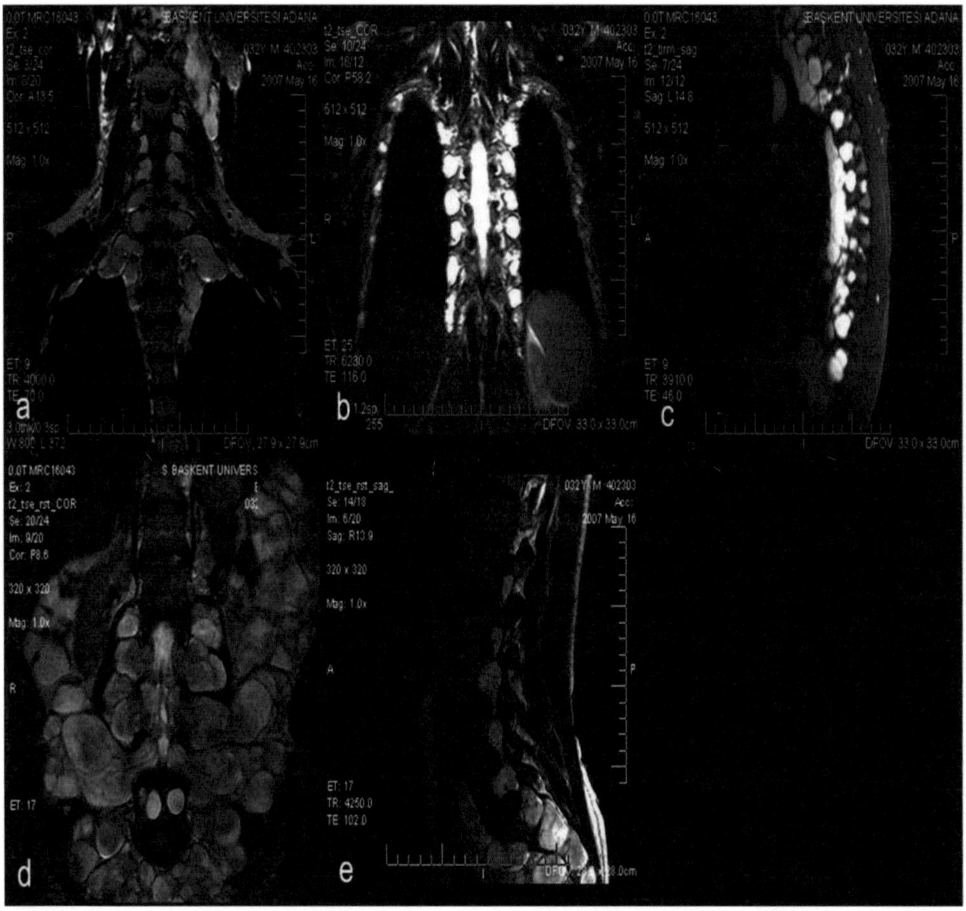

Figure 1.
Preoperative, T2-weighted MRI scan of the patient's spinal axis, revealing multiple, massive, hyperintense lesions displaying heterogenous insignificant contrast enhancement in the paraspinal region. These lesions caused neural foraminal extension by filling all cervical and thoracic neural foramen; they were detectable (a) in the coronal plane in the cervical region, (b) in the coronal plane in the thoracic region, and (c) in the sagittal plane in the thoracic region. (d) View of the coronal plane in the lumbosacral region, showing intra-abdominal dumbbell tumor formation due to multiple, massive, hyperintense lesions causing neural foraminal extension through filling of all neural foramen. The lesions were located paraspinally and showed heterogenous insignificant contrast enhancement. (e) Multiple, massive lesions causing scalloping at the posterior parts of the L3 and L4 sacral vertebrae and in the posterior parts of the sacral vertebrae were detected in the lumbosacral region of the sagittal plane. "This figure is presented with Copyright permission of the Turkish Neurosurgery (Turkish Neurosurgical Society) [22]."

hemorrhage fields can be observed depending on the vascular thrombosis and necrosis developed as long as the tumor grows in the plexiform neurofibromas [32]. Therefore, the big dimensional neurofibromas especially present a heterogeneous appearance in the T1-weighted sequences due to the degenerative variations and pseudocystic fields [33]. Moreover, while the regions are observed as a hyperintense in the T2-weighted sequences since the myxoid degeneration is observed in it, the fields showing the collagenous fibrous tissue give a hypointense appearance. Similarly, the heterogeneous contrast involvement is observed in the big spinal neurofibromas [30].

4. Surgical treatment of the spinal neurofibromas

4.1 General surgical principles of the spinal and dumbbell neurofibromas

The neurofibromas consist of a mixture of the proliferous nerve sheath originating from the perineural fibroblasts. The neurofibromas extend to the fascicules by surrounding the axons. The surgical cleavage plan loss develops between the nerve fibers and tumor as a result of the fascicule's complete involvement with the tumor in the neurofibroma cases. This condition constitutes a foundation of the difficulties in the spinal neurofibroma surgery. The axons surrounded by the tumor are generally taken together with the tumor during the surgery. However, the fascicules, in which the tumor shows an extension but is not completely held, can be most often separated by dissecting the tumor during the surgery, and thus, they can be protected [34, 35]. The MR images of our patient, in which the intraspinal tumor component of the cervical dumbbell neurofibroma was surgically removed, are presented in **Figure 2** [22].

The aim in the spinal neurofibromas' surgical treatments is to remove the tumor totally. The nerve root and nerve showing involvement by the tumor are required to be sufficiently exposed in the first stage of the surgery since the spinal neurofibromas are mostly originated from the nerve root. Then, these neural elements should be separated by the sensitive dissection from the tumor, and the total resection should be made to the tumor in the last stage of the surgery. But, nerve root can be sacrificed especially in the patients, in which neural elements' dissection cannot be achieved.

The total removal of the single solitary neurofibroma surgically is relatively easier. But, the difficulties can be encountered in taking these tumors surgically since they are characterized by the multiple tumors in the plexiform neurofibromas, especially accompanying to the NF1. The postoperative neurologic deficit development risk is much more according to the spinal schwannoma resections in the multiple spinal neurofibroma resections due to more than one nerve fiber involvements. Therefore, the activities in the muscles innerved by the functional nerves should be followed up by using the intraoperative EMG monitorization in order to prevent the postoperative neurodeficit development. Moreover, these fascicules can be enlightened whether they are the motor function with the intraoperative electrical stimulation applied to the fascicules by the tumor. The total tumor resection is rarely applied in the plexiform neurofibroma cases [36]. Therefore, removing the symptomatic tumors primarily is suggested in the multiple spinal neurofibroma cases accompanying to the NF1 [37]. For this purpose, the spinal axis regions, to which the surgical intervention will be applied, should be researched and revealed by both the detailed radiologic imaging methods to be made in the preoperative period and detailed neurophysiologic tests.

Sacrificing the nerve root will not cause an additional neurologic deficit for the patient since the nerve root is already nonfunctional due to the degeneration in the

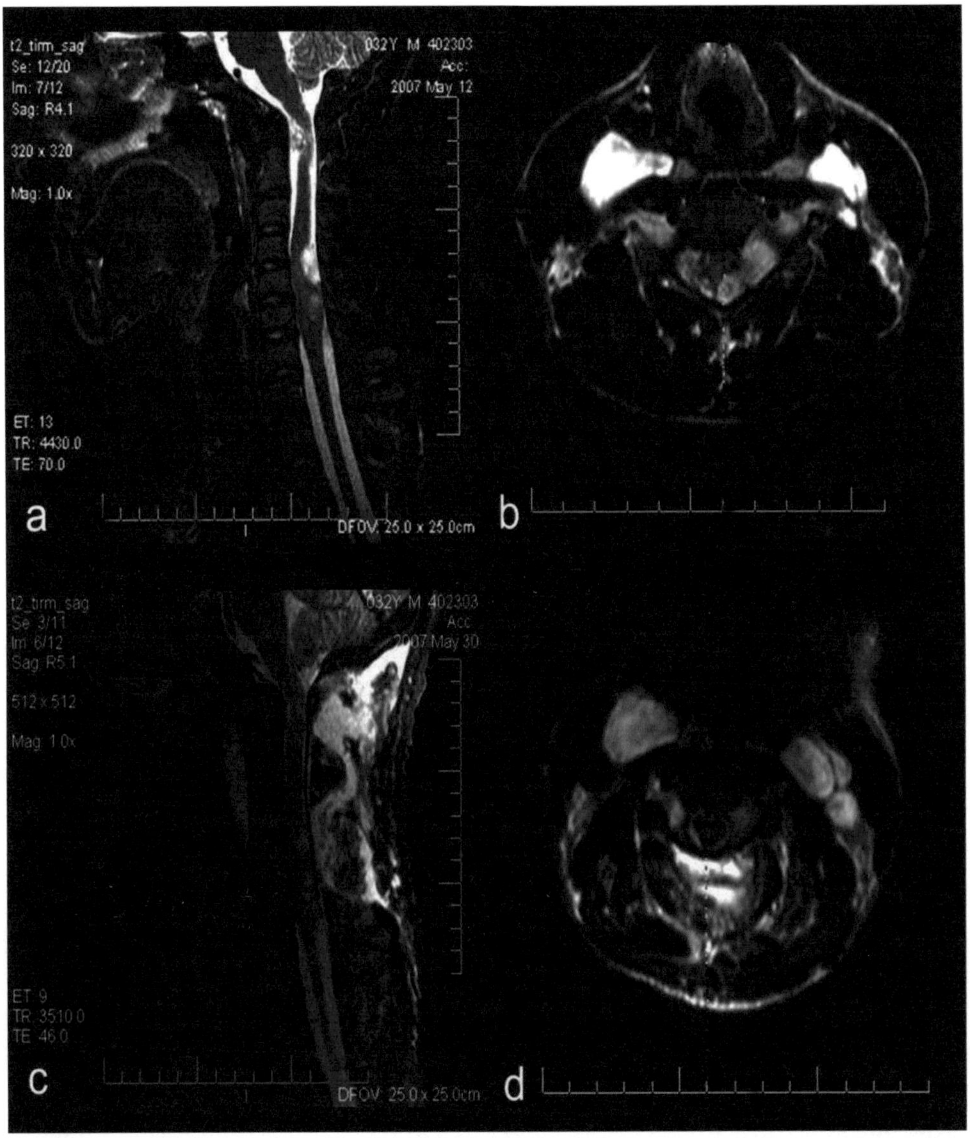

Figure 2.
Detection of massive, hyperintense lesion, located paraspinally and displaying heterogenous insignificant contrast enhancement that was causing significant spinal cord compression at the C4–C5 level by filling in the epidural distance. The lesion was visible in preoperative MRI scans of the patient's cervicospinal area: (a) T2 sagittal sequence, (b) T2 axial sequence. After surgical intervention, removal of the lesions was confirmed in (c) a T2-weighted sagittal sequence and (d) a T2-weighted axial sequence. "This figure is presented with Copyright permission of the Turkish Neurosurgery (Turkish Neurosurgical Society) [22]."

multiple neurofibroma cases accompanying to the NF1 and show a malign degeneration [37]. But, protecting the spinal radicular arteries progressing together with them while sacrificing the nerve root is quite important in order to avoid the spinal cord ischemia that will be preoperatively able to develop [38]. The nerve fibers' large part is held by the tumor, especially in the big or giant dimensional dumbbell neurofibroma cases, and it is unfeasible to take these tumors without sacrificing the root. Consequently, the total resections of these big or huge dimensional dumbbell neurofibromas are surgically concluded by the serious neurologic deficits. Therefore, it should be contented with a partial resection of the tumor, in which the neural structures are protected as far as possible in these cases [27, 31, 37].

On the other hand, even the symptomatic spinal neurofibromas are surgically taken in the cases with NF1; the reoperations can be required in these cases as a result of becoming symptomatic by growing the localized asymptomatic spinal neurofibromas in the other regions [27, 31].

4.2 Surgical approach review

4.2.1 Surgical approach of the cervical spinal neurofibromas

The spinal neurofibromas are generally tumors showing a concentric enlargement throughout the spinal nerve [1]. Especially, the spinal cord and nerve roots should be protected during the cervical dumbbell tumors' surgical resections. Moreover, the vertebral artery is also required to be brought under control, especially during the surgery due to the cervical dumbbell tumors' close relationship. The customized ideal surgical approach should be determined, and the tumor should be totally taken by taking the tumor size and spreading pattern into consideration in order to decrease the recurrence rate to be developed due to the cervical dumbbell tumor's insufficient resection. Moreover, the spinal instability risk to be developed should be preoperatively and/or intraoperatively taken into consideration, and if needed, the cervical fusion should be made in the same session [1, 39].

The important difficulties are encountered in the cervical dumbbell tumors' surgical treatment due to the tumor's close adjacency to the vertebral artery and sheath and the vertebral body's involvement. Therefore, various surgical approaches had been defined in order to take these tumors surgically. McCormick had described a single-stage posterior approach for cervical dumbbell tumors. In this approach, a single segmented facetectomy and hemilaminectomy had been used. However, there are also limitations to the single-stage posterior approach. It had been notified between them that the extraspinal component's extension to the tumor's lateral was not required to be more and the component showing an extension to the lateral was required to be maximum 3 cm beginning from the dural sac margin [40]. But, the tumor is not totally taken by the single-stage posterior approach for the cervical dumbbell tumors exceeding these nerves.

A combined posteroanterior approach is totally required to take the tumors, of which extraspinal extension is big in this manner [41, 42]. The surgery duration is longer in this single-stage approach, and intraoperative hemorrhage is much more observed. The combined posteroanterior approach had been planned as two-stage by Mohd Ariff et al. in order to eliminate the excessive hemorrhage risk arising from the surgery duration's length [43]. The cervical dumbbell tumor's intraspinal component is firstly taken by the posterior approach in this approach. Then, by giving a length of time, it is gained time for the spinal cord edema's resorption. In the second stage, the tumor's extraspinal component is taken by the anterior approach [1]. Jiang et al. had notified the Peking University Third Hospital classification that facilitates the surgical approach planning according to the cervical dumbbell tumors' localization and extension pattern based upon the preoperative MRI or CT images. This classification had been described in two stages. In the first stage of this classification, the regions, in which the tumor is localized, had been divided into five groups, and the regions, in which these tumors extended, had been divided into four groups. In the second stage, seven groups had been constituted according to the tumor localization's combination and extension regions, and the suggested surgical approach patterns had been indicated for these seven groups [41]. In the course of time, the lateral approaches had become to be preferred much more by the neurosurgeons instead of the (single-stage or two-stage) combined (instead of postero-anterior approach) approaches because the lateral approaches provide wider exposure to the spinal axis' lateral, intervertebral foramen and extraforaminal regions in the single session [44].

The first lateral approach had been used by Verbiest in the cervical spondylosis surgery [45]. The various anterolateral approaches had been developed by modifying this lateral approach in the course of time and had been especially used in the cervical tumors' surgical treatments [45–47]. However, these declared anterolateral approaches are the approaches generally and technically containing a difficulty and bearing an injury risk in the adjacent nerves to the vertebral artery and tumor [42]. The transparaspinal approach had been described by Onesti in order to avoid these risk factors and take the paraspinal tumors totally without the necessity of anterior surgery. In this single-stage approach, the vertebra lateral is completely dominated by the combination of cutting the paraspinal muscles with a transverse incision together with the laminectomy. All of the paraspinal tumors localized in the vertebra lateral can be taken by this approach independently from the tumor size. It is a rapid approach that can be used throughout the whole spinal axis as an advantage of this approach. Its disadvantage is that it cannot be used in the dumbbell tumors making an anterior spinal cord pressure since the spinal cord anterior is not seen sufficient with this approach [42].

The extensive posterolateral exposure had been defined by Zhao in 2009 in order to totally take the cervical dumbbell tumors, of which huge extraforaminal component is especially found. It had been notified by this approach that the total tumor resection was made in 16 cases with cervical dumbbell tumor. In this approach, the total lateral mass resection and laminectomy had been used. It had been notified by this approach that the tumors' most lateral part could be reached by the posterolateral wide exposure. Moreover, it had been also notified by this approach that separating tumor from vertebral artery could be easily achieved and tumor component could be resected since it showed an extension to the lateral vertebral body [48, 49].

4.2.2 Surgical approach of the thoracic spinal neurofibromas

The thoracic dumbbell tumors are relatively rarely seen. Taking the thoracic dumbbell tumors surgically shows a difficulty since there are two pieces of extraspinal and intraspinal tumor components connected through the foramen. Therefore, the various approaches had been defined in the course of time in order to take the thoracic dumbbell tumors. The size and position of the thoracic dumbbell tumors and extraspinal components are the most important factors in deciding the surgical approach [50, 51]. In the course of time, although there are various classifications developed by taking these criteria into consideration, nowadays, Eden's classification had been the most frequently preferred one by the neurosurgeons in deciding to the surgical approach [51].

The single-stage posterior approach is frequently preferred in order to take the dumbbell tumor's intraspinal component in the cases having Eden type II and type III tumors according to this classification. The two-stage combined posteroanterior approach is frequently preferred in the cases having a centrally located tumor such as Eden type IV, of which the extraforaminal tumor component is big [51]. The single-stage posterior approach is frequently preferred in the cases, of which extraspinal component is small. The detailed information is obtained about the important peritumoral structures' involvements with the tumor such as the arteries found in the adjacency of the tumor by making 3D-CT scanning in the preoperative period. The patient is taken into surgery under the general anesthesia and in prone position. Then, records of SSEPs and MEPs of patient are monitored by neuromonitorization.

The paraspinal muscles are subperiosteally dissected after a median vertical skin incision in the posterior. The intraspinal component including the tumor's part in the foramen is revealed by making the total facetectomy following the total laminectomy. Then, the costotransverse joint, costa, and transverse process found in the affected side are revealed. The costotransversectomy is made and the tumor's extraspinal component is reached. The dura is opened by the microsurgery method since the tumor's intradural component is firstly required to be taken in the spinal neurofibroma surgery, and the tumor's intradural component is observed. The tumor is firstly separated by the microdissection from the spinal cord and then from the nerve roots. But, the thoracic nerve roots that cannot be separated from the tumor due to the cohesiveness despite the dissection can be sacrificed in this stage of the surgery. Sacrificing the other thoracic nerve roots excluding the T1 nerve root, a part of the brachial plexus, is generally and functionally tolerated better. Nevertheless, when required, the intraoperative stimulation can be also used in this stage in order to evaluate whether the related nerve functions are protected. The tumor's foraminal component is mostly taken by resecting the region together with the surrounding dura. In this stage, the radicular artery's progression coming into existence from the descending aorta's segmental intercostal branches by passing through the foramen toward the spinal cord should be paid attention to, and this artery should be protected in order to avoid the spinal cord damage [52–55].

The combined posteroanterior approach made by the laminectomy and thoracotomy had been described for total resection of the tumor, of which big extraspinal component is found in the chest cavity. This is a two-stage approach, and the laminectomy and costotransversectomy are firstly made by a neurosurgeon with the posterior approach, and the tumor's extraspinal part is taken. Then, the tumor's extraspinal big component is taken by a thoracic surgeon by making the thoracotomy with the anterior approach. An arcuate arc incision is used. One piece of costa part, which is found between the costochondral junction and costotransverse joint, is taken by making it independent from the surrounding tissues. Next, the parietal pleura is opened in the costa bed, and the chest cavity is entered. The lung, which is found on the side in which the surgery is made, is damped with the help of a double-lumen endotracheal tube. The tumor's big extraspinal component found in the chest cavity is taken after providing the sufficient view field [55, 56]. The remaining spinal cord's dura defect is closed as waterproof by the duraplasty made with the help of dura graft after taking the thoracic dumbbell tumor and sacrificing all of the nerve roots affected. Then, the fibrin tissue adhesives are put on it, and the fatty tissue obtained from the subcutaneous tissue is located in this field.

In the course of time, the open thoracotomy gives its place to the thoracoscopic interventions that are more minimally invasive intervention depending on the developments in the endoscopy field. In 1999, it had been firstly notified that the thoracic dumbbell neurofibroma was taken by Citow et al. with the single-stage combined laminectomy and thoracoscopy approach. It had been notified between the advantages of this approach that the potential morbidity observed in the thoracotomy was not observed in this approach and, moreover, the wide muscle dissection observed in the single-stage posterior approach was not needed in this approach, and consequently, the postoperative ache was less often [57]. In 2001, Konno et al. had notified that there were three dumbbell neurofibroma cases and two paraspinal neurofibroma cases that they similarly treated by the single-stage combined laminectomy and thoracoscopy approach. It had been also indicated that the extraforaminal component could be safely and successfully taken by the thoracoscopy and the instability risk following the unilateral laminectomy and medial facetectomy used in this approach was low, and consequently, the fusion was not required. But, it had been notified as a disadvantage of this approach that the chest tubes to be specially used in the postoperative period had many complication risks such as the postoperative ache, pulmonary infection, and pulmonary dysfunction [58].

The T1 nerve root is a part of the brachial plexus and progresses in the adjacency of subclavian artery and vertebral artery. It had been notified that the T1 nerve root dumbbell tumors had a serious hemorrhage risk depending on these big artery injuries during surgically taking the tumor due to the cohesiveness to the big arteries such as subclavian artery and vertebral artery. Also, while sacrificing the other thoracic nerve roots except the T1 can be functionally tolerated due to the tumor cohesiveness, sacrificing the T1 root, a part of the brachial plexus, cannot be functionally tolerated. Therefore, it is especially required to protect the T1 nerve root in dumbbell tumor surgery. As specified above, a standard surgical approach had not been notified in the surgery of dumbbell tumors arising from the T1 nerve root having the different functional and anatomic features rather than the other thoracic nerves [59].

In the course of time, the video-assisted thoracic surgery (VATS), a minimal invasive intervention, had been described by the thoracic surgeons as a result of the developments in the video technology field. In 2015, the T1 nerve root dumbbell tumor had been safely taken by Ohya et al. for the first time with the posterior spinal surgical combination applied after the VATS. In this combined approach, the subclavian artery and vertebral arteries are firstly assured by the thoracic surgeons by making them independent from the T1 nerve root by using the VATS in the anterior approach. Thus, the serious hemorrhages to be developed depending on these artery injuries will have been prevented during the posterior spinal surgery that will be subsequently applied. The tumor is taken by making the partial costotransversectomy in the posterior spinal surgery. It had been indicated that 3D-CT was required to be used in the preoperative period in order to evaluate the tumor's relationship with the structures in the adjacency of it in details in the cases, for which this combined approach was planned [59]. Moreover, in these cases, it had been also notified that the intraoperative stimulation and neuromonitorization were required to be used in order to evaluate whether the T1 nerve function was protected.

In 2018, comparative analyses of the single-stage posterior approach used in those having Eden type II and type III tumors and combined laminectomy and thoracoscopy used in those having Eden type IV tumor had been made in the cases having the thoracic dumbbell neurofibroma in a retrospective study declared by Li YW et al. In conclusion, it had been indicated that the thoracic dumbbell neurofibromas could be effectively and safely taken by both the surgical approaches. However, it had been also notified that the single-stage posterior approach's operative results were better than the combined laminectomy and thoracoscopy approach and the complications related to the approach pattern were less often observed [60].

4.2.3 Surgical approach of the lumbar spinal neurofibromas

The lumbar dumbbell neurofibromas show an extension to the abdomen cavity from the paraspinal muscles and retroperitoneal field and can wrap the surrounding of abdominal organs. These tumors symptomatically make pressure to the abdominal organs with the organ dysfunction findings when they reached the big or huge sizes since they usually show an intraabdominal asymptomatic growth [61, 62]. While the lumbar dumbbell tumors' intraspinal part is taken by posterior approach, big dimensional extraspinal part is especially taken by the anterior approach [62, 63]. But, the common iliac vein laceration, renal pedicle avulsions, and massive hemorrhages had been notified by the single-stage anterior approach, in which the total resection of the dumbbell tumor's intraspinal and extraspinal components was planned [64, 65]. Therefore, the combined posteroanterior approaches had become a current issue, especially for the big or huge dimensional lumbar dumbbell tumors.

The lumbar dumbbell tumors' extraspinal part can reach the big and huge sizes in the retroperitoneal field and intraabdominal region. Park et al. had used the "huge" term for the tumors, of which size exceeds 2.5 cm beginning from the extraspinal component's dural margin [66]. On the contrary, many neurosurgeons had notified that using the "huge" tumor term would be more appropriate in the case where the tumor's extraspinal component caused a pushing or pressure in the retroperitoneal and/or internal organs when they were shown by the radiologic examinations [64]. The surgical approaches used in the conditions, in which the lumbar dumbbell tumors' extraspinal component was big, had been notified in limited number in the literature, and not any guideline describing the surgical approaches to be selected according to the tumor's localization and spreading patterns had been notified. The combined posteroanterior approach had been generally used in taking the big dumbbell tumors. In this approach, the tumor's intraspinal component had been firstly taken by the posterior approach. Then, the anterior approach had been made together with a general surgeon or urologist included in the surgery, and the retroperitoneal and/or intraabdominal components, by which the tumor showed an extraspinal extension, had been taken [67, 68]. There are disadvantages such as being long of the operation duration and being more of the intraoperative hemorrhage amount in the single-stage combined posteroanterior approaches.

Therefore, the single-stage extensive posterior approach, a posterolateral approach pattern, had been developed in the lumbar dumbbell tumors, of which extraspinal component was especially big like in the surgery of cervical and thoracic dumbbell tumors instead of the combined posteroanterior approach. In this approach, a midline skin incision is made like in posterior approach. But, unilateral muscle dissection is made until the transverse process lateral differently from the posterior approach. Then, a wide visual angle is obtained toward the retroperitoneal field from the lateral by making two transverse process resections. In the cases where the visual angle is insufficient despite the transverse process resection, the paraspinal muscles are longitudinally cut by making a second subcutaneous incision in the lateral, and thus, the paraspinal approach is carried out. After revealing the tumor's extraspinal component in this manner, the intraspinal component is also revealed by making the unilateral laminectomy and facetectomy in the second stage. The tumor's intraspinal component is firstly taken following the stages specified in the combined posteroanterior approach. Then, the cohesiveness of the tumor's extraspinal component with the retroperitoneal and intraabdominal organs is tried to be separated as far as possible by making a blunt dissection, and the extraspinal component is taken by resecting gross totally and/or totally. Sometimes, the debulking can be applied in order to minimize the tumor size in the lumbar dumbbell tumors having a huge extraspinal component [64].

4.3 Management of the postoperative complications in the spinal neurofibroma

4.3.1 Spinal deformity and instability

It had been notified that the cervical instability developed in 20% of the cases as a result of the posterior surgical approaches applied in the cervical spinal neurofibromas. Moreover, it had been also notified that scoliosis or kyphoscoliosis developed at the rate of 50% when the fusion is not made in the cases, in which the facetectomy is applied and cervical instability is observed. Therefore, the fusion surgery should be added in the intraoperative period, or the fusion should be made in the essential cases by making a close radiologic follow-up to the patients in the postoperative period in order to prevent the cervical instability to be developed after the posterior approach surgeries [41]. The thoracic instability development risk is quite low even in the combined posteroanterior approaches, in which the total facetectomy and costotransversectomy are made in the thoracic spinal neurofibroma cases. Generally, the fusion is not needed. The principal factor preventing the instability in the thoracic region is originated from a more stable nature of the thoracic spinal axis compared to the cervical and lumbar regions [50, 69]. But, the transpedicular stabilization can be made by putting a pedicle screw following the reconstruction made by putting a cage or bone strut to the defective field when the vertebra destruction developed as a result of the tumor pressure in the adjacency of vertebra body observed in the thoracic paravertebral neurofibroma cases showing an extension to the lateral [64]. The fusion with the similar instrumentation is planned since the postoperative instability development risk is high due to the thoracic vertebra scalloping lesions accompanying to the NF1 [70]. Similarly, making the stabilization with the reconstruction and instrumentation is suggested in over half of the vertebral body in the lumbar spinal neurofibroma cases when the destruction is developed by the tumor [64, 71, 72]. Moreover, the lamina reconstruction is added to the surgical approaches by using an autologous iliac crest bone or allograft in order to prevent the postlaminectomy kyphotic deformity to be developed in the cases, which are the common point of thoracic and lumbar surgical approaches, and to which more than one laminectomy is specially made [73]. In conclusion, the spinal instability risks to be developed should be preoperatively and/or intraoperatively evaluated in the spinal neurofibroma cases, and if needed, making the cervical fusion in the same session will be more appropriate [1, 39].

4.3.2 Recurrence of the tumor

The recurrence rate is quite less for those, for which the total tumor resection is made in the spinal neurofibroma cases. The 5-year and 10–15-year recurrence rates had been notified as 10.7 and 28.2%, respectively, in the localized nerve sheath tumors within the cervical region accompanying the NF1 [39]. It had been also notified by Levy et al. that the recurrence was observed 3 years later in only 1 case of 66 paraspinal neurofibroma cases operated by them [37]. Fifteen patients, to whom the thoracic neurofibroma resection was made by using the single-stage posterior approach with the costotransversectomy, had been followed up for at least 5–10 years, and it had been notified that no recurrence was observed in these cases [53]. Taking the tumor totally has difficulties although the surgical approaches are described in these spinal neurofibroma cases, in which the surgical cleavage plane was lost between nerve fibers and tumor. Moreover, their close relationships with the adjacent important vascular and visceral organs especially affect the dumbbell neurofibromas' total resections in a negative way [1, 34, 35, 39]. Therefore, the tumors' relationships with the peritumoral structures such as the vertebra, costa, and arteries should be researched in details by the MRI and 3D-CT images that will be made in the preoperative period for the spinal neurofibroma cases in order to prevent tumor recurrence, and the appropriate surgical approach should be selected [54]. Although the protection of the held nerve roots is always given precedence, sometimes, the total resection cannot be achieved. Therefore, especially insufficient tumor resections are the most important factor causing the increase in the tumor recurrence. Moreover, it had been notified that the tumor recurrence was generally asymptomatic in the cases accompanying to the NF1. The most important factor in deciding to the surgery in the recurrence cases is whether the patients are symptomatic or not. The surgical tumor resection should be planned in the symptomatic cases [1, 34, 35, 39].

4.3.3 Protection of the nerve roots and fascicules

The fascicules, to which the tumors show an extension but in which they are not completely held in the spinal neurofibroma surgery, can be most often separated and protected by dissecting the tumor during the surgery [34, 35]. However, the nerve roots' protection problems increase, and the nerve root can be sacrificed in the cases, in which dumbbell tumor formation is especially observed. In the literature, in the cases of cervical dumbbell neurofibromas operated with combined posteroanterior approach, the rate of protection of the nerve root has been reported as 18% [44]. Sacrificing the T1 nerve root participated in the brachial plexus together with the cervical and lumbar spinal roots cannot be functionally tolerated better for the patients in the surgery and causes the neurodeficits at the different levels. However, sacrificing the thoracic nerve roots is generally tolerated better in the patients. Therefore, the intraoperative stimulation and neuromonitorization are required to be used in order to detect the functional fascicules during the surgery in the neurofibroma cases, especially arising from the cervical, lumbar, and T1 nerve root [44, 74].

4.3.4 Techniques of the artery protection

The tumor's extraspinal component can show a close adjacency with the vertebral artery in the cervical dumbbell neurofibromas. The vertebral artery is generally pushed toward the anteromedial due to the tumor's extraspinal component. There is mostly a thin periosteum layer and perivertebral venous plexus layer between the tumor and vertebral artery. If the dissection is made from this surgical cleavage region, the ischemic injury probability is much more limited [75, 76]. Adamkiewicz artery should be specially paid attention for not being injured in order to protect it from the serious spinal cord ischemia in the inferior thoracic surgery and upper lumbar region dumbbell neurofibroma cases. Therefore, the enucleation should be made, and the aorta's segmental arteries should be protected in order to minimize the tumor size, especially in the resections of the dumbbell tumors' foraminal and extraforaminal components [64, 77].

4.3.5 Cerebrospinal fluid leakage and intralodge hemorrhage

The incision on the nerve root is taken forward by making a dural incision toward the medial during the dumbbell neurofibroma surgery. Following sacrificing the tumor resection and nerve root, the dura defect is closed to the intervertebral foramen by filling the fibrin tissue adhesive and fat. In this approach, the lateral mass fixation is used by mostly using the lateral mass instrumentation. The cerebrospinal fluid leakage can be observed in the cases, in which the dural defect cannot be successfully made. Moreover, the hemorrhage, hemothorax, and/or intraabdominal hemorrhage can be observed depending on the surgery's duration length, especially in the combined posteroanterior approaches. One piece of a hemorrhagic drain inside of the lodge in the posterior and one piece of an intraabdominal drain in the anterior should be placed at the end of surgery in order to prevent these complications to be developed in the postoperative period [50, 52, 58, 59, 64, 69].

5. Prognosis of the spinal neurofibromas

The patients' lifetimes are quite long depending on the tumor's benign nature in the spinal neurofibroma. The most important factor affecting the prognosis in the spinal neurofibroma cases is tumor's surgical resection pattern. The prognosis is exceptionally good in the cases, in which the total resection is made. The ache complaint is completely recovered in 80% of the cases after the total resection, and the whole remission is provided in 60% of the cases. The tumor recurrence is quite rarely observed in the cases, in which the total resection is made. It had been notified that the recurrence was observed 3 years later on only 1 case of 66 paraspinal neurofibroma cases operated by Levy et al. [37, 40]. Another factor affecting the prognosis is the functional nerve roots' protection during the surgery. In this point, the tumor's localization comes into prominence much more. The thoracic spinal neurofibroma cases' prognosis is better since it is functionally tolerated in most cases by sacrificing the thoracic nerve root [75]. Another prognostic factor is the spinal instability developed depending on the vertebral deformities. Causing the destruction by the tumor's extraspinal component in the intervertebral foramen and the vertebral body lateral leads to spinal instability, especially in the dumbbell neurofibroma cases. Moreover, the total laminectomy, total facetectomy, costo-transversectomy, and multiple costa resections made depending on the surgical approach pattern can also lead to spinal instability. The vertebral scalloping lesions observed in patients with NF1 independent from the spinal neurofibroma also cause spinal instability [53, 77]. Making the fusion surgery with the intraoperative instrumentation will positively affect the prognosis in these tables. Therefore, the customized surgical approach should be planned depending on the tumor's localization and extension pattern in the cases with spinal neurofibroma.

6. Conclusion

In conclusion, a customized ideal surgical approach should be determined, and the tumor should be totally taken by taking the tumor's size and spreading pattern into consideration in order to decrease the recurrence rate to be developed due to the tumor's insufficient resection in the spinal neurofibroma cases. The surgical tumor resection should be carried out in company with the intraoperative stimulation and neuromonitorization. Moreover, if possible, the reconstruction and fusion surgery with instrumentation should be also made in the same session in the cases having a spinal instability risk to be developed.

Conflict of interest

The author reports no conflict of interest concerning the materials or methods used in this study or the findings specified in this paper. And the author has no personal financial or institutional interest in this research described in this article.

Author details

Feyzi Birol Sarica
Department of Neurosurgery, Faculty of Medicine, Giresun University, Giresun, Turkey

*Address all correspondence to: saricafb@gmail.com

References

[1] Hirsch NP, Murphy A, Radcliffe JJ. Neurofibromatosis: Clinical presentations and anaesthetic implications. British Journal of Anaesthesia. 2001;**86**:555-564

[2] DeBella K, Szudek J, Friedman JM. Use of the national institutes of health criteria for diagnosis of neurofibromatosis 1 in children. Pediatrics. 2000;**105**(3 Pt 1):608-614

[3] Abramowicz A. GosM. Neurofibromin in neurofibromatosis type 1—Mutations in NF1gene as a cause of disease. Developmental Period Medicine. 2014;**18**(3):297-306

[4] Ferner RE. Neurofibromatosis 1. European Journal of Human Genetics. 2007;**15**(2):131-138

[5] Weiss SW, Goldblum JR. Benign tumors of peripheral nerve. In: Goldblum JR, Folpe AL, Weiss SW, editors. Enzinger and Weiss's Soft Tissue Tumors. 6th ed. Philadelphia: Elsevier Saunders; 2014. pp. 784-854

[6] Sampson JH, Martuza RL. Neurofibromatosis and other phakomatoses. In: Wilkins RH, Rengachary SS, editors. Neurosurgery. 2nd ed. Vol. IB. New York: Mc-Graw-Hill Book Company; 1996. pp. 673-685

[7] Abramowicz A, Gos M. Neurofibromin in neurofibromatosis type 1—Mutations in NF1gene as a cause of disease. Developmental Period Medicine. 2014;**18**(1):124-133

[8] National Institute of Health Concensus Development Conference: Neurofibromatosis conference statement. Archives of Neurology. 1988;**45**:579-588

[9] Scoles DR, Nguyen VD, Qin Y, Sun CX, Morrison H, Gutmann DH, et al. Neurofibromatosis 2 (NF2) suppressor schwannomin and its interacting protein HRS regulate STAT signaling. Human Molecular Genetics. 2002;**11**(25):3179-3189

[10] Ng HK, Lau KM, Tse JYM, Lo KW, Wong JHC, Poon WS, et al. Combined molecular genetic studies of chromosome 22q and neurofibromatosis type 2 gene in central nervous system tumours. Neurosurgery. 1995;**37**:764-773

[11] Eastwood JD, Florella DJ, Macfall JF, Delong DM, Provenzale JM, Greenwood RS. Increased brain apparent diffusion coefficient in children with neurofibromatosis type 1. Radiology. 2001;**219**:354-358

[12] Hirbe AC, Gutmann DH. Neurofibromatosis type 1: A multidisciplinary approach to care. Lancet Neurology. 2014;**13**(8):834-843

[13] Korf BR. Malignancy in neurofibromatosis type 1. The Oncologist. 2000;**5**:477-485

[14] Goh WH, Khong PL, Leung CS, et al. T2-weighted hyperintensities (unidentified bright objects) in children with neurofibromatosis 1: Their impact on cognitive function. Journal of Child Neurology. 2004;**19**:853-858

[15] Chapparo MJ, Young RF, Moyra S, Shen V, Choi BH. Multiple spinal meningiomas: A case of 47 distinct lesions in the absence of neurofibromatosis or identified chromosomal abnormality. Neurosurgery. 1993;**32**:298-302

[16] Tucker T, Schnabel C, Hartmann M, et al. Bone health and fracture rate in individuals with neurofibromatosis 1 (NF1). Journal of Medical Genetics. 2009;**46**(4):259-265

[17] Agaimy A, Vassos N, Croner RS. Gastrointestinal manifestations of neurofibromatosis type 1 (Recklinghausen's disease): Clinicopathological spectrum with pathogenetic considerations. International Journal of Clinical and Experimental Pathology. 2012;**5**(9):852-862

[18] Russell DS, Rubinstein LJ. Pathology of Tumors of the Nervous System. 5th ed. Baltimore: Williams & Wilkins; 1989. pp. 531-571

[19] Halliday AL, Sobel RS, Martuza RL. Benign spinal nerve sheath tumors: Their occurrence sporadically and in neurofibromatosis type 1 and 2. Journal of Neurosurgery. 1991;**74**(2):248-253

[20] Enzinger FM, Weiss SW. Benign tumors of peripheral nerves. In: Enzinger FM, Weiss SW, editors. Soft Tissue Tumors. 3rd ed. St Louis: Mosby-Year Book; 1995. pp. 821-888

[21] Rao SB. Spinal neurinoma.A study of 80 operated cases. Neurology India. 1975;**23**(1):1-12

[22] Sarica FB, Cekinmez M, Tufan K, Erdogan B, Sen O, Altinors MN. A rare case of massive NF1 with invasion of entire spinal axis by neurofibromas: Case report. Turkish Neurosurgery. 2008;**18**(1):99-106

[23] Webb WR, Goodman PC. Fibrosing alveolitis in patients with neurofibromatosis. Radiology. 1977;**122**:289-293

[24] Conti P, Pascini G, Mouchaty H, Capuano C, Conti R. Spinal neuromas: Retrospective analysis and long-term outcome of 179 consecutively operated cases and review of the literature. Surgical Neurology. 2004;**61**(1):34-43

[25] Hirose T, Sano T, Hizawa K. Ultrastructurel localization of S-100 protein in neurofibroma. Acta Neuropathology (Berl). 1986;**69**(1-2):103-110

[26] D'Alessandro G, Di Giovanni M, Iannizzi L, Guidetti E, Bottachci E. Epidemiology of primary intracranial tumors in the Valle d'Aosta (Italy) during the 6-year period 1986-1991. Neuroepidemiology. 1995;**14**:139-146

[27] Canbaz B, Tanrıverdi T. Nörofibromatozis. In: Aksoy K, Palaoglu S, Pamir TR, editors. Temel Nöroşirürji. Ankara: Turkish Neurosurgery Society Publishing; 2005. pp. 823-829

[28] Leonard JR, Ferner RE, Thomas N, Gutmann DH. Cervical cord compression from plexiform neurofibromas in neurofibromatosis 1. Journal of Neurology, Neurosurgery, and Psychiatry. 2007;**78**(12):1404-1406

[29] Wagenknecht LV, Schumpelick V, Winkler R. Urological aspects of primary retroperitoneal tumors. European Urology. 1976;**2**:15-20

[30] Sakai F, Sone S, Kiyono K, Maruyama A, Ueda H, Aoki J, et al. Intrathoracic neurogenic tumors: MR pathologic correlation. AJR. American Journal of Roentgenology. 1992;**159**:279-283

[31] Unal F. Spinal intradural ekstramedüller tümörler. In: Aksoy K, Palaoglu S, Pamir TR, editors. Temel Nöroşirürji. Ankara: Turkish Neurosurgery Society Publishing; 2005. pp. 1121-1128

[32] Bhatia S, Khosla A, Dhir R, Bhatia R, Banerji AK. Giant lumbosacral nerve sheath tumors. Surgical Neurology. 1992;**37**:118-122

[33] Lin J, Martel W. Cross-sectional imaging of peripheral nerve sheath tumors: Characteristic signs on CT,

MR imaging, and sonography. American Journal of Roentgenology. 2001;**176**:75-82

[34] Donner TR, Vorrhies RM, Kline DG. Neural sheath tumors of major nerves. Journal of Neurosurgery. 1994;**81**:362-373

[35] Haraida S, Nerlich AG, Bise K, Wiest I, Schleicher E. Comparison of various basement membrane components in benign and malignant peripheral nerve tumours. Virchows Archiv A. 1992;**421**(4):331-338

[36] Ozerdem U. Targeting neovascular pericytes in neurofibromatosis type 1. Angiogenesis. 2005;7(4):307-311

[37] Levy WJ Jr, Latchaw J, Hahn JF. Spinal neurofibromas: A report of 66 cases and a comparison with meningiomas. Neurosurgery 1986;**18**:331-334

[38] Iradi G, Peserica L, Salar G. Intraspinal neuromas and meningiomas: A clinical survey of 172 cases. International Surgery. 1971;**56**:289-303

[39] Klekamp J, Samii M. Surgery of spinal nerve sheath tumors reference to neurofibromatosis. Neurosurgery. 1998;**42**(2):279-290

[40] McCormick PC. Surgical management of dumbbell tumors of the cervical spine. Neurosurgery. 1996;**38**:294-300

[41] Jiang L, Lv Y, Liu XG, Ma QJ, Wei F, Dang GT, et al. Results of surgical treatment of cervical dumbbell tumors: Surgical approach and development of an anatomic classification system. Spine. 2009;**34**(12):1307-1314

[42] Onesti ST, Ashkenazi E, Michelsen WJ. Transparaspinal exposure of dumbbell tumors of the spine. Journal of Neurosurgery. 1998;**88**(1):106-110

[43] Mohd Ariff S, Joehaimey J, Ahmet Sabri O, Abdul Halim Y. Two-stage surgery for a large cervical dumbbell tumour in neurofibromatosis 1: A case report. Malaysian Orthopaedic Journal. 2011;**5**(3):24-27

[44] Lot G, George B. Cervical neuromas with extradural components: Surgical management in a series of 57 patients. Neurosurgery. 1997;**41**:813-822

[45] Verbiest H. A lateral approach to the cervical spine: Technique and indications. Journal of Neurosurgery. 1968;**22**:191-203

[46] George B, Zerah M, Lot G, Hurth M. Oblique transcorporeal approach to anteriorly located lesions in the cervical spinal canal. Acta Neurochirurgica. 1993;**121**:187-190

[47] Sen C, Eisenberg M, Casden AM, Sundaresan N, Caalano PJ. Management of the vertebral artery in excision of extradural tumors of the cervical spine. Neurosurgery. 1995;**36**(1):106-115

[48] Zhao B, Xu J. Extensive posterolateral exposure and total removal of the giant extraforaminal dumbbell tumors of cervical spine: Surgical technique in a series of 16 patients. Spine Journal. 2009;**9**(10):822-829

[49] Kyoshima K, Uehara T, Koyama J, Idomari K, Yomo S. Dumbbell C2 schwannomas involving both sensory and motor rootlets: Report of two cases. Neurosurgery. 2003;**53**(2):436-439

[50] Grillo HC, Ojemann RG, Scannell JG, ark v. Combined approach to "dumbbell" intrathoracic and intraspinal neurogenic tumors. The Annals of Thoracic Surgery. 1983;**36**:402-407

[51] Eden K. The dumb-bell tumours of the spine. The British Journal of Surgery. 1941;**28**:549-570

[52] Ando K, Imagama S, Wakao N, Hirano K, Tauchi R, Muramoto A, et al. Single-stage removal of thoracic dumbbell tumors from a posterior approach only with costotransversectomy. Yonsei Medical Journal. 2012;**53**(3):611-617

[53] Ando K, Imagama S, Ito Z, Tauchi R, Muramoto A, Matsui H, et al. Removal of thoracic dumbbell tumors through a single-stage posterior approach: Its usefulness and limitations. Journal of Orthopaedic Science. 2013;**18**:380-387

[54] Takamura Y, Uede T, Igarashi K, Tatewaki K, Morimoto S. Thoracic dumbbell-shaped neurinoma treated by unilateral hemilaminectomy with partial costotransversectomy—Case report. Neurologia Medico-Chirurgica (Tokyo). 1997;**37**:354-357

[55] Akbay A. Torakal anterior yaklaşımlar. In: Aksoy K, Palaoglu S, Pamir, Tuncer R, editors. Temel Nöroşirürji. Ankara: Turkish Neurosurgery Society Publishing; 2005. pp. 994-998

[56] Fager CA. Atlas of Spinal Surgery. London: Lea & Febiger; 1989. pp. 201-213

[57] Citow JS, MacDonald RL, Ferguson MK. Neurosurgery. 1999;**45**(5):1263-1265

[58] Konno SI, Yabuki S, Kinoshita T, Kikuchi SI. Combined laminectomy and thoracoscopic resection of dumbbell—Type thoracic cord tumor. Spine (Phila Pa 1976). 2001;**26**(6):E130-E134

[59] Ohya J, Miyoshi K, Kitagawa T, Sato Y, Maehara T, Mikami Y. Combined video-assisted thoracic surgery and posterior spinal surgery for the treatment of dumbbell tumor of the first thoracic nerve root. Asian Spine Journal. 2015;**9**(4):595-599

[60] Li YW, Wang B, Li L, Lu G. Posterior surgery versus combined laminectomy and thoracoscopic surgery for treatment of dumbbell-type thoracic cord tumor: A long-term follow-up. Clinical Neurology and Neurosurgery. 2018;**166**:31-35

[61] Kao TH, Shen CC, Chen CC, Kwan PH. "Primary" benign retroperitoneal and intraspinal dumbbell-shaped cystic teratoma: Case report. Spine (Phila, PA, 1976). 2005;**30**(15):E439-E443

[62] Yu NH, Lee SE, Jahng TA, Chung CK. Giant invasive spinal schwannoma: Its clinical features and surgical management. Neurosurgery. 2012;**71**(1):58-66

[63] Ravnik J, Potrc S, Kavalar R, Ravnik M, Zakotnik B, Bunc G. Dumbbell synovial sarcoma of the thoracolumbar spine: A case report. Spine. 2009;**34**(10):E363-E366

[64] Yang M, Wang XB, Li J, Xiong GZ, Lu C, Lu GH. Surgical treatment of large abdominally dumbbell tumor in the lumbar region. Journal of Spinal Disorders & Techniques. 2014;**27**(7):E268-E275

[65] Agrawal A, Srivastava S, Joharapurkar SR, Gharde P, Ubeja G. Single stage complete excision of large thoracic dumbbell schwannoma by modified posterior approach. Surgical Neurology. 2008;**70**:432-436

[66] Park SC, Chung SK, Choe G, Kim HJ. Spinal intraosseous schwannoma: A case report and review. Journal of Korean Neurosurgical Association. 2009;**46**:403-408

[67] Pollo C, Richard A, De Preux J. Resection of a retroperitoneal schwannoma by a combined approach. Neuro-Chirurgie. 2004;**50**:53-56

[68] Jankowski R, Szmeja J, Nowak S, et al. Giant schwannoma of the lumbar

spine. A case report. Neurologia i Neurochirurgia Polska. 2010;**44**:91-95

[69] Levy DI, Bucci MN, Weatherbee L, Chandler WF. Intradural extramedullary ganglioneuroma: Case report and review of the literature. Surgical Neurology. 1992;**37**(3):216-218

[70] Chiang ER, Chang MC, Chen TH. Giant retroperitoneal schwannoma from the fifth lumbar nerve root with vertebral body osteolysis: A case report and literature review. Archives of Orthopaedic and Trauma Surgery. 2009;**129**:495-499

[71] Sridhar K, Ramamurthi R, Vasudevan MC, Ramamurthi B. Giant invasive spinal schwannomas: Definition and surgical management. Journal of Neurosurgery. 2001;**94**(2 Suppl):210-215

[72] Theodosopoulos T, Stafyla VK, Tsiantoula P, Yiallourou A, Marinis A, Kondi-Pafitis A, et al. Special problems encountering surgical management of large retroperitoneal schwannomas. World Journal of Surgical Oncology. 2008;**6**:107

[73] Matsuoka H, Itoh Y, Numazawa S, Tomii M, Watanabe K, Hirano Y, et al. Recapping hemilaminoplasty for spinal surgical disorders using ultrasonic bone curette. Surgical Neurology International. 2012;**3**:70

[74] Kwok K, Davis B, Kliot M. Resection of a benign brachial plexus nerve sheath tumor using intraoperative electrophysiological monitoring. Neurosurgery. 2007;**60**(4 Suppl 2):316-320

[75] Schultheiss R, Gullotta G. Resection of relevant nerve roots in surgery of spinal neurinomas without persisting neurological deficit. Acta Neurochirurgica. 1993;**122**:91-96

[76] Sarica FB, Tufan K, Cekinmez M, Erdogan B, Sen O. Dumbbell-shaped neurofibroma of the upper cervical spine: A case report. Journal of Nervous System Surgery. 2008;**1**(3):190-194

[77] Payer M, Radovanovic I, Jost G. Resection of thoracic dumbbell neurinomas: Single postero-lateral approach or combined posterior and transthoracic approach? Journal of Clinical Neuroscience. 2006;**13**:690-693

Section 5

Radiation and Laser Therapy for CNS Tumors

Chapter 7

The Role of Radiotherapy in the Treatment of Primary Central Nervous System Lymphomas

Meral Kurt, Candan Demiröz Abakay and Ali Altay

Abstract

Primary central nervous system (PCNS) lymphomas are rare disease entities, though the incidence is increasing due to various immunosuppressive situations. The brain, eyes, and the spinal cord could be affected without any systemic disease involvement. Untreated PCNS lymphoma has been a rapidly fatal course. However, combined modality treatments have positive impact on overall survival. Pretreatment plan is formed by evaluating the treatment options to be used, disease involvement, and individual comorbidity. The PCNS lymphomas are known to be very sensitive to irradiation and chemotherapy treatments. The treatment plan is also generated according to the neurological condition and functional status of patients. The mainstay of induction therapy has been high dose methotrexate administration for most patients. The addition of radiotherapy as a consolidation treatment increases progression-free survival. The use of reduced irradiation dose and different fractionation schemes has been investigated in different studies to avoid the increased toxicity of high-dose whole-brain radiotherapy. High-dose chemotherapy, autologous hematopoietic cell transplantation, and whole-brain radiotherapy are alternative applications in patients with insufficient response to induction therapy. Stereotactic radiotherapy is another option in case of relapsed or refractory disease. Age and performance are also important indicators of survival and tumor progression.

Keywords: primary central nervous system lymphoma, radiotherapy, new techniques

1. Introduction

Primary central nervous system lymphomas (PCNSLs) are rare disease entities. The brain, eyes, and the spinal cord could be affected without any systemic disease involvement [1]. PCNSL is an uncommon subtype of extranodal non-Hodgkin lymphoma that accounts for ≈ 3–4% of newly diagnosed central nervous system tumors [2]. The overall incidence rate of PCNSL is 0.47 per 100.000 person-years. Its incidence has increased during the last 3 decades and has been reported in both immunocompromised and immunocompetent patients. Immunocompromised patients are affected at a younger age compared with immunocompetent patients. The incidence is significantly higher in males compared with females.

The most significant increase in the incidence rates for PCNSLs over time has occurred in the oldest adults (aged 75+ years) [3]. There is an increase in

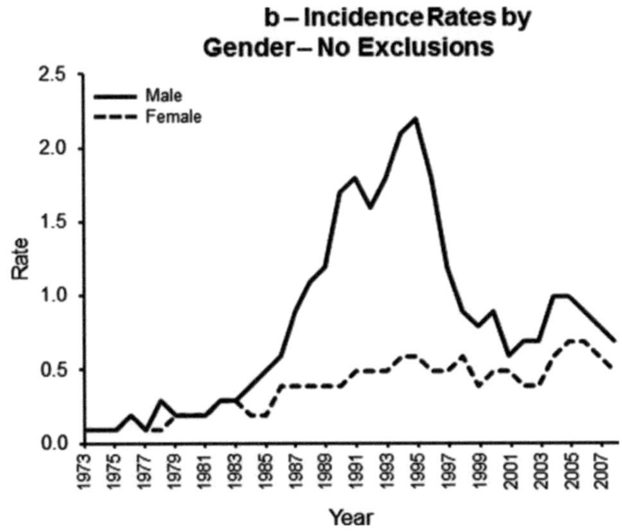

Figure 1.
The incidence rates of PCNSLs by gender from 1973 to 2007 [4].

incidence of PCNSLs in the elderly, and survival remains poor and is negatively dominated by factors associated with HIV infection and advanced age. Such changes were largely driven by PCNSL cases in men between the ages of 20 and 64 years [4]. There has been an overall decline in incidence of PCNSL from 1998 to 2008. Thus the trend has been attributed in large part to changes in HIV/AIDS incidence and management over the same time period. In contrast, the incidence rates continued to increase in women at all ages and men aged 65 and older (**Figure 1**).

In immunocompetent individuals, they occur at a median age of about 55 years [5]. The incidence of this tumor in immunocompetent individuals has risen three-fold during the last decades from 0.027 to 0.075; 100.000 person. Immunodeficient individuals, especially patients with AIDS, transplant recipients, and patients with congenital immunodeficiencies are at increased risk of developing PCNSLs. In patients with such severe immunodeficiencies, survival is heavily influenced by the underlying disease [6]. Autoimmune diseases that predispose to lymphoma include rheumatoid arthritis, systemic lupus erythematosus, Sjögren syndrome, myasthenia gravis, sarcoidosis, and vasculitis [6].

Presenting symptoms and signs vary, depending on the tumor location. Periventricular lesions and related symptoms are common in patients with primary cerebral lymphoma. The majority of the lesions are located in the periventricular area, whereas in a few, they are located in the supratentorial area. In about 60% of cases, PCNSLs originate from periventricular areas such as the thalamus, the basal ganglia, and the corpus callosum, which are followed by the frontal lobe, parietal lobe, temporal lobe, and occipital lobe (20, 18, 15, and 4%, respectively). Immunocompetent patients tend to present predominantly with solitary lesions in 70% of cases, compared with 50% in AIDS patients [1].

2. Pathogenesis

The central nervous system normally lacks lymphoid aggregates. The cellular and molecular events leading to neoplastic lymphocytic infiltration of the central nervous system are seen in PCNSLs [7].

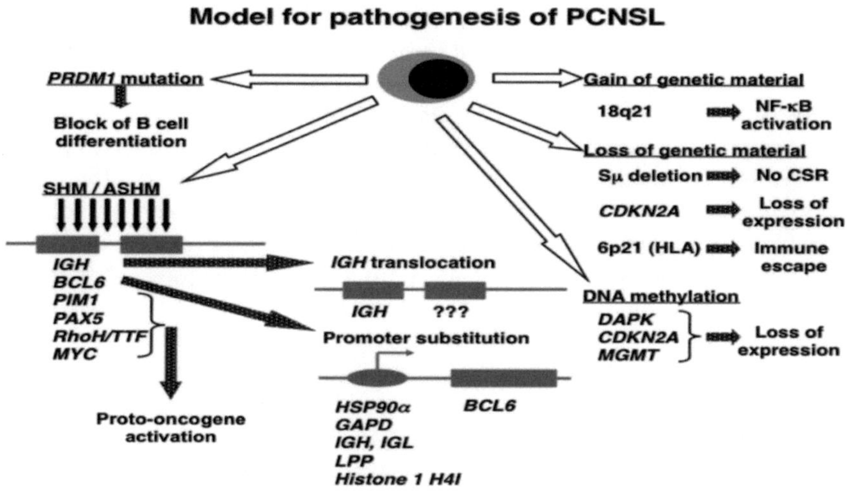

Figure 2.
Model of pathogenesis for PCNSLs. Schematic presentations of several pathways involved in the pathogenesis of PCNSLs, SHM, somatic hypermutation; ASHM, aberrant somatic hypermutation; and CSR, class switch recombination [7].

Primary lymphoma of the central nervous system (CNS) is defined as diffuse large B cell lymphoma confined to the central nervous system. Morphology does not distinguish between PCNSLs and extra-cerebral DLBCL [7]. While most cases of PCNSLs are composed of aggressive lymphoma subtypes, a small number of patients show indolent CNS lymphomas. The median growth fraction is 4% [8]. Three major issues need to be addressed to understand the nature of PCNSLs and develop specific therapeutic regimens (**Figure 2**):

1. The histogenetic origin of the tumor cells.

2. The transforming events.

3. The role of the microenvironment of the CNS.

The underlying molecular pathogenesis of PCNSL has yet to be elucidated.

Because of the fact that PCNSL is closely associated with EBV infection in immunocompromised individuals, involving mechanisms in PCNSL development are directed toward the immunologic reactions against EBV infection. On the other hand, the EBV infected B cells are controlled by T cells in nonimmunocompromised individuals. Therefore, a decline in T cells leads to the proliferation and dissemination of abnormal B cells in immunodeficiency states [6]. In addition, occasionally, patients with EBV DNA in spinal fluid have PCNSL. But EBV DNA is often found together with other microbial findings in CSF of immunocompromised patients [9]. PCNSL may be a consequence of EBV-mediated clonal expansion and malignant transformation of B-lymphocytes, a process that may be regulated by immune mechanisms [10].

3. Clinical presentation

The location of the lymphoma in the CNS determines the clinical presentation. Presenting symptoms and signs vary, depending on the site of involvement PCNSL can manifest in the brain, its coverings, spinal cord, and the eye. Distinct clinicopathologic entities have been described. In a large series with immunocompetent patients with PCNSL, focal neurologic deficits were found to be the most common sign that was seen in 70% of patients. Other important complaints include neuropsychiatric symptoms, the signs of raised intracranial pressure such as headache, nausea, and vomiting, followed by seizures and ocular symptoms [1]. Presenting symptoms may include headaches, blurred vision, motor difficulties, and personality changes. Personality changes are most often associated with lesions of the frontal lobes, periventricular white matter, or corpus callosum. Visual hallucinations may result from infiltration of visual pathways or the brainstem or may result from ocular or leptomeningeal involvement. This may result in delayed diagnosis that usually prompts neurologic evaluation. Cranial neuropathies can occur as a result of either meningeal involvement, infiltration of the brainstem, or invasion of isolated cranial nerves or their roots. Headache, especially late, in the course of the disease, involving the leptomeninges may be indicative of increased intracranial pressure.

In primary leptomeningeal lymphoma, up to 40% of patients with cerebral PCNSL may have evidence of meningeal involvement at the time of diagnosis based on analysis and imaging. The frequency of meningeal dissemination (MD) in primary CNS lymphoma, its prognostic impact, and optimal management have yet to be defined. But involvement of the leptomeninges by high risk systemic lymphoma is also a common relapse pattern. On the other hand, primary leptomeningeal lymphoma without synchronous cerebral/spine or systemic disease is very rare, making up less than 10% of all cases of PCNSLs. MD was concluded in the case of cytological detection of lymphoma cells, or light-chain restricted B cell population demonstrated by immunocytology or flow cytometry, or existence of a dominant amplicon in PCR analysis, or clear evidence of MD on MRI [11].

Major patient's characteristics and therapy did not significantly differ between patients with MD versus those without MD [12]. Progression-free survival (PFS) and overall survival (OS) were not significantly different in patients with MD versus without MD. Median OS, of MD+ and MD- patients, was 21.5 months versus 24.9 months ($p = 0.98$) [12]. Primary leptomeningeal lymphoma is a rare form of primary CNS lymphoma. Patients usually present with multifocal symptoms, with evidence of leptomeningeal enhancement and diagnostic CSF analysis. Presenting symptoms are multifocal in 68%. The most common presenting signs are cranial neuropathies 58%, especially of eye movements and with cranial nerve VI palsy 31%, presented with headache 44%. In another study, leptomeningeal enhancement was seen in 74% and the CSF profile was abnormal in all cases. CSF cytology detected malignant lymphocyte in 67% [13].

The third process neurolymphomatosis (NL) is a rare clinical entity characterized by infiltration of peripheral nerves, nerve roots, plexus, or cranial nerves by malignant lymphocytes. Symptoms include loss of sensation or motor function, for example, weakness of the extremities [14]. These patients showed lymphomatous cell invasion that was more prominent in the proximal portion of the nerve trunk and induced demyelination without macrophage invasion and subsequent axonal degeneration in the portion distal from the demyelination site [14]. NL is poorly localized severe pain in the absence of parenchymal lesions of the brain or spinal cord or obvious lymphoma in the CSF. The process frequently spares the meninges.

The International PCNSL Collaborative Group retrospectively analyzed 50 patients assembled from 12 centers in 5 countries over a 16-year period. NL was related to NHL in 90%. It occurred as the initial manifestation of malignancy in 26% cases. The affected neural structures included peripheral nerves 60%, spinal nerve roots 48%, cranial nerves 46%, and plexus 40% with multiple site involvement 58%. CSF cytology was positive in 40% and nerve biopsy confirmed the diagnosis in 88%. Thus, instead of insufficient CSF cytology studies, could be nerve biopsy [15].

4. Evaluation

The baseline evaluation of any newly diagnosed patient with PCNSL should include a comprehensive physical and neurologic examination. Age and performance status are the two most widely documented prognostic variables and must be recorded in every patient. Evaluation of cognitive function is important at baseline, and follow-up assessments are critical both to determine the benefit of therapy as well as monitor for treatment-related neurocognitive decline.

4.1 Examination of disease extension

Before the initiation of therapy, a careful examination for the disease extension has to be carried out, in order to perform optimal treatment modality. The evaluation processes of patients suspected of having PCNSL should include:

- Optimal imaging of the brain parenchyma requires a gadolinium enhanced MRI scan. Contrast enhanced CT scans may be substituted in patients in whom MRI is medically contraindicated (e.g., cardiac pacemaker) or unavailable. Involvement of the spinal cord parenchyma is sufficiently rare that gadolinium enhanced MRI of the total spine is warranted only in patients with spinal symptoms.

- All patients should have a lumbar puncture for CSF cytology unless medically contraindicated due to elevated intracranial pressure. CSF should be sampled before or 1 week after surgical biopsy to avoid false positive results. CSF protein levels should only be assessed on lumbar puncture samples because ventricular CSF has a lower normal value. Additional CSF studies that may be helpful include cell count, beta-2 microglobulin, immunoglobulin H gene rearrangement, and flow cytometry.

- A detailed ophthalmologic examination, including dilated fundus examination, should be done to exclude vitreous, retinal, or optic nerve involvement. Fluorescein angiography may be helpful to confirm lymphomatous involvement of the retina.

- Testicular ultrasound may be considered in older men to exclude an occult testicular lymphoma metastatic to brain.

Complete systemic staging is warranted in every patient. CT scan of the chest, abdomen, and pelvis and bone morrow biopsy with aspirate are the recommended staging procedures. Body positron emission tomography imaging may be incorporated into the evaluation of systemic disease.

The diagnostic procedure of choice for PCNSL is a stereotactic needle biopsy because patients derive no clinical benefit from surgical resection, and deep seated nature of most lesions increases the risk of surgical complications. Histopathological diagnosis is strongly needed, because of the fact that some intracranial processes, such as multiple sclerosis, sarcoidosis, and occasional gliomas may mimic similar appearance and treatment response to corticosteroids [16]. In general, the use of corticosteroids prior to biopsy should be avoided, as these agents are lymphocytotoxic; a single injection is known to alter proper histopathological evaluation, and a short course of treatment may cause the tumor to disappear temporarily [17].

Whenever possible, the tumor should be characterized by immunophenotyping. Characterizing the basic molecular and genetic abnormalities of PCNSL will foster the future development and application of target specific therapies in this disease [16].

5. Radiographic features

Contrast-enhanced MRI of the brain is the preferred imaging modality. The radiographic lesion tends to be solitary nonhemorrhagic mass, situated in the deep white matter adjacent to the ventricular surface. The borders are sharply circumscribed and supratentorial location in the majority of lesions 87%, but may be ill defined in 15% [1, 18]. Mass effect and tumor edema are seen in over half of the cases. Contrast enhancement is encountered in all lesions but ring enhancement is uncommon [18]. Lesions appear isodense to hyperdense on CT images and isointense to hypointense on T2-weighted MRI images and enhance homogeneously after contrast administration. Diffusion weighted MRI images, sensitive to the intracellular water of masses of lymphoma cells, are frequently abnormal. The role of positron emission tomography scans in diagnosis is unclear. In a study, baseline PET imaging demonstrated hypermetabolism consistent with aggressive lymphoma in 75% of patients [19]. PET scans can be used to distinguish glucose-absorbing neoplastic lesions from areas of radiation necrosis, infection, or inflammation, which may also enhance on conventional CT/MRI [20]. Prompt initiation of therapy is important in patients with PCNSL. Intensive chemotherapy and immunotherapy in patients with PCNSL in study, treatment delay was the most important clinical variable associated with decreased survival, and its independent from baseline performance status or risk score [21].

6. Treatment of PCNSL

PCNSL tends to be highly sensitive to both radiation and selected chemotherapeutic agents, which distinguishes it from most other malignant primary brain neoplasms. Surgery has a limited, mainly diagnostic role. Neurologic deficits and decreased functional status related to the tumor tend to improve rapidly with successful therapy, such as chemotherapy or radiation therapy. The disease can be exquisitely sensitive to glucocorticoids as well and patients will allow functional status particularly if they show an early response to steroids. Methotrexate (MTX), given at sufficiently high dose to penetrate the CNS, is the most active single agent against PCNSL identified. High dose intravenous MTX should therefore be the backbone of induction therapy in most patients. The goal of induction chemotherapy is a radiographic complete response, which can be achieved in over half of the patients with MTX-based therapy and is generally associated with superior outcomes. Most patients, even those in complete response do not achieve long-term disease control or survival with induction chemotherapy alone. The optimal consolidation therapy has not been established, however, and all strategies have the potential for increased toxicity. The three main consolidation approaches being explored include high dose chemotherapy with autologous hematopoietic cell transplant rescue, nonmyeloablative chemotherapy, and whole brain radiation therapy (WBRT).

High dose MTX-based chemotherapy is a standard component of initial therapy for PCNSL. The available data suggest that chemotherapy regimens that include high-dose systemic MTX are more effective against PCNSL than other regimens. WBRT may improve outcome, but is associated with increased risk for neurological side-effects in elderly patients [22]. The optimal high-dose MTX-based regimen for PCNSL is unknown, and there is variation in clinical practice. Most patients with a good performance status suggest using MTX-based combination regimen rather than MTX alone. Examples of reasonable regimens include MTX plus cytarabine, or temozolomide, or procarbazine, or vincristine. Rituximab is included in all regimens, except in rare cases of CD 20 negative or T cell PCNSL. The goal of induction therapy is to achieve a complete radiographic response before proceeding with consolidation therapy in eligible patients. Complete response is achieved in approximately 30 to 60% patients with high-dose MTX-based induction therapy. While high-dose MTX-based induction chemotherapy prolongs survival over WBRT alone, at least half of the patients with PCNSL who achieve a complete response will relapse within 5 years. This late relapse results from residual systemic malignant cell. WBRT remains an alternative consolidation approach in younger patients, particularly those with contraindications, which has been shown to improve PFS compared with induction chemotherapy alone. The consolidation approach in older adults, who are at increased risk for both relapse and toxicities of high dose chemotherapy and radiation, is unknown.

6.1 Radiation therapy

PCNSL is extremely sensitive to radiation therapy, but its use in the initial treatment of PCNSL has waned overtime as chemotherapy-based induction regimens have been optimized. Phase III trial patients with newly diagnosed PCNSL were randomly assigned therapy to six cycles of chemotherapy alone (intravenous MTX+ Ifosfamide) or the same chemotherapy with WBRT (45 Gy in 1.5 Gy fractions) [23–25] (**Figure 3**). A total of 13% patients died during initial chemotherapy; 551 patients were enrolled and randomized, of whom 318 were treated per protocol of these, and 90 patients had a major protocol violation. In the per protocol population, median overall survival was 32.4 months in patients receiving WBRT (n = 154) versus 37.1 months in those not receiving WBRT (n = 164) HR: 1.06. Thus primary hypothesis was not proven. Median progression-free survival was 18.3 months in patients receiving WBRT and 11.9 months in those not receiving WBRT. Treatment-related neurotoxicity in patients with sustained complete response was more common in patients receiving WBRT 49% by clinical assessment and 71% by neuroradiology than in those who did not 26% and 46% (**Figure 4**).

After a median follow up of 81.2 months, patients who received WBRT had a nonsignificant improvement in PFS (18.2 versus 11.9 month HR, 0.83) and significant PFS from last HDMTX (25.5 versus 12 month, HR, 0.65, p = 0.001) but without OS prolongation (**Figure 5**).

This trial prospectively monitored Quality of Life (QoL), to determine whether WBRT might lead to quality of life relevant late neurotoxicity. In year 2 after randomization, cognitive functioning and global health status were reduced in the early WBRT arm as compared to the no early WBRT arm. Also, fatigue, appetite loss, and

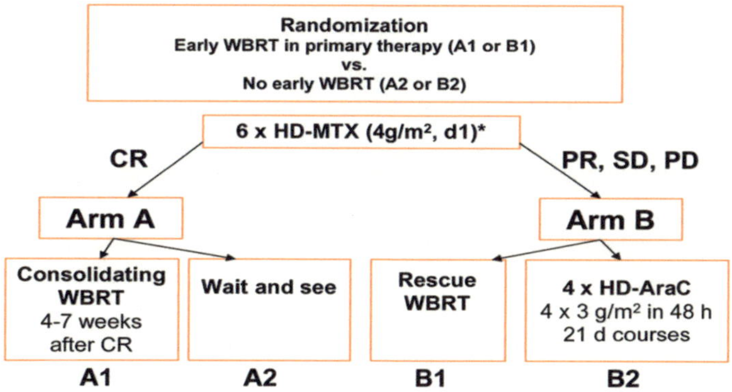

Figure 3.
*The G-PCNSL-SG-1 trial. Abbreviations: WBRT: whole brain radiotherapy; HD-MTX: high-dose methotrexate; CR: complete response; PR: partial response; SD: stable disease; PD: progressive disease; and HD-AraC: high-dose cytarabine. * Combined with ifosfamide 1.5 g/m² daily, d3–5, since 2006 [23].*

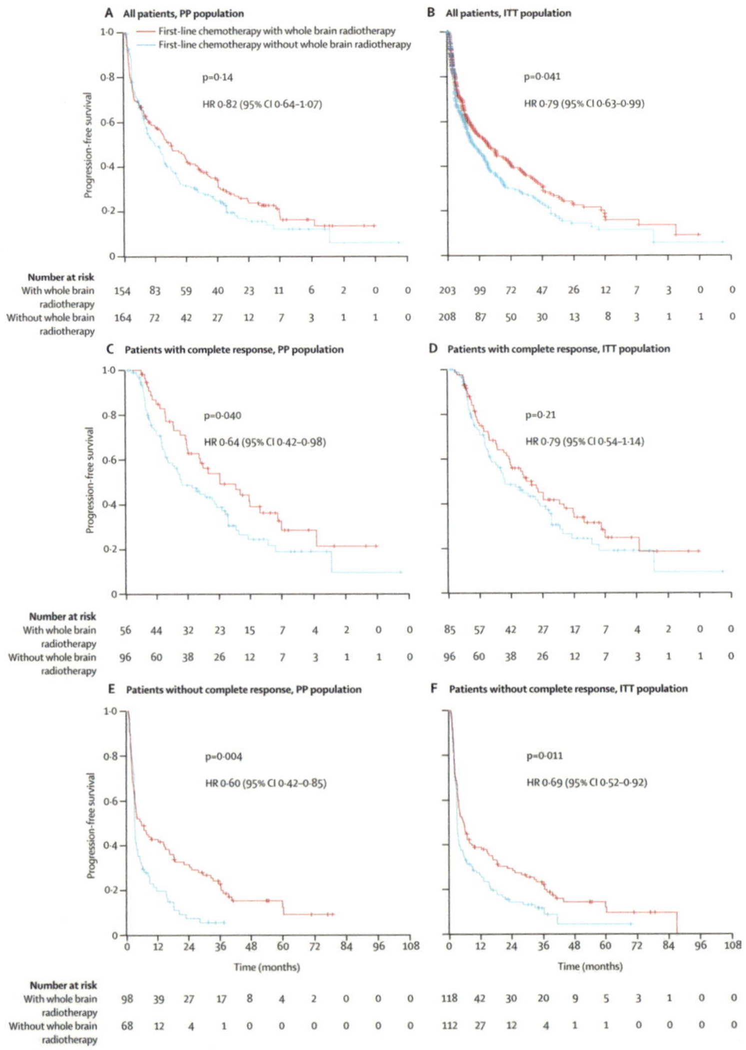

Figure 4.
Progression-free survival in the per-protocol and intention-to-treat populations by treatment group PP = per protocol. ITT = intention to treat. HR = hazard ratio [24].

hair loss were more intense in the early WBRT arm. Mini mental state examination testing revealed lower values (p = 0.002) in the early WBRT arm [25] (**Figure 6**).

As can be seen in **Figure 6**, G-PCNSL-SG-1 trial was the first PCNSL trial documenting a negative influence of early WBRT on QoL parameters. A phase II study combined modality therapy, based on high dose MTX, results in improved survival outcomes in PCNSL. The risk of neurotoxicity for patients aged >60 years is unacceptable with this regimen (1 g/m^2 MTX on days 1 and 8 followed by WBRT 45–50.4 Gy), although survival outcomes for patients aged >60 years were higher than in many other series [26]. At these studies and other demonstrations, the major drawback in the use of WBRT in conjunction with chemotherapy for patients with PCNSL is the high incidence of cognitive worsening and white matter damage [27–29]. Neurotoxicity may present as a rapidly progressive dementia that develops after a variable delay from the end of combined modality treatment. Also, the 5 year cumulative incidence of neurotoxicity was found to be increased over time [27]. Radiological examinations showed diffuse white matter disease as well as cortical-subcortical atrophy. Older age, mental status, changes at diagnosis, and radiotherapy predicted neurotoxicity [27].

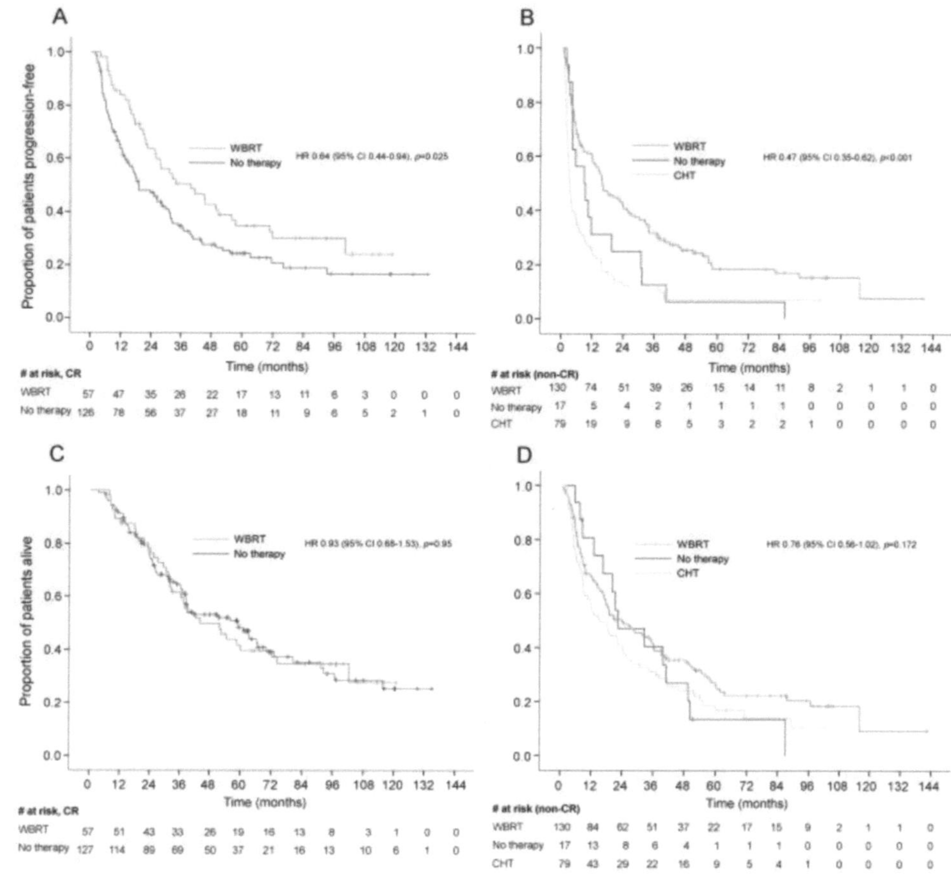

Figure 5.
PFS from last high-dose methotrexate-based chemotherapy and overall survival analyzed as-treated in the ITT population. (A) Progression-free survival (PFS) from last high-dose methotrexate (HDMTX)-based chemotherapy (CHT) in patients with complete response (CR). (B) PFS from last HDMTX-based CHT in patients without CR. (C) Overall survival (OS) in patients with CR. (D) OS in patients without CR. The good outcome of the non-CR patients without further treatment can be explained by the fact that 6 of them probably did in fact have CR after HDMTX-based CHT. They were documented as having CR upon follow-up without further therapy. Moreover, one additional patient received whole-brain radiotherapy (WBRT) without progression 6 months after HDMTX-based CHT. CI = confidence interval; HR = hazard ratio; and ITT = intent-to-treat [25].

Different radiation field and reduced dose WBRT consolidation in responding patients have been explored in studies and appear to be associated with higher response and decreased neurotoxicity rates compared with higher dose WBRT [30–33]. An example of the impact on the outcome and neurologic performance of different radiation fields and doses was assessed in a study in which 33 patients with PCNSL who achieved complete response after MTX-containing chemotherapy were referred to consolidation WBRT [30]. The study demonstrated that higher irradiation doses (≥40 Gy) were not associated with improved disease control compared to lower doses (30–36 Gy). Also, disease control does not significantly differ with regard to irradiation doses to the tumor bed, while functional impairment as assessed by mini mental status examination was significantly more common in patients treated with a WBRT dose ≥40 Gy. Thus, one can consider that consolidation with WBRT 36 Gy is advisable in patients with PCNSL in complete response after HD-MTX based chemotherapy. Higher doses do not change the outcome and could increase the risk of neurotoxicity. The findings of this important study are illustrated in **Figure 7** [30].

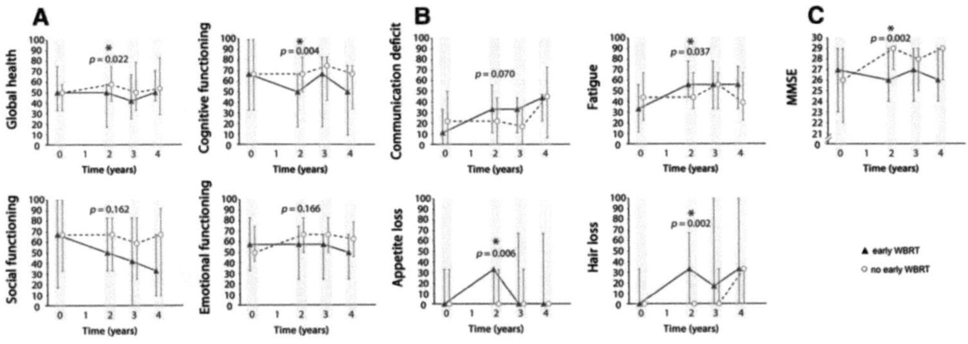

Figure 6.
*Comparison of early-whole brain radiotherapy (WBRT) with no early-WBRT with regard to global health, cognitive-emotional-social functioning using the time course of median scores, interquartile ranges (IQR) for EORTC-QLQ-C30, BN20 dimensions, and the mini mental state examination (MMSE) of the G-PCNSL-SG-1 trial *p < 0.05. (A) scores for emotional and social functioning, (B) symptom scores and (C) Mini Mental State Examination (MMSE) [23].*

As a different radiation fractionation, a phase I/II, NRG Oncology RTOG 0227 study of MTX, Rituximab and Temozolomide, plus hyperfractionated WBRT (36 Gy in twice daily 1.2 Gy fractions) in 66 patients with PCNSL was associated with an objective response rate of 85.7%. This study demonstrated that OS and PFS were improved compared with historical controls from RTOG-9310. Among patients, 66% had grade 3 and 4 toxicities before hWBRT, and 45% of patients experienced grade 3 and 4 toxicities attributable to post hWBRT chemotherapy. Cognitive function and QoL improved or stabilized after hWBRT [31].

Other consecutive prospective studies, the R-MPV (rituximab, MTX, procarbazine, and vincristine) induction chemotherapy followed by consolidation reduced dose WBRT (23.4 Gy/ 1.8 Gy fraction), and cytarabine were found to be feasible and effective. In these studies, patients with ocular involvement were irradiated without orbital shielding to the full dose 23.4 Gy (patients in complete response) or to a dose of 36 Gy (patients with less than a complete response). Response rates were high (79% complete response) allowing a large proportion of patients to receive rdWBRT. These patients achieved durable disease control (2 year PFS 77%) associated with favorable neurocognitive outcomes. Median overall survival could not be reached (median follow-up for survivors, 5.9 years); 3 year OS was 87%. Cognitive assessments showed improvements in terms of executive function and verbal memory after chemotherapy [32, 33].

The mechanisms resulting in radiation-induced neurotoxicity remain to be clarified. However, tissue oxidative stress, vasculopathy, demyelination, and depletion of progenitor oligodendroglial/neural stem cells have been postulated [34].

In addition to its ongoing role as an alternative to second line chemotherapy in younger patients who fail to achieve a complete response with first line systemic chemotherapy alone, WBRT is also a reasonable palliative option in patients who have contraindications to chemotherapy or relapsed, chemotherapy refractory disease.

Stereotactic radiotherapy may be an option for patients who have received WBRT. Prognosis is also influenced by therapy, which may include WBRT or stereotactic radio surgery (SRS). In a study [35], patients who had recurred after WBRT were treated with salvage SRS. The study demonstrated acceptable local control and survival after SRS.

On the other hand, WBRT remains a reasonable salvage therapy in patients who have not responded adequately to induction chemotherapy. In addition, WBRT plus corticosteroids may be used for the palliation of patients who are not candidates

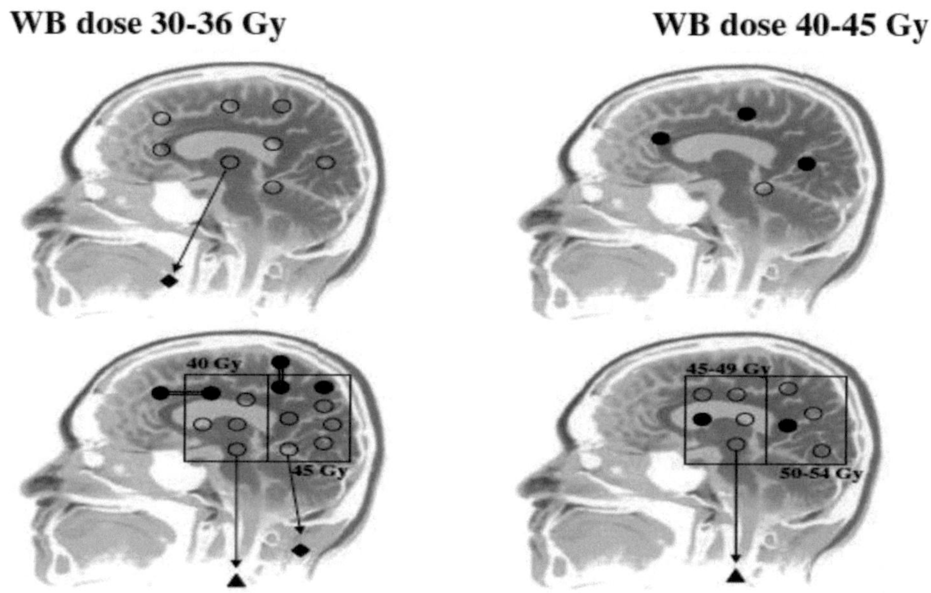

Figure 7.
Pattern of relapse according to radiation therapy fields and doses. Graphics at the left: patients treated with a WBRT dose of 30–36 Gy. Graphics at the right: patients treated with a WBRT dose 40 Gy. Upper graphics: patients treated without a tumor bed boost. Lower graphics: patients irradiated with a tumor bed boost. Symbols: o = irradiated lesion in continuous CR; ● = relapsed lesion; ●==● = relapse with lesions both within and outside the boosted volume; ▲: = relapse in nonirradiated central nervous system areas (i.e., meninges and spinal cord); ♦ = systemic extra-central nervous system relapse. (Adopted from ref. [30]).

for chemotherapy. Complete responses can be obtained in most patients treated with standard fractionation to 20–40 Gy (for a 74% overall response rate). The median survival from initiation of WBRT was 16 months. The median time to PCNSL progression was 10 months. Treatment associated neurotoxicity is more common among those exposed to a total radiation dose >36 Gy, patients treated within 6 months of receiving MTX, and those older than 60 years of age [36, 37]. Treatment-related neurotoxicity was observed in 22% of patients. Salvage WBRT is effective for recurrent and refractory PCNSL.

7. Follow-up and monitoring

After completion of the initially planned treatment of PCNSL, patients should be evaluated to determine the disease response to treatment and should be followed longitudinally for relapse and long-term treatment toxicities.

Patients should be evaluated no more than 2 months after the completion of planned therapy to determine their response to treatment. Gadolinium-enhanced MRI scans are the standard for the evaluation of bulky parenchymal brain disease. Detailed ophthalmologic examination and lumbar puncture for cytology are required only if these studies were initially positive or if clinically indicated by new symptoms or sign. An interdisciplinary, international consensus group has devised the fallowing response criteria [16].

7.1 Response criteria

The following criteria were developed on the basis of anatomic and radiographic definitions.

Complete response requires the following:

1. Complete disappearance of all enhancing abnormalities on gadolinium-enhanced MRI.

2. No evidence of active ocular lymphoma as defined by the absence of cells in the vitreous and resolution of any previously documented retinal or optic nerve infiltrate.

3. Negative CSF cytology. If the CSF is examined, patients with an Ommaya reservoir should have samples taken for the reservoir and lumbar puncture.

4. At the time a complete response is determined, the patient should have discontinued use of all corticosteroids for at least 2 weeks. Patients who met the criteria for CR may have the following features/limitations:

   A. Any patient who otherwise meet all criteria for CR but needs steroid therapy should be regarded as unconfirmed CR.

   B. Some patients will have a small but persistent enhancing abnormality on MRI related to biopsy or focal hemorrhage.

   C. Patients with a persistent minor abnormality on fallow-up ophthalmologic examination.

Partial response (PR) was concluded for patients who met all of the following criteria: equal or more than 50% decrease in the contrast enhancing lesion that was seen on MRI compared to baseline imaging and a decrease in the vitreous cell count or retinal cellular infiltrate. PR was thought to be irrelevant to corticosteroid dose. CSF cytological examination may be negative or continue to show persistent malignant or suspicious cell providing no new sites of disease.

Progressive disease was defined as the following; more than 25% increase in the contrast enhancing lesion that was seen on MRI as compared to the best response, the progression of ocular disease, and the appearance of any new lesion.

Relapsed disease was considered as the appearance of any new lesion. Stable disease is that which does not meet the criteria for CR, CRu, PR, or progressive disease.

8. Prognosis

Untreated PCNSL has a rapidly fatal course, with survival of approximately 1.5 month from the time of diagnosis. Survival increases with combined therapy. In population-based studies, among HIV uninfected cases, a 5-year survival increased from 19.1 (1992–1994) to 30.1% (2004–2006) [38]. Long-term survival is achieved in approximately 15–20% of patients treated with MTX-based therapy and radiation in contemporary clinical trial [39]. In a study on 41 patients treated with MATILDE chemotherapy regimen followed by WBRT, overall response rate was 76% after chemotherapy and 83% after chemotherapy plus radiotherapy. At a median follow-up of 12 years, approximately 75% patients experienced an event, with a 5-year PFS of 24%. At 10 years from diagnosis, no patient showed chronic toxicities, with a mini-mental state examination score of ≥29 in all cases but one.

The most consistent prognostic factors are age and performance status. In order to adequately assess patients with disorder, standardized systems for prognosis have been proposed [40]. Age, PS, LDH serum level, CSF protein concentration, and involvement of deep structures of brain were independent predictors of survival. A prognostic score including these 5 parameters seems advisable in distinguishing different risk groups in PCNSL. The 2 year OS is seen in 80% for patients with zero to one, 48% for patients with two to three, and 15% for patients with four to five unfavorable features.

9. Conclusion

Primary brain lymphoma is an uncommon variant of extranodal NHL. Therapeutic options include treatment with high dose MTX plus combined chemotherapy regimens and WBRT. Patients over age 60 generally succumb to a higher risk of treatment-related neurotoxicity. The optimal consolidation strategy in these patients has yet to be determined, and the best treatment modality should be individualized. By increasing the understanding of the molecular knowledge, and the clinical data originating from new researches, more effective treatment approaches and the best way to the integration of them into the treatment field of PCNSL would be determined.

Thanks

For the endless support, we are thankful to Medical Oncologist Ender KURT.

Author details

Meral Kurt*, Candan Demiröz Abakay and Ali Altay
Faculty of Medicine Radiotherapy Center, Uludağ University, Bursa, Turkey

*Address all correspondence to: mkurt@uludag.edu.tr

References

[1] Bataille B, Delwail V, Menet E, et al. Primary intracerebral malignant lymphoma: Report of 248 cases. Journal of Neurosurgery. 2000;**92**:261. DOI: 10.3171/jns.2000.92.2.0261

[2] Hoffman S, Propp JM, McCarthy BJ. Temporal trends in incidence of primary brain tumors in the United States, 1985-1999. Neuro-Oncology. 2006;**8**:27. DOI: 10.1215/S1522851705000323

[3] Villano JL, Koshy M, Shaikh H, et al. Age, gender, and racial differences in incidence and survival in primary CNS lymphoma. British Journal of Cancer. 2011;**105**:1414. DOI: 10.1038/bjc.2011.357

[4] O'Neill BP, Decker PA, Tieu C, Cerhan JR. The changing incidence of primary central nervous system lymphoma is driven primarily by the changing incidence in young and middle-aged men and differs from time trends in systemic diffuse large B-cell non-Hodgkin's lymphoma. American Journal of Hematology. 2013;**88**:997. DOI: 10.1002/ajh.23551

[5] Herrlinger U, Schabet M, Clemens M, et al. Clinical presentation and therapeutic outcome in 26 patients with primary CNS lymphoma. Acta Neurologica Scandinavica. 1998;**97**:257. DOI: 10.1111/j.1600-0404.1998.tb00647.x

[6] Bhagavathi S, Wilson JD. Primary central nervous system lymphoma. Archives of Pathology & Laboratory Medicine. 2008;**132**:1830. DOI: 10.1043/1543-2165-132.11.1830

[7] Montesinos-Rongen M, Siebert R, Deckert M. Primary lymphoma of the central nervous system: Just DLBCL or not? Blood. 2009;**113**:7. DOI: 10.1182/blood-2008-04-149005

[8] Jahnke K, Thiel E, Schilling A, et al. Low-grade primary central nervous system lymphoma in immunocompetent patients. British Journal of Haematology. 2005;**128**:616. DOI: 10.1111/j.1365-2141.2004.05361.x

[9] Martelius T, Lappalainen M, Palomäki M, Anttila VJ. Clinical characteristics of patients with Epstein Barr virus in cerebrospinal fluid. BMC Infectious Diseases. 2011;**11**:281. DOI: 10.1186/1471-2334-11-281

[10] Rock JP, Cher L, Hochberg FH, et al. Primary CNS lymphoma. In: Yomans JR, editor. Neurological Surgery. 4th ed. Philadelphia: WB Saunders; 1996. p. 2688

[11] Kiewe P, Fischer L, Martus P, et al. Meningeal dissemination in primary CNS lymphoma: Diagnosis, treatment, and survival in a large monocenter cohort. Neuro-Oncology. 2010;**12**:409. DOI: 10.1093/neuonc/nop053

[12] Korfel A, Weller M, Martus P, et al. Prognostic impact of meningeal dissemination in primary CNS lymphoma (PCNSL): Experience from the G-PCNSL-SG1 trial. Annals of Oncology. 2012;**23**:2374. DOI: 10.1093/annonc/mdr627

[13] Taylor JW, Flanagan EP, O'Neill BP, et al. Primary leptomeningeal lymphoma: International primary CNS lymphoma collaborative group report. Neurology. 2013;**81**:1690. DOI: 10.1212/01.wnl.0000435302.02895.f3

[14] Tomita M, Koike H, Kawagashira Y, et al. Clinicopathological features of neuropathy associated with lymphoma. Brain. 2013;**136**:2563. DOI: 10.1093/brain/awt193

[15] Grisariu S, Avni B, Batchelor TT, et al. Neurolymphomatosis: An international primary CNS

lymphoma collaborative group report. Blood. 2010;**115**:5005. DOI: 10.1182/blood-2009-12-258210

[16] Abrey LE, Batchelor TT, Ferreri AJ, et al. Report of an international workshop to standardize baseline evaluation and response criteria for primary CNS lymphoma. Journal of Clinical Oncology. 2005;**23**:5034. DOI: 10.1200/JCO.2005.13.524

[17] Porter AB, Giannini C, Kaufmann T, et al. Primary central nervous system lymphoma can be histologically diagnosed after previous corticosteroid use: A pilot study to determine whether corticosteroids prevent the diagnosis of primary central nervous system lymphoma. Annals of Neurology. 2008;**63**:662. DOI: 10.1002/ana.21366

[18] Bühring U, Herrlinger U, Krings T, et al. MRI features of primary central nervous system lymphomas at presentation. Neurology. 2001;**57**:393. DOI: https://doi.org/10.1212/WNL.57.3.393

[19] Mohile NA, Deangelis LM, Abrey LE. Utility of brain FDG-PET in primary CNS lymphoma. Clinical Advances in Hematology & Oncology. 2008;**6**:818

[20] Karantanis D, O'Neill BP, Subramaniam RM, et al. Contribution of F-18 FDG PET-CT in the detection of systemic spread of primary central nervous system lymphoma. Clinical Nuclear Medicine. 2007;**32**:271. DOI: 10.1097/01.rlu.0000257269.99345.1b

[21] Rubenstein JL, Hsi ED, Johnson JL, et al. Intensive chemotherapy and immunotherapy in patients with newly diagnosed primary CNS lymphoma: CALGB 50202 (Alliance 50202). Journal of Clinical Oncology. 2013;**31**:3061. DOI: 10.1200/JCO.2012.46.9957

[22] Kasenda B, Ferreri AJ, Marturano E, et al. First-line treatment and outcome of elderly patients with primary central nervous system lymphoma (PCNSL)—A systematic review and individual patient data meta-analysis. Annals of Oncology. 2015;**26**:1305. DOI: 10.1093/annonc/mdv076

[23] Herrlinger U, Schäfer N, Fimmers R, et al. Early whole brain radiotherapy in primary CNS lymphoma: Negative impact on quality of life in the randomized G-PCNSL-SG1 trial. Journal of Cancer Research and Clinical Oncology. 2017;**143**:1815. DOI: 10.1007/s00432-017-2423-5

[24] Thiel E, Korfel A, Martus P, et al. High-dose methotrexate with or without whole brain radiotherapy for primary CNS lymphoma (G-PCNSL-SG-1): A phase 3, randomised, non-inferiority trial. The Lancet Oncology. 2010;**11**:1036. DOI: 10.1016/S1470-2045(10)70229-1

[25] Korfel A, Thiel E, Martus P, et al. Randomized phase III study of whole-brain radiotherapy for primary CNS lymphoma. Neurology. 2015;**84**:1242. DOI: 10.1212/WNL.0000000000001395

[26] O'Brien PC, Roos DE, Pratt G, et al. Combined-modality therapy for primary central nervous system lymphoma: Long-term data from a phase II multicenter study (trans-Tasman radiation oncology group). International Journal of Radiation Oncology, Biology, Physics. 2006;**64**:408. DOI: 10.1016/j.ijrobp.2005.07.958

[27] Omuro AM, Ben-Porat LS, Panageas KS, et al. Delayed neurotoxicity in primary central nervous system lymphoma. Archives of Neurology. 2005;**62**:1595. DOI: 10.1001/archneur.62.10.1595

[28] Schuurmans M, Bromberg JE, Doorduijn J, et al. Primary central nervous system lymphoma in the elderly: A multicentre retrospective

analysis. British Journal of Haematology. 2010;**151**:179. DOI: 10.1111/j.1365-2141.2010.08328.x

[29] Doolittle ND, Korfel A, Lubow MA, et al. Long-term cognitive function, neuroimaging, and quality of life in primary CNS lymphoma. Neurology. 2013;**81**:84. DOI: 10.1212/WNL.0b013e318297eeba

[30] Ferreri AJ, Verona C, Politi LS, et al. Consolidation radiotherapy in primary central nervous system lymphomas: Impact on outcome of different fields and doses in patients in complete remission after upfront chemotherapy. International Journal of Radiation Oncology, Biology, Physics. 2011;**80**:169. DOI: 10.1016/j.ijrobp.2010.01.066

[31] Glass J, Won M, Schultz CJ, et al. Phase I and II study of induction chemotherapy with methotrexate, rituximab, and Temozolomide, followed by whole-brain radiotherapy and postirradiation temozolomide for primary CNS lymphoma: NRG oncology RTOG 0227. Journal of Clinical Oncology. 2016;**34**:1620. DOI: 10.1200/JCO.2015.64.8634

[32] Morris PG, Correa DD, Yahalom J, et al. Rituximab, methotrexate, procarbazine, and vincristine followed by consolidation reduced-dose whole-brain radiotherapy and cytarabine in newly diagnosed primary CNS lymphoma: Final results and long-term outcome. Journal of Clinical Oncology. 2013;**31**:3971. DOI: 10.1200/JCO.2013.50.4910

[33] Shah GD, Yahalom J, Correa DD, et al. Combined immunochemotherapy with reduced whole-brain radiotherapy for newly diagnosed primary CNS lymphoma. Journal of Clinical Oncology. 2007;**25**:4730. DOI: 10.1200/JCO.2007.12.5062

[34] Omuro AM, Martin-Duverneuil N, Delattre JY. Complications of radiotherapy to the central nervous system. Handbook of Clinical Neurology. 2012;**105**:887-901. DOI: 10.1016/B978-0-444-53502-3.00030-6

[35] Chao ST, Barnett GH, Vogelbaum MA, et al. Salvage stereotactic radiosurgery effectively treats recurrences from whole-brain radiation therapy. Cancer. 2008;**113**:2198. DOI: 10.1002/cncr.23821

[36] Nguyen PL, Chakravarti A, Finkelstein DM, et al. Results of whole-brain radiation as salvage of methotrexate failure for immunocompetent patients with primary CNS lymphoma. Journal of Clinical Oncology. 2005;**23**:1507. DOI: 10.1200/JCO.2005.01.161

[37] Hottinger AF, DeAngelis LM, Yahalom J, Abrey LE. Salvage whole brain radiotherapy for recurrent or refractory primary CNS lymphoma. Neurology. 2007;**69**:1178. DOI: 10.1212/01.wnl.0000276986.19602.c1

[38] Shiels MS, Pfeiffer RM, Besson C, et al. Trends in primary central nervous system lymphoma incidence and survival in the U.S. British Journal of Haematology. 2016;**174**:417. DOI: 10.1111/bjh.14073

[39] Ferreri AJ, Ciceri F, Brandes AA, et al. MATILDE chemotherapy regimen for primary CNS lymphoma: Results at a median follow-up of 12 years. Neurology. 2014;**82**:1370. DOI: 10.1212/WNL.0000000000000314

[40] Ferreri AJ, Blay JY, Reni M, et al. Prognostic scoring system for primary CNS lymphomas: The international Extranodal lymphoma study group experience. Journal of Clinical Oncology. 2003;**21**:266. DOI: 10.1200/JCO.2003.09.139

Chapter 8

Toxicity of Cranial and Spinal Cord Irradiation

Jason Naziri and Steven J. DiBiase

Abstract

Along with surgery and chemotherapy, radiation therapy is an essential treatment option for metastatic and primary tumors of the central nervous system. Radiation toxicity may be compartmentalized into three subcategories including acute toxicities, early-delayed and late delayed effects. Radiation induced toxicity spans from self-limiting fatigue to more serious delayed side effects of radionecrosis. Stereotactic radiosurgery has recently emerged as a highly focused delivery method of tumoricidal irradiation with promising results compared to whole brain irradiation in many cases. Recognizing and understanding toxicity from cranial irradiation can help guide therapy as ever evolving new technologies develop within this integral component of cancer treatment.

Keywords: cranial irradiation, CNS toxicity, stereotactic radiosurgery, radionecrosis, radiation induced brain toxicity

1. Introduction

Treatment of central nervous system (CNS) tumors involves surgery, chemotherapy, radiation therapy, immunotherapy, or a combination of these modalities. Radiation therapy is a highly effect treatment that plays a role in the management of brain metastases, gliomas, primary central nervous system lymphomas, and meningiomas among other brain tumors.

Radiation toxicity can be divided into three subcategories including acute toxicities, usually arising within 6 weeks of treatment, early-delayed effects (up to 4 months post-irradiation) and late delayed starting 4 months after completion of radiation therapy to several years later.

Central nervous system toxicity can be better understood by compartmentalizing toxicities based on cell biology. Injury to brain parenchyma effected by radiation includes neuronal cells, glial cells, and vasculature. Surprisingly, side effects of radiation are likely not due to damage directly to neuronal cells [1]. This is in part due to the paucity of cell replication of most neurons. As such, radiation toxicity primarily effects glial oligodendrocytes which are the insulating myelin producing cells and glial astrocytes responsible for the essential blood brain barrier. Endothelial vasculature of post-capillary venules within brain parenchyma are also highly susceptible to damaging effects of ionizing radiation. Increased cranial pressure and edema caused by radiation is deemed to be related to damage to endothelial cells [2]. In addition to direct damage to the endothelia, the tight junctions of endothelial cells are another component of the blood-brain barrier. The saliency of

IntechOpen

the blood brain barrier and the susceptibility to damage by irradiation, makes it a point of focus when discussing CNS toxicity.

Not all neuronal cells are uniformly resilient to ionizing radiation. Recent studies have shown extreme sensitivity to even low-dose irradiation to the hippocampus. This is due to damage to highly proliferative neuronal progenitor cells. Specifically, the subgranular zone (SGZ) of the dentate gyrus has been shown to be extremely susceptible to damage to progenitor cells. Research for why these phenomena exists is ongoing. In addition to direct damage to neural progenitor cells, recent studies have linked neuronal damage to endothelial vasculature within the SGZ. Loss of integrity of inter-endothelial tight junctions (and eventually the blood brain barrier) causes edema and an inflammatory response that prevents the proliferation of neuronal progenitor cells. Clinical manifestations of impairment within this very crucial part of the CNS (the dentate gyrus of the hippocampus which is responsible for transitioning short term memories into long term memories) is linked to the irreversible late delayed side effect of cognitive dysfunction [3–5]. It is worth mentioning that these sequelae of radiation to the hippocampus can manifest even with doses as low as 2 Gy or less [6, 7]. Strategies to preserve neurocognitive function in patients receiving whole brain radiation therapy now include hippocampal sparing techniques [8, 9]. Hippocampal avoidance is one of many creative strategies postulated by radiation oncologists to aid in minimizing toxicity. Modern radiation delivery techniques are beyond the scope of this chapter. Some of these modalities used to avoid sensitive anatomic regions and decrease healthy tissue exposure include IMRT, stereotactic radiosurgery, and proton therapy. These novel modalities of radiation therapy continue to be refined in hopes of decreasing brain injury and increasing local control.

Astrocytes also play an important role in support and function of neurons. The cell line responsible for proliferation and differentiation of astrocytes and oligodendrocytes is the oligodendrocyte type-2 astrocyte progenitor cell (O-2A) [2]. In addition to being a crucial component of the BBB, astrocytes have been shown to be homeostatic regulators providing multiple heterogeneous functions including protecting brain parenchyma from reactive oxygen species [10]. Neuroinflammation and reactive astrogliosis caused by irradiation to astrocytes and O-2A, disrupt the BBB and likely play a role in edema.

Therapeutic techniques investigating the loss of neurogenesis are also underway. Inflammation is primarily instigated by microglial cells. Decreasing the inflammatory load within the SGZ by using a nonsteroidal anti-inflammatory, namely indomethacin in this case, helped preserve neuronal progenitor cells [6]. Reducing the inflammatory load caused by radiation may decrease CNS toxicity which in this study was cognitive decline. Prophylactic nonsteroidal anti-inflammatory drugs are not currently standard of care in preventing radiation side effects.

As mentioned earlier, glial cells are by far the most abundant types of cells within the CNS and responsible for neuronal support and protection. Glial progenitor cells which gives rise to oligodendrocytes and astrocytes are vulnerable targets of damage induced by radiation. In addition to glial progenitors, fully differentiated oligodendrocytes are also known to be sensitive to radiation. Enough damage to the DNA of oligodendrocytes can induce a P53 dependent apoptosis [2, 11]. Taking these two cell lines into consideration, damage to myelin producing oligodendrocytes in addition to glial progenitor cells responsible for generating new oligodendrocytes and astrocytes leads to CNS toxicity [2]. Treatment strategies to ameliorate CNS toxicity focused on re-establishing the efficacy of glial progenitor cells are ongoing. To date, optimal treatment for CNS toxicity is still unknown and strategies for managing side effects have yet to be delineated.

When considering the source of CNS toxicities, it is important to take into consideration the timeframe of manifestations, the specific presentation of symptoms, as well as whether the volume treated and dose deliver are compatible with side effects to the CNS. Other modalities of treatment including chemotherapy and immunotherapy as well as tumor progression can also have adverse effects on brain parenchyma on a cell biologic level. Deciphering the cause of CNS injury is not completely understood but should be taken into consideration in guiding treatment options.

2. Acute and early-delayed toxicities of cranial irradiation

Early side effects of radiation treatment are considered to manifest during or within 6 weeks of completion of radiation therapy. Acute side effects are usually transient and self-limiting, due to transient demyelination [3]. Symptoms are rare but may include fatigue, nausea, vomiting, headache, and focal neurologic deficits. These reported side effects were historically common with patients receiving doses >2 Gy per fraction. Reflected in current NCCN guidelines, most clinicians do not deliver conventional doses that exceed 2 Gy in one fraction as to avoid side effects. Acute radiation toxicities are rare with modern techniques with reports of grade 3 and 4 acute toxicities occurring in <5% of patients and are usually self-limiting [12].

Side effects occurring within 4 months of radiation treatment are considered early delayed effects and most commonly involve transient demyelination and somnolence. Similar to acute toxicities, early to late side effects are usually reversible and resolve spontaneously.

2.1 Fatigue

One of the most common side effect of radiation therapy to the central nervous system is fatigue and lethargy. Similar to patterns of irradiation outside of the CNS, side effects are cumulative and initially start to present 2 weeks into therapy [13, 14]. Fatigue usually starts around 2 weeks of therapy, peaks at or around completion of therapy, and resolves within several months. A severe form of fatigue, lethargy, and lack of concentration is known as somnolence syndrome (SS). SS typical occurs as an early delayed toxicity approximately 5–6 weeks after completion of radiation therapy. In one study, patients receiving a hypofractionated treatment plan compared to conventional fractionation experienced more severe fatigue [15].

2.2 Alopecia and radiation dermatitis

Another common side effect of acute radiation toxicity is hair loss. Alopecia from radiation only occurs in areas where hair follicles are exposed to radiation and therefore can be sparse depending on scalp exposure. Alopecia can be permanent or temporary with higher doses to the scalp signifying permanent hair loss [16]. Radiation dermatitis is a desquamating rash that can occur to areas of the scalp exposed to radiation. Most cases are mild and are treated with moisturizing ointments. In severe rare cases of moist desquamation, topical antibiotic ointment may be used.

3. Late-delayed toxicities of cranial irradiation

Late-delayed side effects are of the most concern when discussing radiation toxicity. These effects occur starting after 4 months of treatment up to decades later. Unlike acute and early-delayed side effects, late-delayed side effects are largely irreversible and progressive.

3.1 Cumulative effects

Decline in neurocognitive function in patients with brain tumors is a multifactorial phenomenon. The connection between radiation toxicity and cognitive decline has been well documented. Nevertheless, it is important, however, to consider other factors as well as cumulative effects contributing to cognitive decline. Many patients treated with radiation are also treated in combination with chemotherapy. Multiple new targeted therapies have also been approved for use. Given that each of these individually may cause CNS side effects, it is of utmost importance for healthcare providers to be able to recognize toxicity and delineate whether symptoms are indeed being caused by treatments (either in combination or individually). Furthermore, there are multiple other reasons for why patients may have CNS complications, including tumor progression and advancement of pathologies unrelated to malignancy (dementia, depression, polypharmacy, anxiety, etc.).

3.2 Long term delayed effects

There exist patients who have undergone radiation treatment with an overall survival of multiple years and even decades. For many, cognitive deficits have not arisen even after 6 years of follow-up [6, 13]. Most patients even after 6 years have maintained a stable neurocognitive status. Differences in cognitive deficits were seen, however, in patients with low-grade gliomas who received radiation compared to patients who were radiation naïve after a 12 year follow up [6]. It is worth mentioning however that patients who do receive adjuvant radiation in low grade gliomas are more likely to have local control, better progression free survival and overall survival [14]. Multiple considerations should be taken into account when deciding the correct treatment plan for each individual patient. In the case of low grade gliomas, radiation and chemotherapy with procarbazine, CCNU, and vincristine is recommended by current NCCN guidelines. Given that neurocognitive effects are being reported over a decade after radiation treatment and less so at 6 years, additional long term delayed effects are of more trepidation now compared to years prior.

4. Stereotactic radiosurgery

Advances in the technique and technology of radiation treatment to the brain has given rise to stereotactic radiosurgery. The use of localized radiosurgery in the setting of metastatic disease compared to whole-brain radiotherapy is an ongoing and complex discussion. In general, brain metastases arise from hematologic dissemination and have a poor overall prognosis [17]. Whole brain radiation has been utilized given the assumed likelihood of "seeding" or micrometasis to areas of the brain outside of visible metastasis seen on imaging. As mentioned earlier however, whole brain radiation therapy has high rates of toxicity, the most serious being cognitive impairment without the added benefit of overall survival [18–20]. It is worth mentioning that the concept of oligometastases has arisen among oncologists whereby disease may in fact be truly limited and treated as such. SRS alone, or in combination with whole brain radiation therapy, has thus become a viable option in single lesions or oligometastases. Being a localized modality of treatment, SRS alone has a higher likelihood of intracranial progression when compared with SRS in combination with WBRT. There has not been shown an increase in overall survival nor a better side effect profile with the addition WBRT to SRS vs. SRS alone [19, 20]. Researchers have also concluded that the addition of WBRT results in excess morbidity and a decreased quality-of-life resulting in a 35% increase in neurocognitive deficit compared to SRS alone at 12 months. In one study, there was also a non-statistically significant survival benefit with SRS alone compared to SRS with WBRT [20]. Even with the better distant control of the addition of WBRT to SRS, the increase in morbidity does not outweigh the benefits and thus SRS alone is preferred.

Another viable option for limited brain metastases is surgical resection. Given similar outcomes in overall survival with surgical resection, decreased cost and, most importantly, less invasive nature of treatment compared to neurosurgery, SRS treatment of metastasis is being widely used [19, 21, 22].

The most common long term side effect of SRS is radionecrosis. While in certain cases radionecrosis can cause serious neurocognitive deficits requiring steroids or even surgical resection, certain patients remain asymptomatic and are diagnosed on imaging studies. Only about one third of patients with radionecrosis present with symptomatic neurologic deficits [23, 24]. Image based diagnoses can be difficult to distinguish from other phenomena including self-limiting inflammation [25]. There is a wide range of reported data on the rate of actuarial radionecrosis. In recent studies with adequate follow-up, rates vary from as low as 1.5% [26] to as high 34% [19, 25, 27] The main risk factor of radionecrosis are total dose, maximum tumor diameter and treated volume [25, 27, 28].

Given the variability in data and to help gain a better understanding of risk factors for radionecrosis, it may be salient to delineate the setting in which SRS is being administered. Prevalence of radionecrosis can be divided based on single fraction treatments, hypo fractionated treatments (usually three fractions), and adjuvant SRS after resection.

In patients receiving single fractionation SRS, the risk of radionecrosis are reported to be higher compared to hypofractionated [24]. Additionally, local control in hypofractionated regimens have had similar outcomes. Current NCCN guidelines recommend either single fraction or multi-fractionated SRS for the treatment of brain metastases, with multiple fractions utilized more commonly in patients with larger lesions [25, 29].

Not all patients radiologically diagnosed with radionecrosis are symptomatic. For patients that are symptomatic common manifestations include headache, seizures, motor deficits, sensory deficits, ataxia, and speech deficits [25].

In the past decade, SRS has more frequently been utilized in the post-resection adjuvant setting of brain metastases rather than WBRT. In hopes of optimizing local control and overall survival, SRS is administered to the tumor bed with the goal of covering subtotal resections and unrevealed disease that may have been left behind. In this setting, the prevalence of radionecrosis is varied with trends towards decreased toxicity with hypofractionated schedules compared to single fraction SRS [23, 26, 30]. The region of the brain being irradiated may have implications of morbidity as well. Infratentorial metastases are particularly problematic in that they portend worse outcomes and have a higher rate of radionecrosis [30]. Patients with higher risk of radionecrosis, including large tumors >3 cm, should be considered for hypofractionated treatment.

Another method of predicting radionecrosis in patients being treated with SRS is looking at volumes of brain parenchyma receiving a specific dose. Specifically, volumes receiving 10 Gy (V10) and 12 Gy (V12) have demonstrated strong predictive value in single fraction SRS [24, 25, 31]. The risk of radionecrosis can be predicted using specific volumes that receive certain doses. For example, risk of radionecrosis for V12 of less than 10 cm^3 is 22% compared to more than 10 cm^3

which more than doubles the risk to 55% [32]. Novel studies have proposed using V12 as the standard method of reporting dose to assess toxicity [25]. For patients receiving V12 of <8.5 cm^3, the risk of radionecrosis increase to >10% and patients should be considered for hypofractionated rather than single fraction SRS [25].

Options in the treatment of radionecrosis includes steroids, hyperbaric oxygen, and surgery. There exist novel therapies such as bevacizumab and focused interstitial laser thermal therapy with variable efficacy in treatment [33].

Stereotactic radiosurgery (SRS) is usually well-tolerated and risks of high grade toxicity are low. The most important sequelae of SRS is radiation necrosis. Risks and benefits must be weighed out on an individualized basis using an evidence based and patient centered approach.

5. Hypopituitarism induced by radiation

Endocrine deficiencies have also been reported in lesions irradiated near the hypothalamic-pituitary axis or pituitary gland. The prevalence of endocrinopathies are higher with nasopharyngeal cancers compared to intracerebral tumors, yet there were no differences in the rate of endocrine dysfunction based on underlying tumor type [34]. Endocrinopathies may include panhypopituitarism, hypothalamic hypothyroidism, and hypothalamic hypogonadism among others. A significant portion of the pediatric population treated with radiation therapy are vulnerable to pituitary dysfunction, most commonly growth hormone deficiency revealing short stature and retarded growth [35].

Patients with the pituitary adenomas are commonly treated with either single fraction SRS or hypofractionated SRS with similar rates of efficacy in tumor control and prevalence in new-onset hypopituitarism. Rates of hypopituitarism vary but are reported to be as high as 66% in conventional radiotherapy and significantly lower with stereotactic radiosurgery 5–37% [35–39].

Endocrine dysfunction is considered a late-delay side effect, but current literature is lacking in predicting a timeline for when hypopituitarism can occur. Follow up with dynamic serum hormonal values is of paramount importance given higher likelihood of developing endocrinopathies with longer follow up [35, 37].

6. Radiation induced optic neuropathy and stereotactic radiosurgery

Certain tumor types treated with SRS expose the optic nerves to high doses of radiation that may induce a decrease in visual acuity and blindness. Deterioration of vision may be reversible in an acute setting and is more likely to be permanent >6 months after treatment. Optic neuropathy from radiation is usually painless and can be monocular or biocular depending on whether optic nerves or the optic chiasm are exposed to radiation. Doses of radiation to optic nerves are closely monitored and circumvented as best as possible for patients receiving treatment for meningiomas, pituitary adenomas, and craniopharyngiomas.

Significant risk factors for radiation-induced optic neuropathy include prior radiation re-exposure to the optic chiasm. Prior EBRT and SRS are both risk factors for radiation induced optic neuropathy. Although multiple centers consider <8 Gy to be the upper limit of acceptable tolerability, single fractions of <12 Gy have been validated by recent literature [40–42]. A large recent analysis of pooled data consider the risk of radiation induced optic neuropathy to be 0–2% in patients with no prior irradiation to the optic apparatus and a single fraction <12 Gy [42] and even lower (<1%) for patients with a single fraction of <10 Gy [43].

7. Toxicities of spinal cord irradiation

Radiation myelopathy is the term commonly used for side effects of radiation toxicity to the spinal cord. Late effects of radiation myelopathy are a serious concern for radiation oncologists during treatment planning of CNS as well as extra-neural tumors within the treatment field. This is, in part, due to higher doses of radiation required for certain tumors (lung, certain head and neck, mediastinal tumors). Moreover, metastatic disease to the spine often requires radiation therapy and is becoming more common thanks to the advent of immunotherapy [44]. Long term effects may cause life limiting sequelae and are of paramount concern to radiation planning and treatment.

Adverse facts of spinal cord irradiation are largely determined by the radiation treatment field and can affect both the central and peripheral nervous system. Just as side effects can be subdivided by timeframe in radiation toxicity to the brain, toxicities of spinal cord irradiation are classified as early toxicity, early-delayed effects, and long term effects. Accordingly, the durations are during treatment and up to a couple weeks after treatment, within 3 months of treatment, and more than 3 months after treatment. Although acute central nervous system damage has been reported following acute brain irradiation, there is no clinical or experimental evidence that radiation induces acute spinal cord toxicity. Single doses of up to 100 Gy have been given without acute effects [32].

Significant advances have been made in the treatment of spinal malignancies extrapolating progress made from cranial stereotactic techniques of within millimeter precision high dose focal treatment plans. Recently, SRS has also been utilized for metastasis to the spinal cord. It is important to note that metastasis to the spinal bone, although extremely painful at times, does not carry the risk of neurologic compromise posed by spinal cord tumors or spinal impingement.

Side effects using SRS are extremely rare for spinal tumors. Short-term toxicity although more common, are still at low rates and are usually self-limiting [45]. One study showed no long term side effects with SRS patients with spinal metastasis.

It seems as if long-term toxicity from radiation using SRS and dose sparing techniques to organs at risk is extremely rare with modern treatment techniques and attention to dose volume parameters. The complication of vertebral compression fracture (VCF) is multifactorial including older age portending to higher incidences osteoporosis but may be attributed to, in part, radiation therapy [46]. Doses above 20 Gy in a single fraction have been implicated as a risk factor. The risk of VCF tends to occur in the acute period of toxicity [47].

The main factors associated with risk of neurologic deficit relate to total dose, length of spinal cord irradiated, fractionation scheme and total duration of treatment. An absolute threshold for development of myelopathy cannot be stated. There has not been an established threshold; however the risk of myelopathy varies from 0.2 to 5% at 5 years [39]. Another side effects or radiation to the spine is characterized by acute paralysis presumably secondary to ischemia. Brown-Séquard syndrome is another rare syndrome that has been documented and is characterized by paralysis and loss of proprioception to the ipsilateral side and loss of pain and temperature to the contralateral side. Similar to irradiation to the brain, the greatest concern is delayed-onset radionecrosis of the spinal cord.

Common types of side effects for single dose SRS with 10–16 Gy include: neurologic signs of motor weakness and sensory changes of the extremities [48]. There was no detectable acute or subacute radiation toxicity in this series noted clinically during the maximum follow-up time of 24 months. Other more disabling manifestations of radiation injury, including acute paralysis secondary to ischemia, hemorrhage within the spinal cord, and a lower motor neuron syndrome, are much less common, with only a few case reports in the literature. The treatment of radiation myelopathy has not been well studied. High dose corticosteroids are considered first line therapy.

8. Conclusions

Radiation therapy is highly effective in CNS malignancies. Nevertheless, the rate limiting step in treatment is associated with adverse side effects to healthy tissue. As the treatment of CNS malignancies advance with novel therapies and ever evolving therapeutic combinations, the goal of minimizing treatment side effects remains the same. Significant progress has been made in attempting to understand the dynamic mechanisms of brain injury caused by irradiation to healthy tissue. As patients continue to live longer, central nervous system side effects are of utmost importance to recognize and treat. Radiation oncologists among other cancer specialists are putting keen focus and effort towards increasing and optimizing quality-of-life in addition to overall survival in cancer patients.

Conflict of interest

Authors do not have conflicts of interest to declare.

Author details

Jason Naziri* and Steven J. DiBiase
Weill Cornell Medical College, New York Presbyterian, New York, USA

*Address all correspondence to: Jnaziri2@gmail.com

References

[1] Li YQ, Jay V, Wong CS. Oligodendrocytes in the adult rat spinal cord undergo radiation-induced apoptosis. Cancer Research. 1996;**56**(23):5417-5422

[2] Belka C et al. Radiation induced CNS toxicity—Molecular and cellular mechanisms. British Journal of Cancer. 2001;**85**(9):1233-1239

[3] Kim JH et al. Mechanisms of radiation-induced brain toxicity and implications for future clinical trials. Journal of Neuro-Oncology. 2008;**87**(3):279-286

[4] Limoli CL et al. Redox changes induced in hippocampal precursor cells by heavy ion irradiation. Radiation and Environmental Biophysics. 2007;**46**(2):167-172

[5] Fike JR, Rola R, Limoli CL. Radiation response of neural precursor cells. Neurosurgery Clinics of North America. 2007;**18**(1):115-127, x

[6] Mizumatsu S et al. Extreme sensitivity of adult neurogenesis to low doses of X-irradiation. Cancer Research. 2003;**63**(14):4021-4027

[7] Douw L et al. Cognitive and radiological effects of radiotherapy in patients with low-grade glioma: Long-term follow-up. Lancet Neurology. 2009;**8**(9):810-818

[8] Robin TP, Rusthoven CG. Strategies to preserve cognition in patients with brain metastases: A review. Frontiers in Oncology. 2018;**8**:415

[9] Gondi V et al. Preservation of memory with conformal avoidance of the hippocampal neural stem-cell compartment during whole-brain radiotherapy for brain metastases (RTOG 0933): A phase II multi-institutional trial. Journal of Clinical Oncology. 2014;**32**(34):3810-3816

[10] Baxter PS, Hardingham GE. Adaptive regulation of the brain's antioxidant defences by neurons and astrocytes. Free Radical Biology & Medicine. 2016;**100**:147-152

[11] Chow BM, Li YQ, Wong CS. Radiation-induced apoptosis in the adult central nervous system is p53-dependent. Cell Death and Differentiationr. 2000;**7**(8):712-720

[12] Gore EM et al. Phase III comparison of prophylactic cranial irradiation versus observation in patients with locally advanced non-small-cell lung cancer: Primary analysis of radiation therapy oncology group study RTOG 0214. Journal of Clinical Oncology. 2011;**29**(3):272-278

[13] Harjani RR, Gururajachar JM, Krishnaswamy U. Comprehensive assessment of somnolence syndrome in patients undergoing radiation to the brain. Reports of Practical Oncology and Radiotherapy. 2016;**21**(6):560-566

[14] Powell C et al. Somnolence syndrome in patients receiving radical radiotherapy for primary brain tumours: A prospective study. Radiotherapy and Oncology. 2011;**100**(1):131-136

[15] Faithfull S, Brada M. Somnolence syndrome in adults following cranial irradiation for primary brain tumours. Clinical Oncology (Royal College of Radiologists). 1998;**10**(4):250-254

[16] Lawenda BD et al. Permanent alopecia after cranial irradiation: Dose-response relationship. International Journal of Radiation Oncology, Biology, Physics. 2004;**60**(3):879-887

[17] Nieder C et al. Postoperative treatment and prognosis of patients with resected single brain metastasis: How useful are established prognostic

scores? Clinical Neurology and Neurosurgery. 2011;**113**(2):98-103

[18] Chang EL et al. Neurocognition in patients with brain metastases treated with radiosurgery or radiosurgery plus whole-brain irradiation: A randomised controlled trial. The Lancet Oncology. 2009;**10**(11):1037-1044

[19] Aoyama H et al. Stereotactic radiosurgery plus whole-brain radiation therapy vs stereotactic radiosurgery alone for treatment of brain metastases: A randomized controlled trial. JAMA. 2006;**295**(21):2483-2491

[20] Brown PD et al. Effect of radiosurgery alone vs radiosurgery with whole brain radiation therapy on cognitive function in patients with 1 to 3 brain metastases: A randomized clinical trial. JAMA. 2016;**316**(4):401-409

[21] Frazier JL et al. Stereotactic radiosurgery in the management of brain metastases: An institutional retrospective analysis of survival. International Journal of Radiation Oncology, Biology, Physics. 2010;**76**(5):1486-1492

[22] Rades D et al. A matched-pair analysis comparing whole-brain radiotherapy plus stereotactic radiosurgery versus surgery plus whole-brain radiotherapy and a boost to the metastatic site for one or two brain metastases. International Journal of Radiation Oncology, Biology, Physics. 2009;**73**(4):1077-1081

[23] Dore M et al. Stereotactic radiotherapy following surgery for brain metastasis: Predictive factors for local control and radionecrosis. Cancer Radiothérapie. 2017;**21**(1):4-9

[24] Minniti G et al. Single-fraction versus multifraction (3 × 9 Gy) stereotactic radiosurgery for large (>2 cm) brain metastases: A comparative analysis of local control and risk of radiation-induced brain necrosis. International Journal of Radiation Oncology, Biology, Physics. 2016;**95**(4):1142-1148

[25] Minniti G et al. Stereotactic radiosurgery for brain metastases: Analysis of outcome and risk of brain radionecrosis. Radiation Oncology. 2011;**6**:48

[26] Ahmed KA et al. Fractionated stereotactic radiotherapy to the post-operative cavity for radioresistant and radiosensitive brain metastases. Journal of Neuro-Oncology. 2014;**118**(1):179-186

[27] Kohutek ZA et al. Long-term risk of radionecrosis and imaging changes after stereotactic radiosurgery for brain metastases. Journal of Neuro-Oncology. 2015;**125**(1):149-156

[28] Korytko T et al. 12 Gy gamma knife radiosurgical volume is a predictor for radiation necrosis in non-AVM intracranial tumors. International Journal of Radiation Oncology, Biology, Physics. 2006;**64**(2):419-424

[29] National Comprehensive Cancer Network. Central Nervous System Cancer. 2018. Version 2.2018

[30] Keller A et al. Risk of radionecrosis after hypofractionated stereotactic radiotherapy targeting the postoperative resection cavity of brain metastases. Cancer Radiothérapie. 2017;**21**(5):377-388

[31] Blonigen BJ et al. Irradiated volume as a predictor of brain radionecrosis after linear accelerator stereotactic radiosurgery. International Journal of Radiation Oncology, Biology, Physics. 2010;**77**(4):996-1001

[32] Petrovich Z et al. Survival and pattern of failure in brain metastasis treated with stereotactic gamma knife

radiosurgery. Journal of Neurosurgery. 2002;**97**(5 Suppl):499-506

[33] Chao ST et al. Challenges with the diagnosis and treatment of cerebral radiation necrosis. International Journal of Radiation Oncology, Biology, Physics. 2013;**87**(3):449-457

[34] Lam KS et al. Effects of cranial irradiation on hypothalamic-pituitary function—A 5-year longitudinal study in patients with nasopharyngeal carcinoma. The Quarterly Journal of Medicine. 1991;**78**(286):165-176

[35] Appelman-Dijkstra NM et al. Pituitary dysfunction in adult patients after cranial radiotherapy: Systematic review and meta-analysis. The Journal of Clinical Endocrinology and Metabolism. 2011;**96**(8):2330-2340

[36] Li X et al. Safety and efficacy of fractionated stereotactic radiotherapy and stereotactic radiosurgery for treatment of pituitary adenomas: A systematic review and meta-analysis. Journal of the Neurological Sciences. 2017;**372**:110-116

[37] Toogood AA. Endocrine consequences of brain irradiation. Growth Hormone & IGF Research. 2004;**14**(Suppl A):S118-S124

[38] Paek SH et al. Integration of surgery with fractionated stereotactic radiotherapy for treatment of nonfunctioning pituitary macroadenomas. International Journal of Radiation Oncology, Biology, Physics. 2005;**61**(3):795-808

[39] Stereotactic Radiosurgery and Radiotehrapy of Pituitary Adenomas Clinical White Paper. 2014

[40] Leavitt JA et al. Long-term evaluation of radiation-induced optic neuropathy after single-fraction stereotactic radiosurgery. International Journal of Radiation Oncology, Biology, Physics. 2013;**87**(3):524-527

[41] Stafford SL et al. A study on the radiation tolerance of the optic nerves and chiasm after stereotactic radiosurgery. International Journal of Radiation Oncology, Biology, Physics. 2003;**55**(5):1177-1181

[42] Milano MT et al. Single- and multi-fraction stereotactic radiosurgery dose tolerances of the optic pathways. International Journal of Radiation Oncology, Biology, Physics. 2018

[43] Hiniker SM et al. Dose-response modeling of the visual pathway tolerance to single-fraction and hypofractionated stereotactic radiosurgery. Seminars in Radiation Oncology. 2016;**26**(2):97-104

[44] Thariat J et al. Advances in radiation oncology for metastatic bone disease. Bulletin du Cancer. 2013;**100**(11):1187-1197

[45] Rock JP et al. The evolving role of stereotactic radiosurgery and stereotactic radiation therapy for patients with spine tumors. Journal of Neuro-Oncology. 2004;**69**(1-3):319-334

[46] Wenger M. Vertebroplasty for metastasis. Medical Oncology. 2003;**20**(3):203-209

[47] Faruqi S et al. Vertebral compression fracture after spine stereotactic body radiation therapy: A review of the pathophysiology and risk factors. Neurosurgery. 2018;**83**(3):314-322

[48] Yin FF et al. Dosimetric characteristics of Novalis shaped beam surgery unit. Medical Physics. 2002;**29**(8):1729-1738

Chapter 9

Pediatric Medulloblastoma: A Radiation Oncologist Perspective

Meenu Gupta and Mushtaq Ahmad

Abstract

Pediatric medulloblastomas are radiosensitive and mostly curable tumors if they are non-metastasized. Postsurgery adjuvant radiation therapy remains the cornerstone therapy in the curative intent treatment. In case of children less than three years, pre-irradiation chemotherapy is given to defer radiotherapy till the child is three year old. Introduction of conformal radiotherapy in addition to technical improvements in surgery and radiotherapy, risks definition and molecular analysis of prognostic factors has most likely contributed to the improved survival rates. Children should ideally be referred in time to an appropriate higher center with adequate infrastructure, expertise and radiotherapy facilities for better outcome of the disease.

Keywords: medulloblastomas, radiosensitive, conformal, radiotherapy

1. Introduction

Harvey Cushing and Percival Bailey were the first who described the name medulloblastoma as "Spongioblastoma Cerebelli" in June, 1925 for posterior fossa tumors of preadolescents population. They reported 29 cerebellar vermis tumor in children and young adults. Later they renamed as "medulloblastoma" as the term "Spongioblastoma multiforme" was described by Globus and Strauss in 1925 for various adults cerebral tumors in which feature of considerable cellular differentiation was seen. This picture was found absent in tumors of cerebellar origin [1, 2]. World Health Organization (WHO) defined medulloblastoma as "invasive malignant embryonal tumor of the cerebellum with commonest manifestation seen in children". These neuroepithelial tumors have inherent tendency to spread through the cerebrospinal fluid to cranial and spinal subarachnoid spaces [3].

2. Epidemiology

Injuries followed by malignancy are the second leading cause of mortality among children. After leukaemia's, brain tumors are the most common in children accounting for '25%' of all malignancies in children [4]. Most common malignant CNS tumor in children is medulloblastoma (MB) constituting 20% of primary brain tumors and approximately 40% of all tumors of the posterior fossa [5]. The incidence of *medulloblastoma in adults is relatively low as compared to pediatric population. This constitutes 1% of all CNS tumors and this may be the cause of scanty data available in adult MB group* [6]. U.S data showed the incidence of the medulloblastoma is 1.5–2 cases/100,000 population. Three hundred and fifty new cases in the United States are seen each year. The peak incidence is seen in 1st decade of life and incidence is noted higher in the pediatric age group 3–4 years followed by 8–10 years of age.

CBTRUS (*Central Brain Tumor Registry of the United States*) showed that incidence is higher in males as compared to females (Males: 0.16 vs. Females: 0.12). But this trend is different in children who are less than one year old. There is rising trend of higher incidence (APC: 1.7, 95% CI −0.4, 4.0) and death risk (Hazard Ratio for Survival: 0.74 with p value 0.09) seen in black race compared to whites which is non-significant [7, 8].

3. Clinical presentation

There is rapid initiation of clinical symptoms are secondary to the rapid proliferation of these cellular malignant tumors. Symptoms of medulloblastomas vary with age. Earlier age of onset is associated with behavioral changes. Other symptoms may include listlessness, moodiness or irritability, vomiting, and lack of social interactions. As medulloblastoma is rapidly growing tumor, this results in obstructive hydrocephalus which manifests as raised intracranial pressure (ICP). Children may be seen with macrocephaly, fullness of fontanelle, and delayed developmental milestones. Older children and adults have symptoms of raised intracranial pressure like headache, vomiting, especially upon awakening in the morning hours. Headache usually gets better during the day. As anatomical location of medulloblastoma is cerebellum but symptoms slightly vary within various sites of cerebellum. Truncal ataxia result from tumors located in midline of cerebellum and appendicular ataxia is associated with the hemispheric located tumors [1]. There can be stretching of sixth cranial nerve because of hydrocephalus resulting in double vision. Meningeal irritation causes tilting of head and stiffness of neck due to the tonsillar herniation. Trochlear nerve palsy related to tumor compression is another reason of head tilt. Patients with spinal metastasis had symptoms of backache, weakness of bilateral lower limb and loss of bowel and bladder control. Metastatic disease symptoms depend upon the site involvement [9]. Majority are sporadic cases but there are associated syndromes like *Gorlin syndrome (nevoid basal-cell carcinoma syndrome)*, *Blue rubber-bleb nevus syndrome*, *Rubinstein-Taybi syndrome* and *Turcot syndrome (glioma polyposis syndrome)* [10].

4. Management

Although radiology is good contributor of diagnosis still detailed history and physical examination remained important and has to be done before proceeding for any investigations. Alteration of child behavior, persistent symptoms and focal neurological deficit are warning signs and should be proceeded with neuroimaging for diagnosis.

4.1 Imaging

4.1.1 Computed tomographic

Computed tomographic (CT) appearance of a medulloblastoma is seen as well-defined vermian cerebellar mass which is hyperattenuated with surrounding vasogenic edema and sometimes evidence of hydrocephalus is seen. Contrast enhanced images show homogeneous enhancement.

4.1.2 MRI imaging

MRI imaging of the entire neuraxis, brain and spine is recommended for suspected cases. MRI images show "Low-to-intermediate signal intensity" on T1-weighted images and "moderately high signal intensity" on T2-weighted images, compared to cerebellar white matter. Intratumoral haemorrhage, peritumoral oedema, tonsillar herniation, hydrocephalus and calcification are other associated findings. Multivoxel MR spectroscopy (MRS) of the primary tumor can assess the tumor metabolites like 'elevated Choline peaks and decreased Creatine and N-acetyl acetate peaks'. Even without frank necrosis, a small amount of lipid-lactate peak sometimes observed indicating an increase in metabolic activity. Due to densely packed cells within the tumor and nuclear: cytoplasm ratio is higher, MB causes restriction of diffusion. There is restriction of diffusion of water particles in the tumor. So there is high signal of the tumor in diffusion-weighted MR images [11]. As frequency of spine seeding is 35% at diagnosis, to rule out any leptomeningeal metastases, Sagittal fat-suppressed post- gadolinium contrast MRI of the spine should be performed prior to surgery (**Figure 1**). Guang-Yao Wu et al. published data showed that proton *magnetic resonance spectroscopy* (^{1}H-MRS) and Diffusion Weighted Imaging are helpful for qualitative diagnosis of medulloblastoma [12].

Baseline hearing status with tests like Audiometry, IQ Testing and hormonal levels with Serum TSH and GH can be tested.

4.2 Neurosurgery

Mostly medium and large sized tumors in posterior fossa are associated with hydrocephalus. In routine practice, prior to definitive surgery, ventriculo-peritoneal (VP) shunt should generally be avoided as definitive resection of tumor efficiently relieves the obstruction by opening the CSF pathways. Ideal surgery of any tumor is complete surgical resection, but feasibility and safety is priority. In

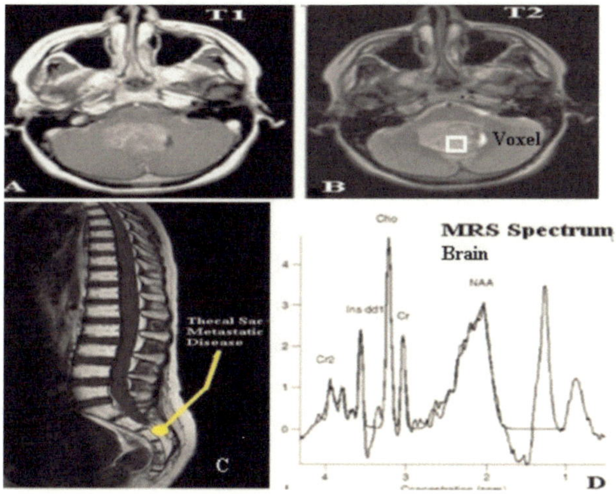

Figure 1.
Showing preoperative MRI. (A) T1 weighted image post- gadolinium with tumor arising from midline of cerebellum. (B) T2 FLAIR with mild hyper intensity and voxel showing the tumor area of interest for spectroscopy. (C) Drop metastasis. (D) Significantly increased choline peaks with decreased NAA and Cr peaks on Spectroscopy.

such circumstances, it is recommended to attempt maximal safe resection and residual disease can be left behind rather than aggressive surgical resection approach that can precipitate significant morbidity. Benefit to risk ratio of complete surgical removal of tumor has to be assessed preoperatively [13, 14].

4.2.1 Post surgery neuroimaging

Ideal timing of post surgery MRI imaging should be obtained immediately, within 24–48 h of tumor resection, for accurately identification of the extent of surgical resection and quantification of the status of the residual tumor. If immediate post surgery MRI imaging has not been obtained, then recommendation is to wait for at least 2–3 weeks, but no more than 4-weeks, for resolution of post surgical changes and this will further prevent false positive results. Recommendations for timing of postoperative CSF analysis for malignant cells are also same, at least 2–3 weeks post surgery to prevent errors like false positive results [15, 16].

4.3 Histopathology

Classification of most of the CNS tumors are still relying on only histopathological features but in medulloblastomas, integration of additional molecular information has updated WHO classification from 2007 to 2016. Medulloblastoma is classified now by an integrative diagnosis including a histologically as well as genetically defined compound as shown in **Table 1** [17].

Molecular classification provides additional clinical and prognostic information which has the potential for identification of innovative strategies and research for the management of this disease (**Table 2**) [18, 19].

4.4 Staging

Medulloblastomas originally were staged only on surgical basis but "Modified Chang Staging" is the current standard and there is addition of imaging [20] explained in **Figure 2**.

Risk stratification based on clinico-radiological analysis is still widely practiced and remains valid for Radiation planning in institutions. COG and SIOP Group accepted the clinical prognostic variables [21] shown in **Figure 3**. Although with the inclusion of molecular sub-grouping and genetic analysis of disease, more robust information about risk stratification and outcome of disease can be concluded to some extent but this required availability of these facilities with expertise in institutions. Incomplete neuraxis staging should be classified as high risk disease.

Histopathologically defined MB	Genetically defined MB
Medulloblastoma, classic	• Medulloblastoma, WNT-activated
Desmoplastic/nodular medulloblastoma	• Sonic Hedgehog (SHH) activated and *TP53*-mutant • Sonic Hedgehog (SHH) activated and *TP53*-wildtype
Medulloblastoma of extensive nodularity	• Non-SHH/Non-WNT
Large cell/anaplastic medulloblastoma	• Medulloblastoma, group 3
Medulloblastoma, not otherwise specified (NOS)	• Medulloblastoma, group 4

Table 1.
WHO 2016 updated classification of medulloblastomas.

	Wingless activated (*WNT*) MB	**Sonic hedgehog (*SHH*) subgroup**	**Group 3**	**Group 4**
Cell of origin	Dorsal brainstem (*lower rhombic lip*) neuronal progenitors	Cerebellar external granular layer, neuron precursors	Ventricular zone neural progenitors	Cerebellum progenitors (*upper rhombic lip*)
Prevalence	10%	30%	25%	35%
Male:female	1:1	1:1	2:1	3:1
Common age	Older children	<3 year and >16 year, adult group	Infants and children <16 year	Infants/children/adults
Histopathology	Classic. In few case, large cell and anaplastic	Nodular desmoplastic histology, classic, large cell and anaplastic	Classic, large cell and anaplastic	Classic, large cell and anaplastic
Genetic aberrations	*CTNNB1 DDX3X SMARCA4*	*MYCN, GLI2, PTCH1, SUFU, MLL2, SMO, TP53, BCOR1, LDB1, GABRG1*	*MYC, PVT1, OTX2, MLL2, SMARCA4, CHD7*	*OTX2, DDX31, CHD7, SNCAIP, MYCN, CDK6 GFI1/GFI1B, MLL2, KDM6A, MLL3, ZMYM3*
Chromosome	*−/6*	*3q gain, 9q loss, 10q loss*	*1q gain, 5q loss, 10q loss*	*Isochromosome 17q chr X loss, 17p loss*
Molecular markers	Beta-catenin	SFRP1or GAB1	MYC activation in 50% of this subtype	Unknown
Metastasis	Rarely present	Not common	High	35–40% at presentation
Recurrence	Rarely seen	Local	Metastasis	Metastasis
5 year overall survival	95%	75%	50%	75%
Future strategy	Reduction in therapy	SHH pathway inhibitors	Intensified therapy, novel therapeutics	Robust and large data research

Table 2.
Medulloblastoma as a group of molecularly distinct subtypes.

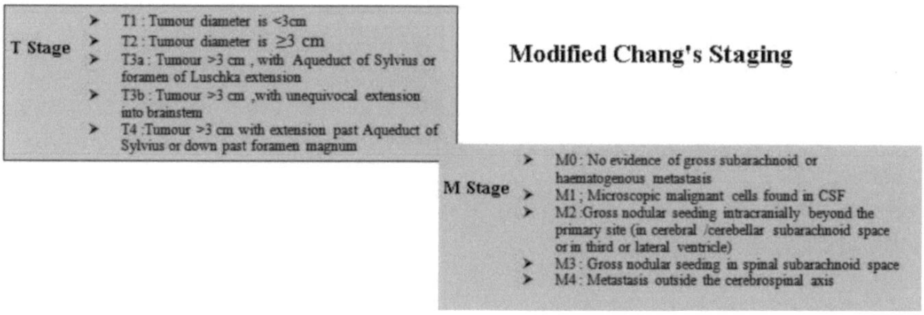

Figure 2.
Modified Chang's staging system.

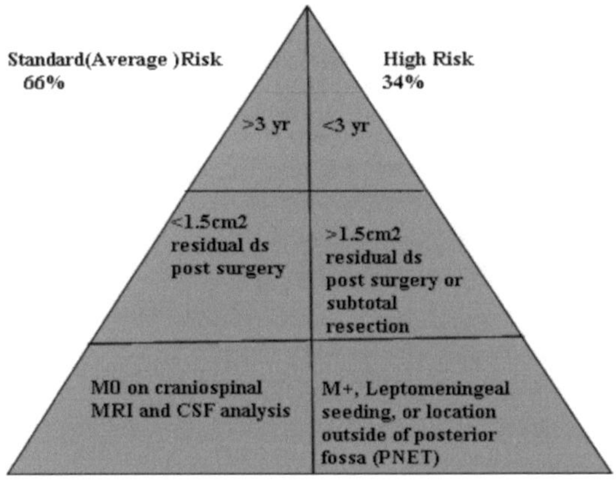

Figure 3.
The stratifying medulloblastoma patients clinically into high risk and standard (average) risk based on variables like age, resection and metastasis.

5. Radiation therapy

Medulloblastoma, the embryonal tumors of the central nervous system, are highly radiosensitive tumors. After 200 cGy, the survival fraction has been reported to be 27%. Although Dargeon in 1948 stated that "medulloblastomas ... have a consistently unfavourable prognosis" but later careful observation of Edith Paterson regarding pattern of disease spread brings hope to this disease. Radiating brain and spinal cord in one undivided volume principle mentioned by Edith Paterson and Farr. was based on the post-mortem findings of brain and spinal cord deposits in untreated cases. In 1953, at the Christie Hospital a five-year survival rate for children who were treated with kV irradiation reported by Paterson and Farr was 41%. Since then the practice to irradiate the entire craniospinal axis is universally adopted [22, 23].

After resection of tumor, entire craniospinal axis irradiation followed by whole posterior fossa or tumor bed boost irradiation is recommended irrespective of clinically detectable disease. Being Radiosensitive, Radiotherapy is curative up to 70% of standard risk patients. For this pediatric age group disease, linear accelerators are better than telecobalt machines and these children should preferably be referred in time to well equipped higher center with radiotherapy facility and infrastructure to prevent unnecessary side effects. As treatment delays beyond 6–7 weeks result in worse outcome, cobalt-60 therapy may be offered in those areas where linacs are not available. To prevent the adverse effects of radiotherapy in the developing nervous system, radiotherapy is avoided initially in children up to 3 years of age. CSI technique required accurate reproducibility and complex field matching techniques. Long and complex shaped target volume homogeneity is a technically challenging process.

Timing of radiotherapy

Improved survival for patients is associated with a shorter interval from surgery to the start of radiation therapy. After definitive surgery, treatment should be started within 4–7 weeks. International Society of Paediatric Oncology (SIOP) trials showed that increase in the risk of relapse is seen if radiotherapy treatment is delivered after 7 weeks [24].

5.1 Radiotherapy planning techniques

Younger brains are much more sensitive to damage caused by radiotherapy. CT based conformal radiation therapy, 3DCRT, is standard of care exists for many years. Patient can be in the supine or prone position during CSI treatment. Over the years, prone position was used universally. Nowadays supine position is used increasingly.

Advantages of supine position [25]

- Target volume coverage is more easily assured and delivery more reproducible.
- Patient is more comfortable due to stable position.
- Technically, there is better shielding of cribriform plate and inferior temporal lobes.
- For younger pediatric patients who require anaesthesia, there can be better management of airways and cardiopulmonary complications can be reduced.

Limitations of supine position

- Without adequate portal imaging, setup accuracy is difficult.
- Old couches contain metal inserts and beam entrance posteriorly through the head rest and treatment couch is not possible.

Advantages of prone position is the junction between the spinal and cranial fields can be better visualized.

For younger children, good sedation may be required. Expert play therapist may help in treatment for radiotherapy without sedation.

5.1.1 Conventional planning

In 2-dimensional planning, fluoroscopic guidance two-dimensional simulation is done. Immobilization is done with thermoplastic cast and universal prone head-rest is used. CSI board with Lucite base plate having semicircular Lucite structures are available for head rest and chin rest. Various degrees of neck extensions is possible which will prevent the exit of superior border of spinal field through the oral cavity. Chest wall can be supported by thermocols.

This complex 2-dimensional CSI technique fundamentals are:

- Two parallel opposed lateral portals for cranium and upper cervical spinal cord.
- Posterior spinal field matching with the cranial fields.
- In case of adults or larger children, matching of upper posterior spinal field with the separate lower posterior spinal field.

Craniospinal junction can be placed at higher level: C1/C2 interspace or lower level C5-C7. At higher level, overdose to spinal cord is low. Shoulders are excluded from the lateral fields by keeping the craniospinal junction at lower level (C5-C7). Also the exit dose to mandible, thyroid, pharynx and larynx is lowered. Inferior edge of S2 is mostly the anatomical landmark where lower border of spinal field (SF) is set. Single Craniospinal junction is set for smaller children. If length is >36 cm, two junctions are required which are craniospinal and spinal-spinal (SS) junction. Mostly SS junction is place at L2-L3 interspace. Multi-leaf collimators or custom made lead blocks are utilized for orofacial region shielding. In order to know the divergence of spinal fields, the spinal fields are simulated first.

Various techniques used for matching craniospinal junction are:

- For matching the beam divergence of the lateral head portals with the superior beam edge of SF, Collimator rotation is done 7–10°.
- Couch rotation 6°.
- Half beam blocks
- Asymmetric jaws
- Penumbra trimmers

The craniospinal junction should be feathering/moving weekly during craniospinal irradiation for homogenous dose distribution and further minimizing the hot or cold spots resulted from the gap-junction or set-up errors. With each shift, spinal field can be extended superiorly, and cranial fields can be decreased inferiorly by 0.5–1 cm. Similarly LB (lower border) of "superior spinal field" and SB (superior border) of "inferior spinal" field can be shifted superiorly. This all is done for spread out of dose homogeneity. Still the contribution of human errors is seen in many studies. As there is direct visualization of the optical field light on the skin surface in prone position, verification of beam delivery of CSI is relatively simple (**Figure 4A**) [26, 27].

The posterior fossa (PF) boost volume

Depending on the risk-stratification of the disease, volume of the posterior fossa boost is decided. Those cases which are considered low risk and standard risk medulloblastomas, posterior fossa target volume includes pre-operative tumor bed with adequate margins. Most institutions add 1–1.5 cm margin to the tumor bed. Cases of high risk and very high risk disease require irradiation of the entire posterior fossa. Posterior fossa irradiation can easily be planned based on fluoroscopic imaging in low and middle income countries where there is no availability of multileaf collimators.

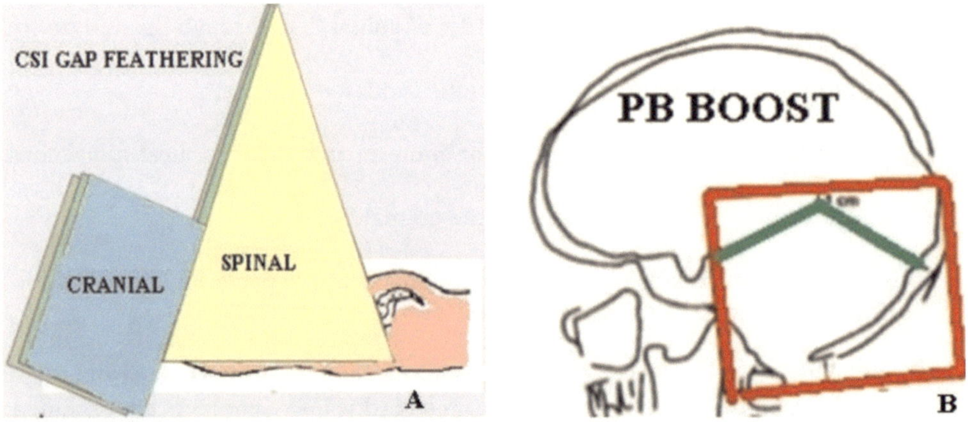

Figure 4.
(A) Gap feathering during craniospinal irradiation (CSI). Junction movement across the long treatment length allows homogenous dose distribution by reducing the overlap hot spot and gapping cold spots. If field length < 35 cm, 100 cm SSD is used and for field length >35 cm, 120 cm SSD is used. (B) Posterior fossa boost volume including whole infratentorial compartment.

Conventional portals for PF boost

The PF boost is given using two lateral opposing fields. Anterior radiotherapy borders are formed by the posterior clinoids, posteriorly by internal occipital protuberance, superiorly extended up to mid-point of *foramen magnum* and *vertex* (or 1 cm above tentorium) and inferiorly extended up to C2-C3 interspace (**Figure 4B**) [28].

5.1.2 Conformal radiotherapy planning

In case of pediatric patients who are potential long term survivors, critical structures are better spared by conformal techniques.

Immobilization is done in supine position and patient is aligned straight keeping neck in the neutral position. A 4-clamp thermoplastic immobilization cast for the head and shoulder region along with appropriate neck rest should be used. A five point orfit for immobilization along with hyperextended head and depressed both shoulders can result in optimal sparing of the upper esophagus and laryngeal structures.

Traditionally, axial planning images of 5 mm thickness on CT simulator from the vertex till the upper thigh region were preferred. But in this era of high precision radiotherapy where CTV accuracy is important for optimal outcome, CT slice thickness is reduced in some anatomical sites of CSI field. Slice Thickness of 1–2.5 mm from the vertex to the inferior border of third cervical vertebrae (C3) and 2–5 mm from the lower border of third cervical vertebrae (C3) to the upper anatomical region of the femur should be obtained. Skull base foramina delineation is of utmost important and for their identification, "1 mm slice thickness at the base of skull" is preferred. To improve better identification of cranial nerves dural sheaths, co-registration of planning imaging CT to MRI can be done [29]. CSF extensions within the dural reflections are better demonstrated by FIESTA (Fast Imaging Employing Steady-State Acquisition) MRI sequences [30].

Treatment volumes

Due to the risk of CSF dissemination, entire arachnoid space is included in the clinical target volume (CTV).

5.1.2.1 Whole brain treatment volume

The frontal lobe and the cribriform plate must be included in the clinical target volume. Inclusion of superior orbital tissue is must in the radiation field for the adequate coverage of the frontal lobe and cribriform plate. As per SIOPE guidelines, "the geometric edge of shielding should extend at least 0.5 cm inferiorly below the cribriform plate and at least 1 cm elsewhere below the base of the skull".

Delineation of $CTV_{cranial}$

a. Brain along with its covering meninges are contoured till second cervical vertebrae (C_2). For outlining the inner table of the skull, CT bony window setting is used with window/level: 1500–2000/300–350 suggested by SIOPE group.

b. The most critical sites are the 'cribriform plate', the 'most inferior parts of the temporal lobes', and the 'whole pituitary fossa'. They all to be included in the $CTV_{cranial}$ delineation. For cribriform plate CT window/level suggested is 3000/400.

c. For inclusion of CSF within the dural sheath of cranial nerves, CTVcranial is modified. For second cranial (optic) nerve, window width 350/level 40 is to be used

Foramina or canals of skull base which are significant for delineation of $CTV_{cranial}$ are cribriform plate, optical canal of sphenoid, superior orbital fissure, foramen ovale, internal auditory meatus (IAM), jugular foramen and hypoglossal canal. Entire components length of the optic nerves in the $CTV_{cranial}$ is included in most institutions where photons are used. But in those institutions where medulloblastomas are treated by protons, for prevention of any potential optical retinopathy risk, only the posterior length components of the optic nerves is included [31, 32].

As CSF flows up to the posterior aspect of eyeball which is better observed in MRI images, it is better to include whole optic nerves in CTV in routine practice of photon beam based radiotherapy in these cases. The cranial nerves which are wrapped without dural cuff are the third, fourth and sixth (oculomotor, trochlear and abducens) nerves. Nobel et al. studied the flow of cerebrospinal fluid beyond the inner table of skull into the IAM (internal auditory meatus), juglar foramen (JF) and hypoglossal canal (HC). Their study (on basis of 96 FIESTA MRI sequences) concluded that the CSF extension was up to '16 mm' in the internal auditory meatus which is not very far away from the cochlea. So the cochlear sparing by CSF exclusion within the internal acoustic canal should not be attempted. Their data also showed that the CSF extension was up to 11 mm in the juglar fossa from inner table of skull. There is no extension of CSF within these dural sheaths outside the outer table of the skull. It is not so easy to delineate dural sheath CSF on MRI but CT images with 1 mm thickness along the base of skull can show skull foramina and canals and they can easily be contoured on bony windows (**Figure 5**) [29].

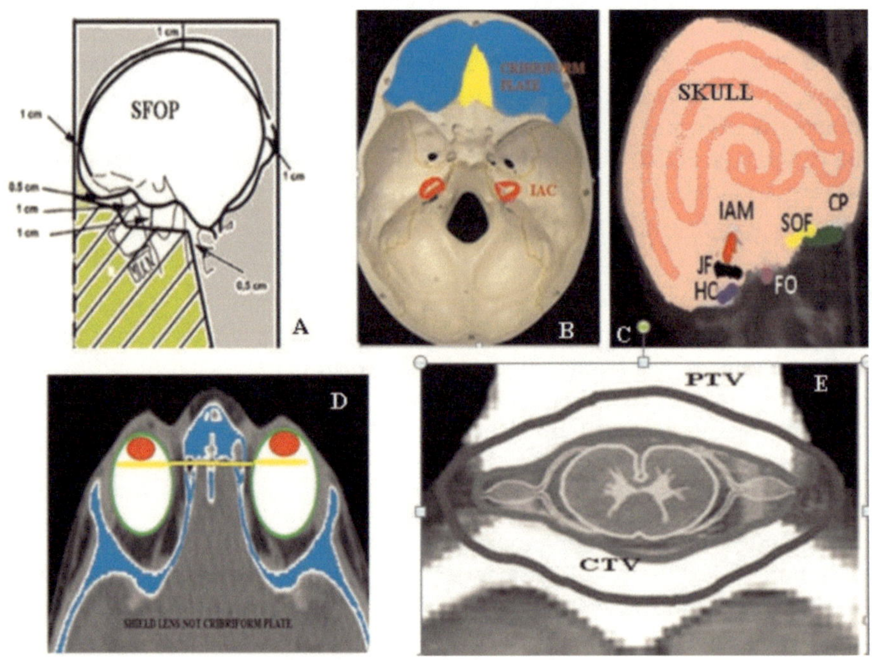

Figure 5.
Showing conformal planning. (A) Cribriform plate is in close proximity to ocular structures. Shielding edge should be at least 0.5 cm below the cribriform plate and 1 cm elsewhere below base of skull to cover the temporal fossa and skull base foramina. (B) The petrous part of temporal bone showing Internal acoustic canal (IAC). (C) Various skull base foramina contoured in $CTV_{cranial}$ including dural cuffs of cranial nerves. (D) Cribriform plate must be in target volume. (E) Entire subarachnoid space, including nerve roots laterally must be included in CTV_{spinal}. SFOP, French Paediatric Oncology Society; CP, cribriform plate; SOF, superior orbital fissure; FO, foramen ovale.

CTV brain: brain and its covering meninges till lower border of C2.
PTV brain: 5 mm isotropic margin around CTV brain.
CTV spine: entire arachnoid space with nerve roots.
PTV spine: 5–8 mm isotropic margin is recommended around the CTV-spine

Issues of the cribriform plate (CP)

According to a 1982 report from MSKCC, 15% of recurrences are subfrontal in medulloblastomas [33]. Hypothesis given by Donnal et al. was that the pooling of cells secondary to gravitational effect of prone position with maximum shielding of eyes can result in the recurrences at the region of cribriform plate [34].

5.1.2.2 CTV_{Spinal}

The CTV_{Spinal} (spinal target volume) includes the complete dural or thecal sac. Lateral extension of delineation is must to cover the intervertebral or neural foramina with their exiting nerve roots from the C2 cervical spine till the lower end of the thecal sac. Lower border of CTV_{Spinal} is appreciated by the latest spinal MRI imaging. Children Oncology Group (ACNS0332, ACNS 0331, ACNS 0122) recommended the inferior border of CTV_{Spinal} is '*2 cm below the termination of the subdural space*' which is usually at bottom of second sacral vertebrae. The other SIOPE group trials recommended that the lower border of CTV_{Spinal} must be determined by the spinal MRI imaging of the termination of the thecal or dural sac. This border should be kep. 1 cm inferior to this. Root canals in the Sacral CTV_{Spinal} can be excluded. This recommendation is based on a MRI study conducted on ten volunteers who were healthy proved that there was no CSF around the nerve roots of sacral segments.

If patients are to be treated by protons, then for skeletally immature patients, CTV_{Spine} should include the vertebral bodies. This will decrease the risk of unequal vertebral growth. In skeletally mature patients, spinal TV should include the sub-arachnoid space of spine with a margin of 3–5 mm is summed up to the body of vertebrae for set up uncertainties/variation (interfraction) [29].

Delineation of posterior fossa boost volume

High Risk and Very High Risk disease: The clinical target volume PF (CTV_{PF}) boost encompassed the whole PF. The boost CTV_{PF} extends superiorly up to the tentorium cerebelli, inferiorly to the foramen magnum, and posterolaterally to the occipital bony walls and temporal fossa. BS (Brain Stem) anterior border and mid-brain cover the components of the posterior fossa anteriorly. The geometric margin of 0.5 cm around the CTV_{PF} is taken for delineation of the PTV posterior fossa (PTV_{PF}). PTV_{PF} is limited to the bony confines of the skull, except at the foramen magnum where it extended to the level of C1. The PTV_{PF} contoured anteriorly up to the posterior clinoids and inferiorly to the C1-C2 junction. PTV is modified at sella and pituitary gland is excluded from anterior extension of PF boost planning.

For low risk and standard risk, tumor bed, as defined on CT images, delineation with a margin of 1–2 cm is recommended. For three-dimensional planning, two lateral opposing portals with editing/shaping using the multileaf collimators (MLCs) is recommended. Finally, these craniospinal and boost plans must be summated to produce a composite treatment plan and final dose-distribution is calculated [35, 36].

5.2 Intensity modulated radiotherapy for CSI

Children and adults are two different groups as far as radiotherapy treatment in medulloblastoma is concerned. Proliferating tissues are more in children as compared to the adults. IMRT for adult population is a used as a routine practice for numerous malignancies but for pediatric patients, IMRT has to be used with great caution in view of low dose volumes. Spinal irradiation during CSI results in increased doses delivered to anterior thoracic and abdominal structures with conventional plans. Parker et al. published data showed that the PTV and dose homogeneity was better for the medulloblastoma CSI, IMRT plans. Dosimeteric analysis showed $V_{95\%}$ for IMRT was 100%, 3D planning was 96% and 2D planning was 98%. Also $V_{107\%}$ for IMRT was 3%, 3D planning 38% and 2D was 37%. The IMRT plans provided better sparing of heart and liver in terms of V (10 Gy) and above. Integral Dose analysis showed the IMRT plans were superior for liver and heart and the 3D plan were better for the body contour. Tomotherapy may be helpful in reducing high dose regions in OAR, but low dose of radiation to a large volume is a concern for pediatric patients [37].

IMRT planning

IMRT for craniospinal irradiation in adult medulloblastomas is delivered after summation of PTV brain plan and PTV spine plan. Usually the spinal PTV planning is done first with 'inverse planning technique' using the 5 posterior fields with 0°, ±20° and ± 50°gantry angles. For the craniocaudal direction, the isocenter is kept at the "geometrical center of the PTV_spine". For the depth and lateral position, it is usually set at the "midline and midplane" at the level of the interphase of second and third cervical vertebral body. Dose prescription and normalization is to the isocenter of the spine. For the cranial target, a separate plan is created. Cranial fields isocenter is set at the inferior most slice of the PTV brain. MLC positions can be modified for dose reduction to the nearby OARs and adequate coverage of the target volume. The geometric center of the PTV_brain is defined as the reference point for dose prescription and normalization. Final composite plan for the whole cranio-spinal axis is obtained after dosimetrically summation of spinal and cranial plans. For taller patients, for upper and lower spine, IMRT plans are created separately [38].

Intensity modulated radiotherapy for posterior fossa boost

Meenu et al. re-planned seven previously irradiated patients of MB with seven field inverse planning IMRT for whole posterior fossa boost. Equidistant gantry angles (0°, 50°, 100°, 150°, 210°, 260°, 310°) were used with step and shoot IMRT on 6MV energy LINAC. Treatment isocenter was set at the geometrical center of the planning target volume. They compared with 3DCRT plan delivered by two lateral opposing beams with multileaf collimators for shaping. Their dosimeteric results showed there were decreased mean dose to most critical organ at risk, cochlea, with IMRT compared to the three dimensional radiotherapy plans with significant p values i.e. 0.032 for the cochlea of right ear and 0.020 for the left sided cochlea (**Figure 6**) [35] Similar results are found in published clinical studies conducted by Huang et al. where 13% of the IMRT group had grade 3 or 4 hearing loss as compared to 64% for the conventional group [39].

Organ at risk

OAR as demarcated on axial CT images include brain, eyes, lens, optic nerves, optic chiasma, cochlea, parotids, mandible, thyroid, esophagus, lungs, heart, breasts, liver, kidneys, bowel bag, rectum, bladder, gonads (ovary or testes), vertebral bodies, uterus plus pelvis (red bone marrow).

5.3 Radiotherapy doses

Berry et al. reported a five year survival rate of 47% with lesser doses and ten year DFS of 77% once the posterior fossa doses delivered were >52 Gy [40]. Abacioglu et al. showed in adult medulloblastomas, control rate was 33% at 5 year

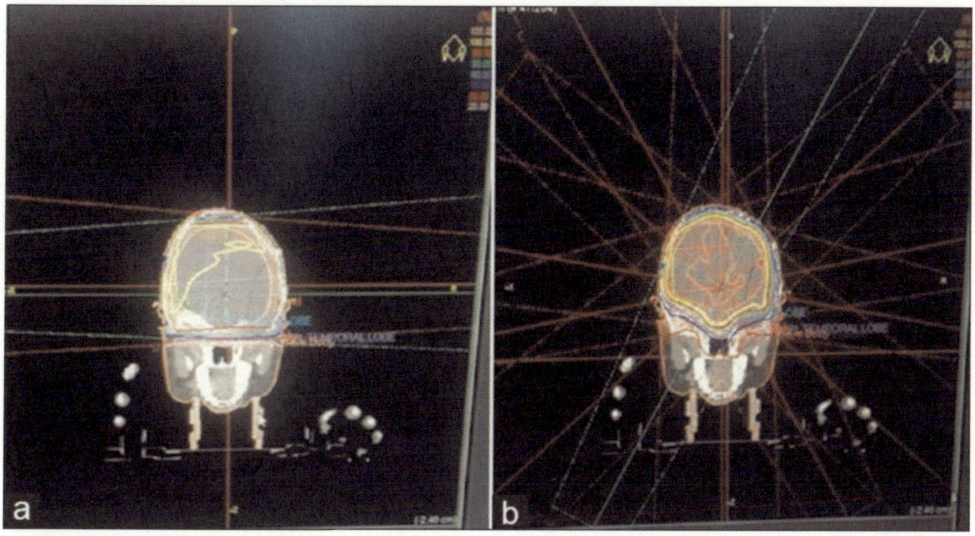

Figure 6.
Coursey JCRT. Meenu et al. mid-axial dose distributions with (a) 3DCRT (b) IMRT for one of the representative case of entire posterior fossa boost. Yellow represents 100%, red 95% and blue 70% of the isodose lines. IMRT is advantageous over 3DCRT for cochlear sparing. 3DCRT, three dimensional conformal radiotherapy; IMRT, intensity modulated radiotherapy.

with doses <54 Gy native to 91% in those patients on whom higher doses were delivered [41]. CSI dose reduction is feasible with the addition of chemotherapy as level 1 evidence based data released by Children's Cancer Study Group showed that the reduction of doses from 36- to 23.4 Gy resulted in significantly higher risk of recurrences outside the posterior fossa [42].

Radiotherapy doses to CSI depends upon the risk stratification of the disease at presentation. If risk stratification or accurate staging is incomplete then patient can be treated as high-risk disease. Radiation therapy doses according to the risk stratification are shown in **Table 3** [43]. There are different long term toxicities between the adult and children. CSI dose reduction approach is avoided for adult patients. Still big data is required to justify the addition of adjuvant chemotherapy to radiotherapy in average risk adult patients as data showed that 70–80% of these patients have no progression of disease at 5 years when RT is used as a sole modality. Also there are issues of hematological toxicities in adult patients.

5.4 Proton therapy

Pediatric age is more sensitive to radiation induced carcinogenesis as compared to adults by a factor of at least 10 [44].

As children anatomy is small so critical organs are very much close to the target volume. Also the scatter from the treatment volume is highly significant in children having small body area as compared to large body of adults. Particle beam therapy is a potential powerful tool for improving the therapeutic ratio. Goal of pediatric radiation oncologists is integral dose minimization to whole body and organs at risk. Advantage of protons over the photons is that they can modulate the dose to avoid very close OARs. For CSI, advantages of protons are because of absorption of low dose on tissue entry and the point of maximum dose deposition at the Bragg-peak. This results in the avoidance of dose deposition to anterior organs like thyroid, lungs, heart, gut, liver, esophagus, kidneys and urinary bladder. Also critical brain structures such as the lens, optic chiasma, pituitary, cochleae are better spared.

Various risk stratification	Volume and doses of radiation therapy	Concurrent or adjuvant chemotherapy
High risk and very high risk disease	CSI: 36 Gy/ 20 fractions, 5 days a week Boost to posterior fossa: 19.8 Gy/ 11 fractions, 5 times/week Gross metastatic deposits: Boost dose of 5.4–9 Gy/3–5 fractions	Concurrent carboplatin followed by adjuvant six cycles of systemic chemotherapy
Standard risk	Children <18 year CSI: 23.4 Gy/13 fractions, 5 days a week Boost to whole posterior fossa (or tumor bed): 30.6 Gy/17 fractions, 5 times/week Adults CSI: 36 Gy/20 fractions, 5 days a week Boost to posterior fossa: 19.8 Gy/11 fractions, 5 times/week	Children <18 year Weekly vincristine followed by adjuvant six cycles of systemic chemotherapy
Low risk	CSI: 23.4 Gy/13 fractions, 5 days a week Boost to whole posterior fossa (or tumor bed): 30.6 Gy/17 fractions, 5 times/week	Reduced intensity chemotherapy

Table 3.
Radiotherapy doses according to risk stratification.

In grown up children, sparing the anterior portion of the vertebral body results in minimization of bone marrow dose (**Figure 7**).

Consensus report from the Stockholm pediatric proton therapy conference showed that treatment of choice for medulloblastoma is proton therapy [45]. Based on the review of the existing theoretical and early clinical outcomes evidence, results showed that proton craniospinal irradiation provide similar control of tumor with potentially decreased doses to the normal structures thus reduces the risk of side effects when compared with photon existing data [46]. Spot-scanned intensity-modulated proton therapy (IMPT) is advantageous over the photon therapy in terms of all radiobiological risk estimation [47].

Weight changes in medulloblastoma and adaptive proton therapy are coming up but at present there is scanty data available. Patient selection is of utmost important in proton therapy. Limitations of patients with their families to travel in these

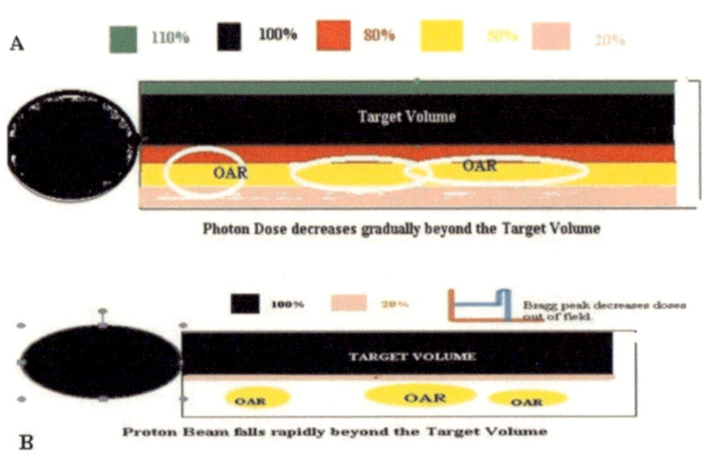

Figure 7.
CSI Schematic Model. (A) Photons are absorbed and secondary electrons have large range in mm resulting in doses beyond the target volume. (B) Advantage of stopping of protons is due to the Bragg peak curve resulting in lower doses to OARs with proton therapy.

centers, the proton center capacity to treat children and the availability of expertise and support structures must be evaluated by the referral physicians.

6. Chemotherapy

Chemotherapy is integral part of treatment and in standard risk cases CSI doses can be reduced. Children less than 3 years, chemotherapy is recommended till the child will attain the age of 3 years. Drugs like carboplatin, cyclophosphamide and etoposide is recommended. There are various regimens recommended (**Box 1**). In a published database analysis of medulloblastoma children (n = 816) age 3–8 years who received adjuvant chemotherapy after surgery, overall rate of RT deferral after surgery was 15.1%. Their practice was associated was decreased overall survival in this pediatric population even in the well-established era of chemotherapy. [48] At present, recommendations of chemotherapy are:

- Following RT as adjuvant settings
- In Infant medulloblastoma, to defer RT, till the age of 3-years
- Autologous stem-cell rescue accompanied with high-dose chemotherapy with
- Concurrent chemotherapy with radiotherapy
- As a salvage therapy in cases of relapsed of recurrent medulloblastoma.

Box 1.
Chemotherapy regimens (adjuvant) in MB children >3 years of age [49, 36].

Packer's Regimen 1	Regimen II	Regimen III
Cisplatin, Lomustine, Vincristine	Cisplatin, Cyclophosphamide , Vincristine	(Days of administration are different from Regimen II) Cisplatin, Cyclophosphamide , Vincristine

A detailed discussion about the chemotherapy and late effects of radio-chemotherapy, management of adverse effects are outside the scope of this chapter. It is recommended and important *to have* multidisciplinary follow-up with pediatric radiation oncologists and endocrinologists.

7. Follow up

Follow up counseling is mandatory prior to initiation of treatment. MRI brain may be performed every three months and MRI spine may be obtained every six months in standard risk category of standard risk patients for the initial two years. These two investigations can be performed every 6 months up to five years, and then repeated every year. In high-risk group, MRI of whole brain and spine may be repeated every three months for the initial two years. Thorough clinical examination with every visit is necessary. In case of pediatric or adolescence groups following radiotherapy, neuroendocrine follow-up with evaluation of serum hormonal levels should be performed every six months.

Acknowledgements

Authors are grateful to Prof. Sunil Saini, Director Cancer Research Institute, Swami Rama Himalayan University for providing motivation and necessary facilities for writing this book chapter.

Conflict of interest

The authors declare that this chapter was written in the absence of any commercial or financial relationships that could elucidate as a potential conflict of interest.

Author details

Meenu Gupta* and Mushtaq Ahmad
Cancer Research Institute, Swami Rama Himalayan University, Dehradun, India

*Address all correspondence to: meenugupta.786@rediffmail.com

References

[1] Millard NE, De Braganca KC. Medulloblastoma. Journal of Child Neurology. 2016;**31**(12):1341-1353

[2] Nelson JS et al. Embryonal tumors of the central nervous system. In: Principles and Practice of Neuropathology. 2nd ed. Oxford University Press; 2003. p. 384

[3] Adesina AM, Yachnis AT. Medulloblastoma Pathology. 2015

[4] Gregory JJ. Overview of pediatric cancer. In: Pediatrics. Merck Manual; Global Medical Knowledge. 2015

[5] Huang MA . Pediatric Medulloblastoma. 2017

[6] Lassaletta A, Ramaswamy V. Medulloblastoma in adults: They're not just big kids. Neuro-Oncology. 2016; **18**(7):895-897

[7] Jallo GI, Osburn BR, Shimony N. Medulloblastoma, 2018

[8] Khanna V, Achey RL, Ostrom QT, Block-Beach H, Kruchko C, Barnholtz-Sloan JS. Incidence and survival trends for medulloblastomas in the United States from 2001 to 2013. Journal of Neuro-Oncology. 2017;**135**(3):433-441

[9] Wilne S, Collier J, Kennedy C, Jenkins A, Grout J, Mackie S, et al. Progression from first symptom to diagnosis in childhood brain tumors. European Journal of Pediatrics. 2012;**171**(1): 87-9310. DOI: 1007/s00431-011-1485-7

[10] Krishna V. The nervous system. In: Text Book of Pathology. Chennai, India: Orient Longman Private Limited; 2004. p. 1035

[11] Koeller KK, Rushing EJ. Medulloblastoma: A comprehensive review with radiologic-pathologic correlation. Radiographics. 2003;**23**(6): 1613-1637

[12] Wu G-Y, Haopeng P, Ghimire P, Liu G. H magnetic resonance spectroscopy and diffusion weighted imaging findings of medulloblastoma in 3.0T MRI: A retrospective analysis of 17 cases. Neural Regeneration Research. 2012;**7**(32):2554-2559

[13] Muzumdar D, Deshpande A, Kumar R, Sharma A, Goel N, Dange N, et al. Medulloblastoma in childhood—King Edward Memorial hospital surgical experience and review: Comparative analysis of the case series of 365 patients. Journal of Pediatric Neurosciences. 2011;**6**(Supp. 1):S78-S85

[14] Spennato P, Ruggiero C, Cinalli G. Medulloblastoma—Surgery. In: Ozek MM, Cinalli G, Maixner W, Sainte-Rose C, editors. Posterior Fossa Tumors in Children. Switzerland: Springer; 2015. pp. 313-332

[15] Meyers SP, Wildenhain SL, Chang JK, Bourekas EC, Beattie PF, Korones DN, et al. Postoperative evaluation for disseminated medulloblastoma involving the spine: Contrast-enhanced MRI findings, CSF cytologic analysis, timing of disease occurrence, and patient outcomes. AJNR. American Journal of Neuroradiology. 2000;**21**:1757-1765

[16] Harreld JH, Mohammed N, Goldsberry G, Li X, Li Y, Boop F, et al. Postoperative intraspinal subdural collections after pediatric posterior fossa tumor resection: Incidence, imaging, and clinical features. AJNR. American Journal of Neuroradiology. 2015;**36**: 993-999

[17] Louis DN, Perry A, Reifenberger G, von Deimling A, Figarella-Branger D, Cavenee WK, et al. The 2016 World Health Organization classification of tumors of the central nervous system: A summary. Acta Neuropathologica. 2016; **131**:103-120

[18] Sengupta S, Krummel DP, Pomeroy S. The evolution of medulloblastoma therapy to personalized medicine. F1000Research. 2017;**6**:490

[19] Kijima N, Kanemura Y. Molecular classification of medulloblastoma. Neurologia Medico-Chirurgica. 2016; **56**(11):687-697

[20] Hayat MA, editor. Pediatric Cancer. Diagnosis, Therapy, and Prognosis. Vol. 42013. Springer. pp. 93-95

[21] DeSouza R-M, Jones BRT, Lowis SP, Kurian KM. Pediatric medulloblastoma —Update on molecular classification driving targeted therapies. Frontiers in Oncology. 2014;**4**:176

[22] Paterson E, Farr RF. Cerebellar medulloblastoma: Treatment by irradiation of the whole central nervous system. Acta Radiologica. 1953;**39**(4): 323-336

[23] Paulino AC. Radiotherapeutic management of medulloblastoma. Oncology. 1997;**11**:813-823

[24] Lannering B, Rutkowski S, Doz F, Pizer B, Gustafsson G, Navajas A, et al. Hyperfractionated versus conventional radiotherapy followed by chemotherapy in standard-risk medulloblastoma: Results from the randomized multicenter HIT-SIOP PNET 4 trial. Journal of Clinical Oncology. 2012; **30**(26):3187-3193

[25] Tai P, Koul R, Khanh V, Edwards T, Buwembo J, Teles AR, et al. A simplified supine technique expedites the delivery of effective craniospinal radiation to medulloblastoma—Comparison with other techniques in the literature. Cureus. 2015;**7**(12):e404

[26] Athiyaman H, Mayilvaganan A, Singh D. A simple planning technique of craniospinal irradiation in the eclipse treatment planning system. Journal of Medical Physics. 2014;**39**(4):251-258

[27] Parker WA, Freeman CR. A simple technique for craniospinal radiotherapy in the supine position. Radiotherapy and Oncology. 2006;**78**:217-222

[28] Taqaddas A. Oncological management of medulloblastoma and new viral therapeutic targets. International Journal of Medical and Health Sciences. 2015;**9**(1):27-30

[29] Ajithkumar T, Horan G, Padovani L, Thorp N, Timmermann B, Alapetite C, et al. SIOPE—Brain tumor group consensus guideline on craniospinal target volume delineation for high-precision radiotherapy. Radiotherapy & Oncology. 2018;**128**(2):192-197

[30] Noble DJ, Scoffings D, et al. Fast imaging employing steady-state acquisition (FIESTA) MRI to investigate cerebrospinal fluid (CSF) within dural reflections of posterior fossa cranial nerves. The British Journal of Radiology. 2016;**89**(1067):20160392

[31] Siddiqui JD, Loeffler JS, Murphy MA. Radiation optic neuropathy after proton beam therapy for optic nerve sheath meningioma. Journal of Neuro-Ophthalmology. 2013;**33**:165-168

[32] Ferguson I et al. Risk factors for radiation-induced optic neuropathy: A casecontrol study. Clinical & Experimental Ophthalmology. 2017;**45**: 592-597

[33] Jereb B, Reid A, Ahuja RK. Patterns of failure in patients with medulloblastoma. Cancer. 1982;**50**:2941-2947

[34] Donnal J, Halperin EC, Friedman HS, et al. Subfrontal recurrenceof medulloblastoma. Journal of Neurology Research. 1992;**13**:1617-1618

[35] Gupta M, Kant R, et al. A dosimetric comparison between three-dimensional conformal radiation therapy and intensity-modulated radiation therapy in the treatment of posterior fossa boost in medulloblastoma. Journal of Cancer

Research and Therapeutics. 2017;**13**: 1027-1031

[36] Gupta T, Sarkar C, et al. Indian society of neuro-oncology consensus guidelines for the contemporary management of medulloblastoma. Neurology India. 2017;**65**:315-332

[37] Parker W, Filion E, et al. Intensity-modulated radiotherapy for craniospinal irradiation: Target volume considerations, dose constraints, and competing risks. International Journal of Radiation Oncology • Biology • Physics. 2007;**69**(1):251-257

[38] Sharma DS, Gupta T, Jalali R, Master Z, Phurailatpam RD, Sarin R. High-precision radiotherapy for craniospinal irradiation: Evaluation of three-dimensional conformal radiotherapy, intensity-modulated radiation therapy and helical tomotherapy. The British Journal of Radiology. 2009 Dec;**82**(984): 1000-1009

[39] Huang E, Teh BS, Strother DR, Davis QG, Chiu JK, Lu HH, et al. Intensity-modulated radiation therapy for pediatric medulloblastoma: Early report on the reduction of ototoxicity. International Journal of Radiation Oncology, Biology, Physics. 2002;**52**:599-605

[40] Pierotti MA, van Harten W, editors. European Options and Recommendations for Cancer Diagnosis and Therapy. Vol. 12011. Brussels, Belgium: Organisation of European Cancer Institutes European Economic Interest Grouping c/o Fondation Universitaire (OECI-EEIG); ISBN: 9789080625679

[41] Abacioglu U, OmerUzel MS, SedatTurkan AO. Medulloblastoma in adults: Treatment results and prognostic factors. International Journal of Radiation Oncology • Biology • Physics. 2002;**54**(3):855-860

[42] Thomas PR, Deutsch M, Kepner JL, et al. Low-stage medulloblastoma: Final analysis of trial comparing standard-dose with reduced-dose neuraxis irradiation. Journal of Clinical Oncology. 2000;**18**:3004-3011

[43] Parkes J, Hendricks M, Ssenyonga P, Mugamba J, Molyneux E, Meeterenet A S-v, et al. Clinical practice guidelines SIOP PODC. Adapted treatment recommendations for standard-risk medulloblastoma in low and middle income settings. Pediatric Blood & Cancer. 2015;**62**:553-564

[44] Kutanzi KR, Lumen A, Koturbash I, Miousse IR. Pediatric exposures to ionizing radiation: Carcinogenic considerations. International Journal of Environmental Research and Public Health. 2016;**13**(11):1057

[45] Indelicato DJ, Merchant T, Laperriere N, Lassen Y, Vennarini S, Wolden S. Consensus report from the stockholm pediatric proton therapy conference. International Journal of Radiation Oncology, Biology, Physics. 2016;**96**(2):387-392

[46] Mahajan A. Proton craniospinal radiation therapy: Rationale and clinical evidence. International Journal of Particle Therapy. 2014;**1**(2):399-407

[47] Brodin NP, Munck Af Rosenschöld P, Aznar MC, et al. Radiobiological risk estimates of adverse events and secondary cancer for proton and photon radiation therapy of pediatric medulloblastoma. Acta Oncologica. 2011;**50**:806-816

[48] Kann BH, Park HS, Lester-Coll NH, Yeboa DN, Benitez V, Khanet AJ, et al. Postoperative radiotherapy patterns of care and survival implications for medulloblastoma in young children. JAMA Oncology. 2016;**2**(12):1574-1581

[49] Packer RJ, Gajjar A, Vezina G, Rorke-Adams L, Burger PC, Robertson PL, et al. Phase III study of craniospinal radiation therapy followed by adjuvant chemotherapy for newly diagnosed average-risk medulloblastoma. Journal of Clinical Oncology. 2006;**24**: 4202-4208

Chapter 10

Laser Ablation for Gliomas

Alexa Semonche, Daniel Eichberg, Ashish Shah and Michael E. Ivan

Abstract

Laser interstitial thermal therapy (LITT) is a novel minimally invasive neurosurgical procedure in which laser light is delivered through a stereotactically positioned probe to an intracranial lesion for controlled thermal ablation of the pathological tissue. LITT is considered for patients who are poor candidates for open surgical resection due to (1) location of lesion (e.g., deep-seated or near critical structures), (2) history of intracranial interventions or medical comorbidities that increase surgical risk, or (3) lesion refractoriness to prior conventional therapies. The use of LITT was initially limited by concerns over off-target thermal damage; however, recent advances in magnetic resonance imaging-based thermal imaging have enabled real-time monitoring of tissue ablation dynamics, thereby improving its safety profile. Accordingly, the past two decades have seen a rapid expansion in the use of LITT for a variety of intracranial pathologies, including neoplasms, radiation necrosis, and epilepsy. This chapter focuses on the novel application of LITT to both newly diagnosed and recurrent glioblastoma multiforme (GBM). We first review the technological developments that enabled the safe use of LITT for GBM. We then review recent evidence regarding the indications, outcomes, and limitations of LITT as a novel adjuvant treatment for GBM.

Keywords: LITT, laser, glioma, glioblastoma, astrocytoma, ablation

1. Introduction

1.1 Glioblastoma multiforme: standard-of-care and prognosis

World Health Organization (WHO) grade IV glioma (glioblastoma multiforme) is the most common and most lethal malignant primary brain tumor. The incidence in the United States is estimated to be 3.12 per 100,000 persons with a median age of 64 years at diagnosis [1]. Current standard-of-care guidelines for initial treatment for grade III or IV gliomas (high-grade gliomas (HGG)) are maximal safe surgical resection followed by adjuvant temozolomide chemotherapy and radiation [2]. Although standard-of-care treatment improves median survival from 3 months in untreated patients to 14.8 months, GBM remains a terminal diagnosis as tumors inevitably recur [2, 3]. There are few positive prognostic factors. In a minority of patients, certain tumor molecular phenotypes correlate with improved prognosis. For example, methylguanine methyltransferase (MGMT) promoter hypermethylation is associated with an increased median survival of 21.7 months. Isocitrate dehydrogenase 1 (IDH) mutation-positive tumors, especially in combination with MGMT hypermethylation, also correlate with a survival benefit [4]. Other favorable prognostic factors include younger age at diagnosis, pre-treatment functional status, and extent of surgical resection of the tumor mass [5].

1.2 Rationale for use of LITT for glioblastoma

Recent studies have improved our understanding of how the extent of surgical resection impacts progression-free survival and overall survival for GBM patients [6, 7]. Although GBM is a diffusely infiltrative disease, gross total resection (GTR) is associated with increased progression-free survival and overall survival compared to subtotal resection (STR), which itself confers a survival benefit compared to biopsy alone [7]. Studies aiming to quantify a threshold extent of resection have concluded that a threshold at 78% resection of radiographic tumor is necessary to confer a survival benefit compared to radiation and chemotherapy alone [8–11]. Other recent studies have found an additional survival benefit from supra-total resection (i.e., resection beyond the contrast-enhancing tumor margins) to include any fluid-attenuated inversion recovery (FLAIR) abnormalities or a total right frontal or parietal lobectomy compared to GTR [12, 13]. These findings support the current standard-of-care guidelines for maximal safe surgical resection and reinforce the primary role of cytoreduction in GBM treatment.

However, some patients may not be able to undergo conventional open surgical resection. Factors contributing to this include medical comorbidities that increase surgical risk, low preoperative functional status, inability to tolerate general anesthesia, and history of radiation therapy or prior craniotomy that may impair wound healing and increase risk of postoperative neurological worsening [14]. Up to 40% of GBM tumors are considered surgically "unresectable" based on their location in deep or eloquent brain regions or adjacent to critical neurovascular structures [15]. Postoperative neurological deficits from injury to eloquent brain regions during open surgical resection are associated with reduced overall survival and functional status [16]. When open surgery is not an option, patients may simply receive a needle biopsy for diagnosis and chemoradiation. For these patients, laser interstitial thermal therapy is a minimally invasive alternative approach for cytoreductive intervention.

2. Laser interstitial thermal therapy: Principles and technological developments

2.1 Technological principles

LITT is a minimally invasive neurosurgical procedure that delivers laser light to an intracranial target to thermally ablate pathological tissue [17]. Laser light is a form of non-ionizing radiation and is emitted from a power source as a coherent beam of electromagnetic radiation. Laser light is delivered intracranially through a fiber optic ensheathed in a rigid laser probe that can be stereotactically inserted along a linear trajectory from a single skull entry point to the lesion. The primary mechanism of thermal damage occurs when laser light is absorbed by tissue water and hemoglobin molecules, causing excitation and release of heat. In LITT, laser light in the near-infrared range (980–1064 nm) is used to maximize tissue penetrance (up to 10 mm). Tissue heating to at least 43°C for several minutes is sufficient to cause irreversible tissue damage; heating to 60°C rapidly induces protein denaturation and damage to DNA and lipid membranes, resulting in coagulative necrosis [18]. At 100°C, tissue vaporization occurs, which can result in increased intracranial pressure. Tissue charring at temperatures >90°C can also damage healthy brain and impair laser penetration to further target regions. Therefore, the ideal temperature range for thermal ablation is 50–90°C [19].

The first use of LITT in neurosurgery was reported in the early 1980s [20]; however, concerns were raised over how to limit thermal injury to pathological tissue only [21]. Although early LITT users could stereotactically position a laser optical fiber to the center of a lesion, they did not have an accurate method for measuring heat distribution throughout the target and to surrounding off-target areas. Two advances in LITT technology have improved its safety: (1) real-time magnetic resonance (MR) thermometry and (2) the development of commercially available LITT systems that successfully integrate MR thermometry data and enhanced control over laser energy delivery into a standard workflow.

MR thermometry was introduced in the 1990s as a way to monitor real-time changes in tissue temperature on an MR imaging sequence [22, 23]. T2-weighted MRI images are taken intraoperatively; changes in tissue temperature affect the water proton resonance frequency signal in a linear relationship and can be mapped onto pixels of the MRI image. The result is a heat damage map that can be updated throughout the procedure and used to guide the boundaries of laser ablation [24].

The NeuroBlate laser ablation system (Monteris, Inc.) and the Visualase Thermal Therapy System (Medtronic, Inc.) received Food and Drug Administration (FDA) approval in 2007 and 2009, respectively. These commercial LITT platforms use MR thermometry software that allows the surgeon to define a maximum temperature threshold at the periphery of the target lesion; surpassing this threshold automatically triggers laser shutdown to protect off-target regions [24]. The Visualase and NeuroBlate LITT systems also improved procedure safety in designing a cooling sheath to surround the laser fiber along the length of laser probe, thereby limiting thermal damage to the tip of the probe [18].

2.2 Overview of the LITT setup and workflow

The LITT setup consists of four components: (1) laser energy source, (2) laser applicator probe, (3) cooling mechanism, and (4) computer workstation with software for processing real-time MRI thermometry data and controlling laser energy delivery. The patient is induced under general anesthesia or monitored anesthesia care (MAC). In the operating room, the laser trajectory from a skull entry point to the target lesion is planned using standard neuronavigation (e.g., Stealth system, Medtronic Inc.) technology. The laser applicator probe is stereotactically positioned along this trajectory through a single burr hole at the entry point. The surgeon may opt to perform stereotactic needle biopsy prior to implantation of the applicator probe to obtain a histopathological diagnosis. The patient is then transferred to an MRI suite under anesthesia. Laser energy is delivered through the probe to the target lesion in controlled doses lasting several minutes each. Concurrent real-time MRI thermal imaging (MRTI) of the treatment region allows the user to adjust laser output parameters so that thermal ablation of the target is achieved while avoiding thermal damage to normal surrounding brain tissue. Following LITT treatment, the applicator probe is removed, and the small skin opening overlying the entry point is closed.

2.3 LITT system platforms and surgical technique

2.3.1 LITT system platforms

The NeuroBlate system consists of a 12-Watt (W) pulsed-output 1064 nm wavelength neodymium-doped yttrium aluminum garnet (Nd-YAG) laser with a side-firing laser probe design, allowing some control over the direction of ablation. Temperature at the tip is controlled with a CO_2 gas cooling mechanism with a built-in thermocouple for feedback control. The Visualase system consists of a 15 W 980 nm diode laser with diffusing-tip probe design. Within the probe, the laser fiber optic is ensheathed within catheter circulating cooled saline. Both systems have a computer workstation with software for MR thermal imaging analysis and control over laser treatment parameters [25]. The 1064 nm wavelength laser used in the NeuroBlate system allows for deeper tissue penetration and potentially larger ablation zone, while the Visualase 980 nm wavelength laser produces more efficient heating [9].

2.3.2 Surgical procedure

After the patient is induced under anesthesia, stereotactic registration is performed to plan laser probe trajectory. If a stereotactic headframe is used to set the laser probe trajectory, then a preoperative T1-weighted MRI with contrast and neuronavigation technology is used to plan the trajectory. If the surgeon is using a frameless setup for registration, then an initial computed-tomography (CT) head with fiducial markers is obtained; this is merged with preoperative T1-weighted MRI with contrast studies, and then registration proceeds using neuronavigation. Once registration is complete, a linear trajectory is planned connecting a single entry site at the skull to the lesion that avoids critical brain structures. A trajectory that is orthogonal to the skull surface in all three dimensional planes helps to prevent skiving during drilling and catheter placement and should be utilized. After image registration, the entry point is found with the navigation wand and marked. Local anesthetic is infiltrated at the scalp over the entry site. A precision aiming device and Stealth navigation wand are aligned along the planned trajectory. A 4-mm incision is made to bring the navigation wand tip onto the skull surface entry point. A small burr hole is made with a 3.2-mm drill bit. After the dura is punctured, a reducing cannula is used to pass a rigid stylet, which maintains alignment during placement of the plastic bone anchor. The plastic bone anchor is screwed into the skull with the rigid stylet as a guide. The laser probe is placed into the cooling catheter and fixed in place (**Figure 1**). The patient is then transported under sterile draping and with continued general anesthesia to the MRI suite, where a T2-weighted MRI imaging is then performed to confirm placement of the laser probe in the lesion.

The LITT system software is used to set maximum temperature thresholds of 90°C in the immediate ablation zone around the laser probe tip and 50°C at the target periphery to ensure tissue ablation throughout the target zone (**Figure 2A–D**). Additional maximum temperature thresholds are set in the normal parenchyma surrounding the lesion that, if reached, trigger automatic shutoff to avoid off-target tissue damage [19]. Under real-time MR thermography guidance, a 30–60-second, 3–4 W-test dose is administered to localize the distal end of the laser probe. Once localization of the laser probe to the target is confirmed, the lesion is treated with 10–15 W doses of laser light in 1–3 minute intervals. Ablation is considered complete when the region of tissue reaching 50°C is covered (**Figure 2E**). After ablation is complete, the LITT apparatus is removed through the burr hole craniotomy, and the skin is closed. Typical length of hospital stay is under 48 hours [19, 24, 26, 27].

Postoperative MRI imaging is typically obtained on the first day following LITT. On T1-weighted MRI with contrast, the thermal ablation zone has a thin enhancing rim with potential surrounding edema and enhancing residual blood products and protein coagulation [19]. Residual tumor remaining after subtotal ablation can be

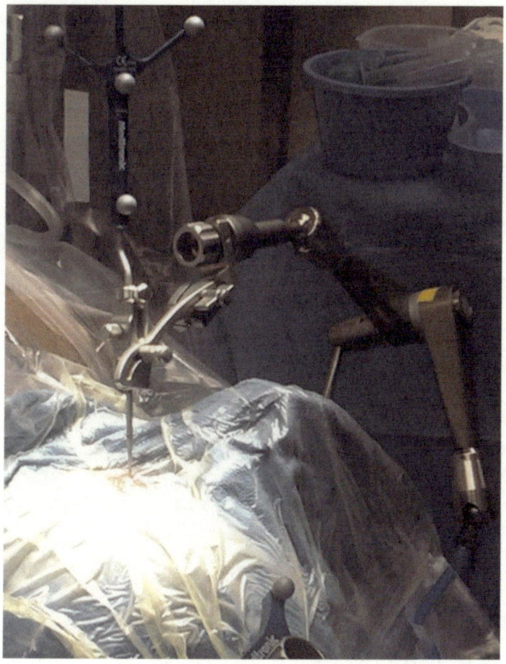

Figure 1.
Intraoperative setup for laser interstitial thermal therapy. The laser probe trajectory is planned under neuronavigation. The skin overlying the skull entry point is incised, a small burr hole is drilled, and a small incision in the dura is made. A cannula is inserted and used to guide the rigid stylet and bone anchor in the correct orientation along the planned trajectory.

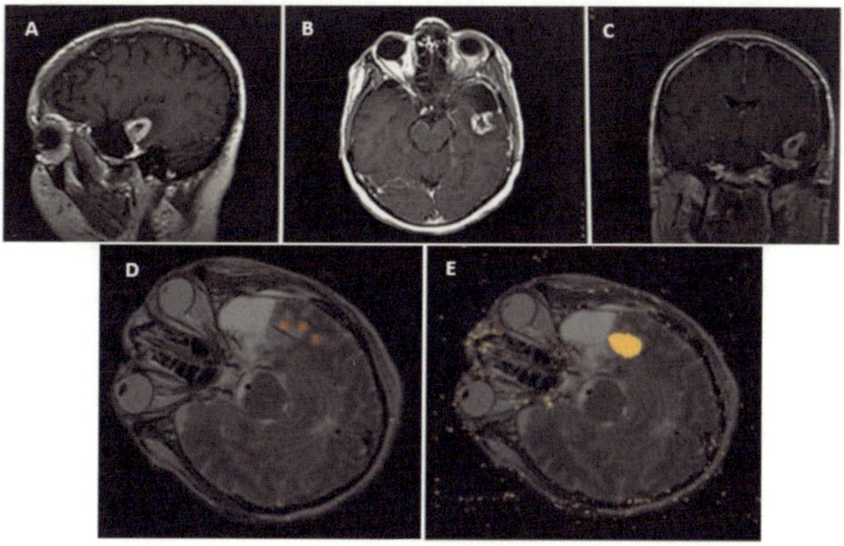

Figure 2.
Representative results of MR thermometry, which acquires real-time temperature data for each pixel of an M2-weighted MRI image. Representative preoperative sagittal (A), axial (B), and coronal (C) T1-weighted MRI with contrast images are suggestive of high-grade glioma. In planning a course of LITT, markers for temperature thresholds to achieve ablation while avoiding off-target damage or tissue vaporization are set by the user (D). During LITT, a damage zone of tissue achieving temperatures sufficient for ablation is represented by orange pixels (E).

detected on this first postoperative scan. The extent of ablation can be determined using volumetric analysis volume of the ablation zone postoperatively to the volume of the lesion on the preoperative MRI obtained for surgical planning [28].

Additional follow-up MRI studies are obtained 1–3 months postoperatively and then at longer intervals depending on clinical status, pathology, and radiology findings.

3. Patient selection

3.1 Indications

The development of commercially available stereotactic LITT systems that allow highly controlled delivery of laser light and real-time MRTI monitoring has enabled the routine use of the LITT. Currently, LITT is a treatment option for a variety of intracranial pathologies, including neoplasms (e.g., dural-based lesions, gliomas, metastases), epileptogenic foci (e.g., medial temporal sclerosis, focal cortical dysplasia), radiation necrosis, and chronic pain syndromes. The application of LITT to both newly diagnosed and recurrent gliomas has developed over the past decade; reports from initial institutional experiences demonstrate that LITT can be safely used for both supratentorial and infratentorial gliomas [28].

3.2 Criteria for patient selection

Identifying suitable candidates for LITT is important to ensure procedural safety and to optimize target lesion ablation. We propose that LITT is a viable alternative to open surgical resection in patients who meet the following criteria:

1. Lesion size of <3 cm diameter in any dimension. This size restriction reduces the risk of damage to critical brain regions.

2. The surgeon can reasonably predict to achieve an extent of ablation of at least 80%. This threshold is generalized from previous studies of the extent of tumor resection necessary to confer a significant survival benefit in open surgical resection [8–11].

3. Lesions that are inaccessible via conventional open surgery (e.g., lesions located adjacent to deep structures such as the basal ganglia, thalamus, splenium, etc., in eloquent motor or speech areas or near critical neurovascular structures).

4. Treatment refractory lesions (i.e., failure of previous craniotomy or radiation).

5. Patients with medical comorbidities, low preoperative functional status, or history of previous craniotomy/radiation therapy who are unable to tolerate prolonged anesthesia and blood loss or who are at high risk of surgical morbidity and impaired wound healing. Of note, patients should still have a preoperative functional status appropriate for a minimally invasive surgical procedure under anesthesia; in our institutional experience, patients are eligible if they have a Karnofsky Performance Score (KPS) of at least 70.

Therefore, LITT offers a minimally invasive cytoreductive therapy for patients with surgically inaccessible or treatment refractory tumors who would not benefit more from open surgical resection.

3.3 Illustrative case series

Here we present three cases of GBM tumors treated with LITT at our institution (University of Miami, Miller School of Medicine). Case 1 illustrates the use of LITT for recurrent GBM. Case 2 demonstrates the use of LITT in treating primary GBM and the utility of performing stereotactic needle biopsy during the same operative setting to yield diagnostic information. In Case 3, we provide an example of subtotal ablation of a recurrent GBM tumor.

3.3.1 Case 1

A 55-year-old gentleman with a 1-year history of GBM presented with focal nodular enhancement in the right temporal lobe on surveillance MRI. One year prior, he underwent surgical resection followed by temozolomide chemotherapy and radiation. Upon presentation to our surgical neuro-oncology service, the patient was asymptomatic; neurological exam was non-focal. Because of the surgeon's judgment that LITT would be able to achieve gross total ablation, the small size of the lesion, and the patient's history of treatment failure with surgical resection and chemoradiation, the patient was consented for LITT. After the stereotactic placement of the Visualase laser probe and confirmation of its location on intraoperative MRI imaging (**Figure 3A**), LITT was performed according to the following treatment parameters:

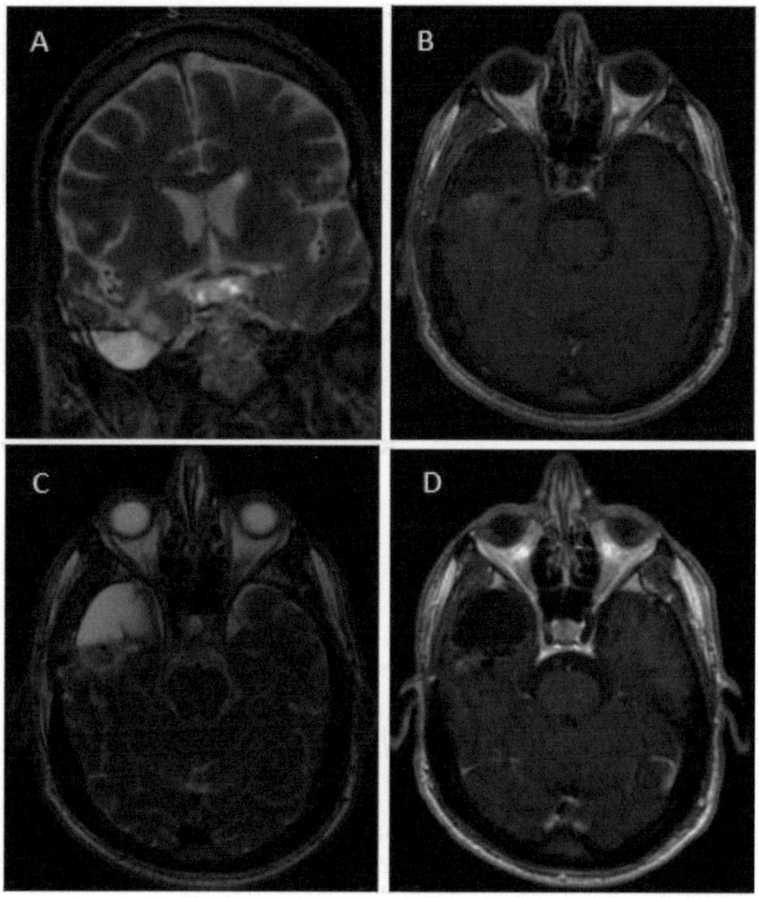

Figure 3.
A 55-year-old gentleman presenting with asymptomatic GBM recurrence. Intraoperative T2-weighted sagittal MRI showing stereotactic placement of laser probe at target lesion (A). Postoperative day 1 of T1-weighted axial MRI with contrast demonstrates gross total lesion ablation; hyperintense signal most likely represents blood products (B) instead of residual tumor, as the same region does not enhance on T2-weighted MRI (C). At 22-months follow-up, T1-weighted axial MRI imaging with contrast showed the patient was recurrence-free (D).

1. Test dose at 4 W for 7 seconds. Concurrent real-time MRI thermometry data confirmed total coverage of the target lesion.

2. Ablation dose at 10 W laser power for 3 minutes. Because MRI thermometry data confirmed target area ablation and ablation temperature threshold was reached (without reaching the maximum temperature threshold in off-target zones), the treatment was considered complete.

T1-weighted MRI on postoperative day 1 showed gross total (100%) lesion ablation (**Figure 3B** and **C**). The hyperintense signal in the tumor region represented blood products. On follow-up, the patient remained recurrence-free for over 2 years (26 months) (**Figure 3D**). The patient's family reported his death 3 months following tumor recurrence.

3.3.2 Case 2

A 60-year-old gentleman with progressive gait instability and confusion for 2 weeks and worsening headache for 2 days presented to the emergency department. MRI demonstrated a deep-seated left mesial temporal lobe lesion (**Figure 4A**). Due to the location of the lesion and progression of his symptoms, the patient was consented for stereotactic needle biopsy and LITT. In the operating room, a trajectory for the stereotactic biopsy needle and laser probe was planned, taking care to avoid critical cortical structures, ventricles, tentorium, arteries, and veins, targeting the center of the lesion volume (**Figure 4B**). To perform stereotactic needle biopsy, a preoperative and intraoperative computed-tomography scan was obtained using an O-Arm (Medtronic) to register and confirm intralesional biopsy. Two frozen cores of tissue were sent for pathological analysis, which confirmed the presence of necrotic brain tissue. Following biopsy, the laser probe was targeted to the lesion using neuronavigation with preoperative MRI registration. Follow-up T1-weighted MRI with contrast demonstrated gross total (100%) ablation (**Figure 4C**). At 1.4-year follow-up, the patient remains recurrence-free.

3.3.3 Case 3

A 58-year-old female with history of GBM initially diagnosed 2 years prior presented with focal recurrence in the left frontoparietal lobe on MRI imaging. The recurrence had recently been treated with stereotactic radiosurgery, after which the patient noticed new-onset right-hand weakness that did not improve with steroids.

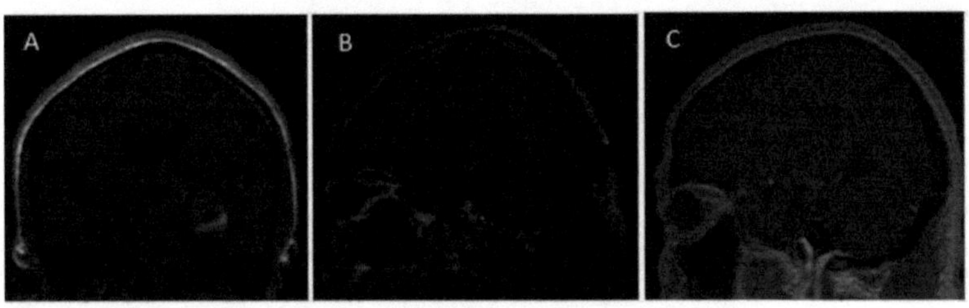

Figure 4.
A 60-year-old gentleman found to have a new, deep-seated lesion on T1-weighted coronal MRI with contrast suspicious for glioma (A). Intraoperative T2-weighted sagittal MRI shows stereotactic positioning of the laser probe to access the lesion while avoiding critical brain structures (B). Postoperative T1-weighted sagittal MRI with contrast demonstrates gross total ablation of the lesion (C).

Neurological exam was positive for 4/5 strength in the right hand, but was otherwise non-focal. MRI studies re-demonstrated the recurrence and extensive surrounding edema (**Figure 5A, B**). Because the lesion was small (2.0 cm maximum diameter) and failed both prior surgical resection and radiosurgery, the patient was consented for LITT. The patient was induced under general anesthesia, and a laser probe entry site and trajectory angle to the target lesion were planned using preoperative MRI imaging and Stealth neuronavigation (Medtronic, Inc.). The Visualase thermal therapy system laser probe was inserted stereotactically along the planned trajectory as described above (**Figure 5C**). The ablation procedure began with a test dose of laser energy at 3 W (20% of maximum power) for 3 minutes. Concurrent real-time MRI thermometry data was used to confirm target lesion coverage by the developing ablation zone. Next laser power output was increased to 7.5 W (50% maximum power) for 3 minutes, with successive 3-minute doses at 3 W stepwise increases in power. Once target area coverage was maximized and ablation temperature threshold reached (without reaching the maximum temperature threshold in off-target zones), the laser power was increased to 90% maximum power output for maximal ablation in 3-minute intervals. The final ablation zone was confirmed with MRI thermometry.

There were no complications. The patient was discharged the following day on a course of dexamethasone with steroid taper over 2 weeks. T1-weighted MRI with contrast on postoperative day 1 showed subtotal ablation of 70% of the pre-treatment volume (**Figure 5D**). Follow-up MRI imaging showed tumor recurrence at 9-week post-LITT (**Figure 5E**). The patient died 10 months following the procedure.

We present this case to illustrate how a subtotal ablation <80% may not be sufficient to confer a clinical benefit.

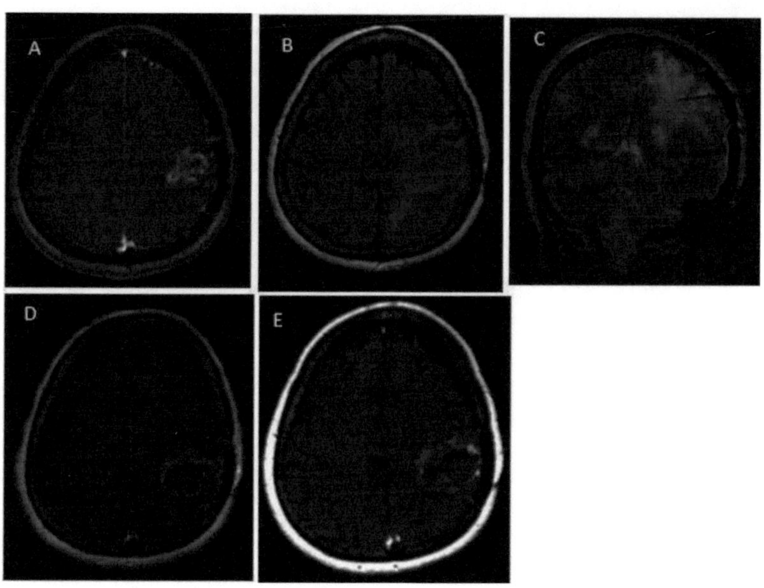

Figure 5.
A 58-year-old female with left frontoparietal ring-enhancing lesion T1-weighted axial MRI with contrast suspicious for tumor recurrence (A) with surrounding peripheral edema on T2-weighted FLAIR sequence (B). Intraoperative sagittal T2-weighted MRI showing correct positioning of the laser probe to the lesion (C). Postoperative day 1 of axial T1-weighted MRI (D) demonstrates subtotal (~70%) thermal ablation of the lesion. Follow-up T1-weighted MRI with contrast approximately 9-week post-LITT demonstrates tumor progression (E).

4. Clinical outcomes

The first case series reporting the use of LITT in gliomas were published in 1990 by Sugiyama et al., which described the successful total ablation of five deep-seated gliomas [37]. The advent of MRI thermography and the Visualase and NeuroBlate systems enabled institutional centers to publish data on larger case series over the past decade. These initial experiences provide valuable evidence supporting the safety and efficacy of LITT in select patient. In **Table 1** we present a comprehensive review of the literature of studies evaluating clinical outcomes in patients treated with LITT for either newly diagnosed or recurrent GBM tumors. To accurately represent the current use of LITT, only studies that included the use of real-time MR thermography are included in our review.

Abbreviations: M, male; F, female; NR, not reported; LITT, laser interstitial thermal therapy; STA, subtotal ablation; SupA, supra-ablation

5. Discussion

5.1 Current role of LITT in neurosurgery

The use of laser-based ablation technology in neurosurgery began with the treatment of movement disorders, chronic pain syndromes, and epilepsy. Technological advances over the past two decades in laser interstitial thermal therapy delivery platforms and real-time MR thermal imaging of tissue ablation dynamics have made LITT a viable minimally invasive therapy for a variety of intracranial and spinal lesions, including metastases, epileptogenic foci, radiation necrosis, dural-based lesions, and gliomas.

The advantage of LITT in treating gliomas includes:

1. Achieving cytoreduction in poor open surgical candidates: because laser light is delivered through a 1–3-mm diameter laser probe inserted through a single burr hole and dural opening, LITT reduces the risk of morbidity associated with craniotomy for surgical resection. This is especially relevant in GBM patients as the risk of neurological morbidity and poor wound healing or infection increases with repeat craniotomies and radiation therapy. The ability to tightly control the ablation zone using real-time MR thermography means that LITT is well suited for treatment of lesions in deep-seated locations or near critical structures.

2. Shorter procedure time and quicker recovery: the small incision required may result in fewer wound-healing complications, particularly in patients with impaired wound healing due to prior craniotomies or radiation therapy. Finally, a minimally invasive approach enables a quicker recovery and transition to continue chemotherapy or initiate another adjuvant therapy [26, 39].

3. The use of non-ionizing radiation: unlike ionizing radiation therapy, LITT thermal therapy can be used repeatedly without the risk of radiation necrosis [9]. Moreover, LITT can be used as a salvage therapy in treatment refractory tumors and may avoid increased risk of secondary malignancy-associated ionizing radiation [18].

4. Treatment of lesions that are inaccessible via open surgery: gliomas located in deep or eloquent regions of the brain (e.g., insula, thalamus, corpus callosum)

Reference	# Cases	Newly-diagnosed or recurrent GBM lesions	Age, Gender	Location of lesion	LITT system used, Extent of ablation	Mean/median Recurrence-free survival; Overall survival
Schwartzmaier et al. 2005 [29]	2	Recurrent	47 M 67 M	1 Temporal 1 Parietooccipital	1064 nm laser, STA	1 recurrence; 13-16 months
Schwartzmaier et al. 2006 [30]	16	Recurrent	Median age 62, range 44-69, 10 men, 6 women	3 Frontal 1 Frontoparietal 1 Frontotemporal 1 Temporal 1 Parietal 3 Parietooccipital 1 Corpus callosum 1 Parasagittal	1064 nm laser; NR	6.9 months; NR
Carpentier et al. 2012 [26]	4	Recurrent	40-58 years, 3 men, 1 woman	1 temporo-polar 1 corpus callosum 1 frontal 1 temporal	Visualase; SupA of 1 mm diameter or more	1.25 months; 10 months
Jethwa et al 2012 [19]	4	Newly-diagnosed	Media n 60 years, range 56-81	right frontal right frontal left temporal right midbrain	Visualase, NR	NR; NR
Hawasli et al., 2013 [31]	6	Newly-diagnosed	Media n 50 years, range 34-78, 6 men, 2 women	thalamus left thalamus basal ganglia left thalamus right corpus callosum thalamus	Neuroblate; median 90.3% ablation	Recurrence in 3 of 6 patients at median 3.2 months (range 2.5-15 months); 3 of 6 patients alive at last follow-up, 3 of 6 patients died at median 1.7 months
Sloan et al. 2013 [27]	10	Recurrent	Media n 54 years, range 34-69. 8 men, 2 women	2 temporal 1 temporoparietal 1 temporooccipital 3 parietal 3 frontal	NR	10.5 months;
Mohammadi et al. 2014 [32]	24	Recurrent (14) and new (10) lesions	Media n age 56 (range 19-79), 38% female	15 tumors in frontal lobe, 7 in thalamic region, 5 parietal, 5 temporal, 2 insular, 1 corpus callosum.	Neuroblate; Median ablation volume at yellow line: 98%, at blue line: 91% (includes non-GBM tumors included in study)	5.1 months; 68% survival at 1 year
Thomas et al. 2016 [33]	21	Recurrent (13) and new (8) lesions	Mean age 49 years	8 in eloquent regions (62%): 3 in motor cortex, 3 in speech, 1 temporal, 2 splenium, 2 cingulate, 2 insular	NeuroBlate; NR	5 months; 7 months

Reference	# Cases	Newly-diagnosed or recurrent GBM lesions	Age, Gender	Location of lesion	LITT system used, Extent of ablation	Mean/median Recurrence-free survival; Overall survival
Shah et al., 2016 [34]	7	Newly-diagnosed	Mean age 59, 3 male, 4 female	1 splenium 1 orbitofrontal 1 parieto- occipital 1 post. Cingulate 1. precuneus 1 Genu	Visualase; mean 98.5%	14.3 months; 6 of 7 patients alive at last follow-up, 1 death at 14 months
Schroeder et al. 2014 [35]	5	Newly-diagnosed	Mean age 47		94%	11.5 months; NR
Kamath et al. 2019 [36]	54	Recurrent (41) and Newly-diagnosed (17)	Mean age 59 years	14 frontal 8 temporal 9 parietal 1 occipital 4 pareito-occipital 4 temporo-parietal 8 corpus callosum 2 insular 8 thalamic	Neuroblate; 93.2% (yellow boundary), 88.0% (blue boundary)	6.6 months; 11.5 months

Abbreviations: M, male; F, female; NR, not reported; LITT, laser interstitial thermal therapy; STA, subtotal ablation; SupA, supra-ablation.

Table 1.
Literature review of case series describing LITT for GBM (adapted from: [9, 38]).

may increase open surgical risk to a degree that patients only receive stereotactic needle biopsy and adjuvant chemoradiation, thus losing the survival benefit associated with aggressive cytoreduction. Because LITT is delivered through a thin laser probe, lesions that are typically considered "surgically inaccessible" can now be treated with reduced risk of neurological morbidity [39].

The use of LITT for gliomas was initially limited to treating recurrences that failed conventional first-line therapies (i.e., surgical resection and adjuvant chemoradiation). Recently, LITT has been applied as a primary treatment for newly-diagnosed gliomas. Preliminary institutional experiences report local control and overall survival times of several months—over 1 year.

Patient selection is of critical importance in ensuring safe and effective use of LITT. To summarize, lesions should be <3 cm in diameter, in a region that can be accessed via a linear laser catheter trajectory without injury to critical structures and in patients who are able to tolerate a minimally invasive surgical procedure under anesthesia. In addition, the lesion should have identifiable margins such that at least 80% of the target area can be feasibly ablated with a roughly spherical ablation zone.

5.2 Limitations of LITT

The increasing use of LITT has revealed it to be an overall safe, well-tolerated procedure. The most common adverse events associated with the procedure include:

1. Intracranial hemorrhage: despite the use of neuronavigation and stereotaxy for trajectory planning, the laser probe may be malpositioned, resulting in injury to vessels and bleeding [40]. Estimates of overall rates of accurate implantation range from 85.7 to over 95%, with only three reported cases of resulting intracranial hemorrhage resulting from malpositioning [19, 40]. The risk of

hemorrhage may be reduced by obtaining a computed-tomography angiography (CTA) showing the location of critical vessels to avoid during laser trajectory planning.

2. Transient neurological deficit: neurological deficits such as weakness, hemianopsia, seizures, and dysphagia are often attributed to direct thermal injury to functional brain areas or cerebral edema. Estimates of transient neurological deficits have been reported to occur in 13–15% of patients [19, 40]. Permanent neurological morbidity is less common (5.6% of cases according to a recent literature review) [40]. Cerebral edema is frequently observed in the immediate postoperative period following LITT. A recent volumetric and time-course analysis found that edema volume has been shown to increase on average 41.5% immediately postoperatively, followed by a gradual decline resulting on average an 80.9% decrease in preoperative edema volume [28]. Although cerebral edema is common, it is unlikely to cause permanent neurological deficits and may be controlled with a course of steroids. Treatment of large (>3cm) lesions, use of multiple laser probes, or use of multiple laser trajectories is associated with a higher risk of significant cerebral edema [41].

Less common (<5% of all cases) complications include permanent neurological deficit, infection (e.g., ventriculitis, meningitis, or brain abscess), deep venous thrombosis, diabetes insipidus, hyponatremia, and intracranial hypertension. There is one reported case of gliosarcoma tumor seeding along the laser probe tract [27]. Finally, there are only two recorded deaths attributed to LITT in the literature, from postoperative meningitis and intracranial hemorrhage [32].

Our discussion of patient selection also reveals specific limitations of LITT. Multiple reviews cite a lesion size limit of 3 cm to reduce the chance of intracranial hypertension secondary to edema [18, 31]. As discussed previously, preoperative functional status, lesion accessibility by a laser trajectory, and anticipated extent of ablation are also factors that limit the use of LITT to particular lesions.

5.3 Future directions

In discussing complication rates, it is important to emphasize that LITT is a novel procedure, and so practitioners and institutions operate with a learning curve [18]. Recently, more institutional case series have proposed modifications to improve safety, for example, staging the treatment of larger (>3 cm) lesions to over multiple procedures to avoid morbidity or employing algorithms to optimize laser trajectory planning [42].

Along with further improvements in procedural safety, the future of LITT may lie in combination therapies to enhance tumor control and overall survival. Previous studies have shown that LITT induces a temporary increase in blood-brain barrier (BBB) permeability, which may offer a window of opportunity to deliver adjuvant chemotherapy more effectively [42, 43]. Another line of investigation is the use of gold nanoparticles, which may enhance tissue energy absorption and increase ablation efficacy [45].

Finally, future investigations will require prospective and randomized-controlled trials to evaluate the clinical outcomes of LITT compared to other therapies.

6. Conclusion

LITT is a novel adjuvant therapy for treatment of a wide variety of intracranial pathologies. In this chapter we review the evidence supporting the safety and efficacy of LITT as a primary or adjuvant treatment for glioblastoma. Thus far, LITT is a safe, minimally invasive approach to cytoreduction in patients with gliomas that are poor open surgical candidates.

Acknowledgements

The authors have no source of financial support to report.

Conflict of interest

Michael Ivan is a consultant for Medtronic. The other authors have no financial, personal, or institutional interests in any of the materials, devices, or drugs described in this article. Laser ablation is the only Food and Drug Administration-approved procedure for the ablation of soft tissue.

Author details

Alexa Semonche, Daniel Eichberg, Ashish Shah and Michael E. Ivan*
Department of Neurological Surgery, University of Miami Miller School of Medicine, Miami, United States

*Address all correspondence to: mivan@med.miami.edu

References

[1] Ostrom QT, Gittleman H, Farah P, Ondracek A, et al. CBTRUS statistical United States in 2006–2010. Neuro-Oncology. 2013;**15** Suppl 2:ii1-i56. DOI: 10.1093/neuonc/not151

[2] Stupp R, Hegi ME, Mason WP, Van den Bent MJ, et al. Effects of radiotherapy with concomitant and adjuvant temozolomide versus radiotherapy alone on survival in glioblastoma in a randomised phase III study: 5-year analysis of the EORTC-NCIC trial. The Lancet Oncology. 2009; **10**(5):459-466. DOI: 10.1016/S1470-2045(09)70025-7

[3] Johnson DR, O'Neill BP. Glioblastoma survival in the United States before and during the temozolomide era. Journal of Neuro-Oncology. 2012;**107**(2):359-364. DOI: 10.1007/s11060-011-0749-4

[4] Yang P, Zhang W, Wang Y, Peng X, et al. IDH mutation and MGMT promoter methylation in glioblastoma: Results of a prospective registry. Oncotarget. 2015;**6**(38):40896-40906. DOI: 10.18632/oncotarget.5683

[5] Lamborn KR, Chang SM, Prados MD. Prognostic factors for survival of patients with glioblastoma: Recursive partitioning analysis. Neuro-Oncology. 2004;**6**(3):227-235. DOI: 10.1215/S1152851703000620

[6] Sanai N, Polley MY, McDermott MW, Parsa AT, Berger MS. An extent of resection threshold for newly diagnosed glioblastomas. Journal of Neurosurgery. 2011;**115**(1):3-8. DOI: 10.3171/2011.2.JNS10998

[7] Brown TJ, Brennan MC, Li M, Church EW, et al. Association of extent of resection with survival in glioblastoma: A systematic review and meta-analysis. JAMA Oncology. 2016; **2**(11):14560-11469

[8] Chaudhry NS, Shah AH, Ferraro N, Snelling BM, Bregy A, Madhavan K, et al. Predictors of long-term survival in patients with glioblastoma multiforme: Advancements from the last quarter century. Cancer Investigation. 2013; **31**(5):287-308. DOI: 10.3109/07357907.2013.789899

[9] Ivan ME, Mohammadi AM, De Deugd N, Reyes J, et al. Laser ablation of newly diagnosed malignant gliomas: A meta-analysis. Neurosurgery. 2016;**79** (Suppl 1):S17-S23. DOI: 10.1227/NEU.0000000000001446

[10] Oppenlander ME. An extent of resection threshold for recurrent glioblastoma and its risk for neurological morbidity. Journal of Neurosurgery. 2014;**120**(4):846-853

[11] Laws ER, Parney IF, Huang W, Anderson F, et al. Glioma outcomes I: Survival following surgery and prognostic factors for recently diagnosed malignant glioma: Data from the glioma outcomes project. Journal of Neurosurgery. 2003;**99**(3):467-473. DOI: 10.3171/jns.2003.99.3.0467

[12] Roh TH, Kang SG, Moon JH, Sung KS, et al. Survival benefit of lobectomy over gross-total resection without lobectomy in cases of glioblastoma in the noneloquent area: A retrospective study. Journal of Neurosurgery. 2019;**1**: 1-7. DOI: 10.3171/2018.12.JNS182558

[13] Pessina F, Navarria P, Cozzi L, Ascolese AM, Simonelli M, Santoro A, et al. Noninvasive MRI thermometry with the proton resonance frequency method: Study of susceptibility effects. Magnetic Resonance in Medicine. 1995; **34**:359-367

[14] Chang SM, Parney IF, McDermott M, Barker FG 2nd, Schmidt MH, Huang W, et al. Perioperative complications and

neurological outcomes of first and second craniotomies among patients enrolled in the glioma outcome project. Journal of Neurosurgery. 2003;**98**(6): 1175-1181

[15] Fazeny-Dörner B, Wenzel C, Veitl M, Piribauer M, Rössler K, Dieckmann K, et al. Survival and prognostic factors of patients with unresectable glioblastoma multiforme. Anti-Cancer Drugs. 2003;**14**:305-312

[16] McGirt MJ, Chaichana KL, Gathinji M, Attenello FJ, et al. Independent association of extent of resection with survival in patients with malignant brain astrocytoma. Journal of Neurosurgery. 2010;**110**(1):156-162. DOI: 10.3171/2008.4.17536

[17] Schober R, Bettag M, Sabel M, Ulrich F, Hessel S. Fine structure of zonal changes in experimental Nd:YAG laser-induced interstitial hyperthermia. Lasers in Surgery and Medicine. 1993; **13**(2):234-241

[18] Patel NV, Mian M, Stafford RJ, Nahed BV, et al. Laser interstitial thermal therapy technology, physics of magnetic resonance imaging, thermometry, and technical considerations for proper catheter placement during magnetic resonance imaging–guided laser interstitial thermal therapy. Neurosurgery. 2016;**79** (Suppl 1):S8-S16

[19] Jethwa PR, Barrese JC, Gowda A, Shetty A, Danish SF. Magnetic resonance thermometry-guided laser-induced thermal therapy for intracranial neoplasms: Initial experience. Neurosurgery. 2012;**71**(1 Suppl Operative):133-144, 144-135). DOI: 10.1227/NEU.0b013e31826101d4

[20] Beck OJ. The use of the Nd-YAG and the CO_2 laser in neurosurgery. Neurosurgical Review. 1980;**3**:261-266

[21] Missios S, Bekelis K, Barnett GH. Renaissance of laser interstitial thermal ablation. Neurosurgical Focus. 2015; **38**(3):E13

[22] De Poorter J. Noninvasive MRI thermometry with the proton resonance frequency method: Study of susceptibility effects. Magnetic Resonance in Medicine. 1995;**34**(3): 359-367

[23] Rieke V, Butts Pauly K. MR thermometry. Journal of Magnetic Resonance Imaging. 2008;**27**(2):376-390

[24] Medvid R, Ruiz A, Komotar RJ, Jagid JR, et al. Current applications of MRI-guided laser interstitial thermal therapy in the treatment of brain neoplasms and epilepsy: A radiologic and neurosurgical overview. American Journal of Neuroradiology. 2015;**36**(11): 1998-2006. DOI: 10.3174/ajnr.A4362

[25] Langman C, Chung LK, Pelargos PE. Laser neurosurgery: A systematic analysis of magnetic resonance-guided laser interstitial thermal therapies. Journal of Clinical Neuroscience. 2017; **36**:20-26. DOI: 10.1016/j.jocn.2016.10.019

[26] Carpentier A, Chauvet D, Reina V, Beccaria K, et al. MR-guided laser-induced thermal therapy (LITT) for recurrent glioblastomas. Lasers in Surgery and Medicine. 2012;**44**(5): 361-368. DOI: 10.1002/lsm.22025

[27] Sloan AE, Ahluwalia MS, Valerio-Pascua J, Manjila S, et al. Results of the NeuroBlate system first-in-humans phase I clinical trial for recurrent glioblastoma: Clinical article. Journal of Neurosurgery. 2013;**118**(6):1202-1219. DOI: 10.3171/2013.1.JNS1291

[28] Eichberg DG, VanDenBerg R, Komotar RJ, Ivan ME. Quantitative volumetric analysis following magnetic resonance-guided laser interstitial thermal ablation of cerebellar metastases. World Neurosurgery. 2018; **110**:3755-3765

[29] Schwarzmaier HJ, Eickmeyer F, von Tempelhoff W, Fiedler V, et al. MR-guided laser irradiation of recurrent glioblastomas. Journal of Magnetic Resonance Imaging. 2005;**22**(6): 799-803. DOI: 10.1002/jmri.20446

[30] Schwarzmaier HJ, Eickmeyer F, von Tempelhoff W, Fiedler V, et al. MR-guided laser-induced interstitial thermotherapy of recurrent glioblastoma multiforme: Preliminary results in 16 patients. European Journal of Radiology. 2006;**59**(2):208-215. DOI: 10.1016/j.ejrad.2006.05.010

[31] Hawasli AH, Bagade S, Shimony JS, Miller-Thomas M, Leuthardt EC. Magnetic resonance imaging-guided focused laser interstitial thermal therapy for intracranial lesions: Single-institution series. Neurosurgery. 2013; **73**(6):1007-1017. DOI: 10.1227/NEU. 0000000000000144

[32] Mohammadi AM, Schroeder JL. Laser interstitial thermal therapy in treatment of brain tumors—The NeuroBlate system. Expert Review of Medical Devices. 2014;**11**(2):109-119. DOI: 10.1586/17434440.2014.882225

[33] Thomas JG, Rao G, Kew Y, Prabhu SS. Laser interstitial thermal therapy for newly diagnosed and recurrent glioblastoma. Neurosurgical Focus. 2016;**41**(4):E12

[34] Shah AH, Burks JD, Buttrick SS, et al. Laser interstitial thermal therapy as a primary treatment for deep inaccessible gliomas. Neurosurgery. 2018;**0**(0):1-10. DOI: 10.1093/neuros/ nyy238/5033265

[35] Schroeder JL, Missios S, Barnett GH, Mohammadi AM. Laser interstitial thermal therapy as a novel treatment modality for brain tumors in the thalamus and basal ganglia. Photonics and Lasers in Medicine. 2014;**3**(2): 151-118. DOI: 10.1515/plm-2013-0053

[36] Kamath AA, Friedman DD, Akbari SHA, Kim AH, et al. Glioblastoma treated with magnetic resonance imaging-guided laser interstitial thermal therapy: Safety, efficacy, and outcomes. Neurosurgery. 2019;**84**(4):836-843. DOI: 10.1093/neuros/nyy375

[37] Sugiyama K, Sakai T, Fujishima I, Ryu H et al. Stereotactic interstitial laser-hyperthermia using Nd-YAG laser. Stereotactic and Functional Neurosurgery. 1990;**54**:501-505

[38] Banerjee C, Snelling B, Berger MH, Shah A, Ivan ME, Komotar RJ. The role of magnetic resonance-guided laser ablation in neurooncology. Br J Neurosurg. 2015;**2**:192-6

[39] Diaz R, Ivan ME, Hanft S, Vanni S, et al. Laser interstitial thermal therapy: Lighting the way to a new treatment option in neurosurgery. Neurosurgery. 2016;**79**(Suppl 1):S3-S7

[40] Pruitt R, Gamble A, Black K, Schulder M, et al. Complication avoidance in laser interstitial thermal therapy: Lessons learned. Journal of Neurosurgery. 2017;**126**:1238-1245

[41] Ashraf O, Patel NV, Hanft S, Danish SF. Laser-induced thermal therapy in neuro-oncology: A review. World Neurosurgery. 2018;**112**:166-177. DOI: 10.1016/j.wneu.2018.01.123

[42] Li K, Vakharia VN, Sparks R, Franca LGS, et al. Optimizing trajectories for cranial laser interstitial thermal therapy using computer-assisted planning: A machine learning approach. Neurotherapeutics. 2019;**16**(1):182-191

[43] Sabel M, Rommel F, Kondakci M, Gorol M, Willers R, Bilzer T. Locoregional opening of the rodent blood-brain barrier for paclitaxel using Nd:YAG laser-induced thermo therapy: A new concept of adjuvant glioma therapy? Lasers in Surgery and Medicine. 2003;**33**(2):75-80

[44] Leuthardt EC, Duan C, Kim MJ, et al. Hyperthermic laser ablation of recurrent glioblastoma leads to temporary disruption of the peritumoral blood brain barrier. PLoS One. 2016; **11**(2):e0148613

[45] Baek SK, Makkouk AR, Krasieva T, Sun CH, et al. Photothermal treatment of glioma; an in vitro study of macrophage mediated delivery of gold nanoparticles. Journal of Neuro-Oncology. 2011;**104**:439-448

Section 6

Chemo/Immunotherapies for CNS Tumors

Chapter 11

Neoplastic Brain, Glioblastoma, and Immunotherapy

Annabelle Trojan, Heliodor Kasprzak, Oscar Gutierrez, Pedro Penagos, Ignacio Briceno, Heber O. Siachoque, Donald D. Anthony, Alvaro Alvarez and Jerzy Trojan

Abstract

IGF-I, insulin-like growth factor 1, is present in normal fetal/neonatal brain development and reappears in the mature brain participating in the development of malignant tumor, glioblastoma multiforme. Targeting the IGF-I system has emerged as a useful method to reduce glial malignant development. Downregulation in the expression of IGF-I using antigene anti-IGF-I technology (antisense, AS, and triple helix, TH) applied in glioma cell culture established from glioblastoma biopsies induces the expression of B7 and MHC-I antigens in transfected cells (immunogenicity). The transfected cancer cells, "vaccines," after subcutaneous injection, initiated an immune response mediated by T CD8+ lymphocytes, followed by tumor regression (immunotherapy). The median survival of patients treated by surgery followed by radiotherapy and immunotherapy was 21–24 months. On the other side, the experimental work has demonstrated that IGF-I AS or TH transfected tumor cells fused with activated dendritic cells, DC, showing more striking immunogenic character. Using IGF-I TH/DC "vaccination," the efficiency in suppressing rat glioma tumors is not only relatively higher than that obtained using IGF-I TH cells but is also more rapid.

Keywords: brain neoplastic development, glioblastoma, IGF-I, antisense, triple helix, immunogene therapy, cell hybridomas, dendritic cells, CD8

1. Introduction

There is a convergence between onto-genesis and onco-genesisgenesis and the same specific oncoproteins like alpha-fetoprotein (AFP) or growth factors, such as IGF and TGF-beta, are present in embryo/fetal tissues and in neoplastic developing tissues and particularly in the central nervous system (CNS). As far as AFP and IGF-I are considered, there is an important remarque: the first antigen is present in both neural and glial developing and cancerous cells, whereas the second one is only present in glial developing and tumoral cells. This striking difference has oriented our studies toward the most malignant brain tumor expressing IGF-I gene: glioblastoma.

In this chapter, we have described our scientific approach coming from the analysis of neoplastic CNS development conducted to glioblastoma malignancy up to the establishment of immunogene therapy of this tumor: the first cancer immunogene therapy. The strategy of therapy consisted of blocking IGF-I synthesis in cancer cells inducing apoptotic and immunogenic phenomena. Both phenomena, related to the arrest of IGF-I expression in neoplastic glial cells, were used to prepare antitumor cell vaccines for therapy of glioblastoma. Successful clinical results were obtained in USA, EU, and China and the therapy is introduced in Colombia (Wikipedia—Gene therapy, History 1990s–2010s).

2. Neoplastic brain

To understand the morphology of CNS neoplastic development, the model of mouse teratocarcinoma derived from PCC3 and PCC4 embryonal carcinoma cell lines was investigated. Thanks to this unique model reproducing "caricatural" development of the normal CNS, after examining histologic and electron microscopy sections, the different stages of abnormal nervous tissue histogenesis [1–4] were established as follows: 1. undifferentiated carcino-embryonic structures; 2. medulloepithelial structures (composed of a mixture of ectoblastic and neuroectoblastic components); 3. neuroblastic structures; and 4. neuroepithelial structures. The final differentiation was the encephaloid tissue. These results were confirmed by studying the localization of oncoproteins as alpha-fetoprotein (AFP), serum-albumin (SA), and IGF-I directly included in normal and neoplastic histogenesis, the last using teratocarcinoma model [3, 5–8].

As to the application of these observations in the pathology of human central nervous system (CNS) tumors, the model of mouse teratocarcinomas, containing neuroglial structures [3, 6, 9, 10] (described in the first studies of Stevens and then by his followers during almost 40 years of investigations [11–20]), should be useful as well in understanding human embryonic tumors of the CNS, which are able to differentiate into both neuronal and glial lineages [1, 10, 21–23], as in future gene therapies, including CNS malignant tumors [24–27].

3. IGF-I

In 1992, Trojan and his coworkers demonstrated that another oncodevelopmental antigen, an insulin like-growth factor, IGF-I [28–32], is present in glioma cells but absent in neuroblastoma cells [33]. Using the teratocarcinoma model, Trojan and his coworkers showed that neoplastic neuroblastic cells express IGF-II [34]. These observations permitted to study separately, using IGF-I and IGF-II as the oncoprotein markers, different tumors, especially glial and neural tumors [28–31, 35–40].

Comparative studies of the presence of AFP, IGF-I, and IGF-II in neoplastic cells [3, 33, 40–49] have demonstrated that IGF-I constitutes an essential target for genetic testing and therapy purpose. IGF-I, similar to AFP, is involved in tissue development and differentiation, especially in the development of the nervous system [6, 50, 51] as a mediator of growth hormone and glucose metabolism and acting locally with autocrine/paracrine, with a predominant role compared to other growth factors [29, 39, 51–55]. IGF-I is currently considered as one of the most important growth factors related to normal and neoplastic differentiation, and its overproduction is considered to be a participating factor in cancer development [32, 54, 56–58] (**Figure 3**). IGF-I reconstitutes the first step of the following signal transduction pathway: IRS/PI3K-PKC/PDK1/AKT-Bcl2/GSK3/GS [59, 60]. The elements of the said IGF-I-related transduction pathway were also considered as targets for diagnostic and therapeutic purposes [51, 59, 61–70].

Considering the IGF-1 gene, an overexpression of this gene in mature tissues is a sign of neoplastic processes, especially brain tumors [40]. IGF-I becomes useful in the molecular diagnosis of neonatal CNS malformations and tumors [9, 21, 38, 51, 71, 72]. Diagnosis and treatment should logically be related, at first using IGF-I gene testing for diagnosis [73–75] and then targeting IGF-I gene through special therapy, such as cancer gene therapy, especially therapy of gliomas [40, 76–79].

4. Gene therapy

4.1 Introduction

IGF-I and -II are expressed at high levels in nervous system–derived tumors, for example, astrocytomas and meningiomas [37, 44, 80]. In contrast, the block of IGF-I synthesis in these tumors induces apoptotic and immunogenic phenomena [81].

Our experimental approach of gene therapy has centered on the comparative use of IGF-I RNA antisense and IGF-I RNA–DNA triple helix [82, 83], to stop the translation and transcription of the IGF-I gene, respectively. Triple helix strategy [84, 85] and antisense strategy [86–88] have been applied successfully to a growing number of genes in cultured cells. However, the antisense approach has sometimes been not completely efficient due probably to insufficient antisense RNA levels [89].

We have applied the antisense strategy by employing a self-amplifying episomal vector that replicates to high copy numbers extrachromosomally [33]. The utility of episome-based expression vectors for the effective inhibition of cellular RNA expression has been subsequently confirmed by others [90]. C6 rat glioma cells expressed MHC-I [91, 92] and B7 [55, 93, 94] antigens when transfected with vectors producing IGF-I antisense RNA (IGF-I AS) or inducing IGF-I triple helix RNA-DNA (IGF-I TH) [95, 96]. IGF-I AS or IGF-I TH blockade of IGF-I syntheses changes the phenotype of transfected CNS-1 and PCC-4 cells. Moreover, it was demonstrated that transfected C6 cells become pro-apoptotic [96]. The AS and TH cells lost tumorigenicity and were able to induce a T-cell–mediated immune response in syngeneic animals against both themselves and the nontransfected tumorigenic parental cells [34, 40, 82, 97]. The experiment described here has permitted us to prepare human "vaccine" for a Phase 1 clinical trial.

4.2 Material and methods

Cell culture. The CNS-1 cell line was offered by the Dartmouth Medical School, Hanover, NH, USA (Dr W. Hickey) and then cultivated in the Laboratory of INSERM, Salpetriere Hospital, Paris (Dr M. Sanson). The PCC-4 cell line was provided by Institut Pasteur, Paris (Dr J.F. Nicolas). The cell lines were cultivated as described earlier [97]. Primary cell cultures of human glioma derived from tumors of glioblastoma multiforme patients were established (Clinical Laboratory of Collegium Medicum, UJ University, and School of Medicine, CWRU) according to the technique described earlier [96, 98–100] (**Figure 1**).

Plasmids. The vector pMT-EP [6, 26] was described earlier [33] (**Figure 2**). IGF-I "antisense" and "triple helix" technology was used to construct episome-based plasmids expressing IGF-I RNA antisense, pMT-anti IGF-I [26], or IGF-I triple helix–inducing vector, pMT-AG TH [33, 82]. The vector pMT-EP containing cDNA expressing IGF-II antisense RNA as insert was used in control experiments [34]. In parallel, using the vector pMT-EP, the vectors expressing MHC-I and B7, as well as vectors "antisense" MHC-I and B7, were prepared [96].

Transfection. The FuGENE 6 Transfection Reagent (Boehringer Mannheim) was used. Hygromycin B (Boehringer Mannheim) at a concentration of 0.05 mg/ml was added 48 h after transfection to select for transfected cells.

Northern blot. The content of IGF-I antisense RNA was determined in 50% confluent cell cultures. Northern blot and hybridizations were done according to Maniatis [98]; the 770 bp human IGF-I cDNA and 500 bp rat IGF-I cDNA were used as probes (**Figure 3**).

Flow cytometric analysis. Cells were incubated (30 min, 40°C) with saturated amounts of monoclonal antibodies, rat or human MHC-I (HLA ABC), MHC- II, CD80, and CD86 (Becton Dickinson Pharmingen). Cells were collected (10.000 events per sample) in FACScan BD cytometer (**Figure 4**).

Ex vivo generation of dendritic cells. Two techniques for the generation of dendritic cells were used:

1. CD34+ hematopoietic progenitor cells were isolated, using the MACS CD34 Cell Isolation Kit, and functional DC cells were generated by culturing CD34+ cells in the presence of GM-CSF, TNFalpha, and SCF for 10 days [101].

2. Monocytes were isolated, using MACS CD14 MicroBeads. Monocytes were cultured in the presence of GM-CSF and IL-4 generated activated DCs [102].

Hybridomas of transfected cells with dendritic cells. The fusion of dendritic cells with tumor transfected cells was obtained as follows [103]: activated DCs (one of the two techniques mentioned above) were fusioned with tumo IGF-I antisense or triple helix transfected cells using polyethylene glycol—PEG [104]. Fusions were carried out with 40% PEG in PBS without Ca^{2+} and Mg^{2+}.

In vivo experiment. For the determination of tumorigenicity, 5 x 10^6 rat CNS-1 cells were injected subcutaneously into Lewis rats. Experimental sets were injected with: (a) parental cells; (b) IGF-I "triple helix" transfected cells expressing MHC-I; and (c) IGF-I "triple helix" transfected cells expressing both MHC-I and B7 molecules.

4.3 Results and discussion

Northern blot analysis is shown in **Figure 3**. The RNA of nontransfected cells is distributed in 7.5 and 1.0 kb bands. The RNA of anti-IGF-I transfected cells shows

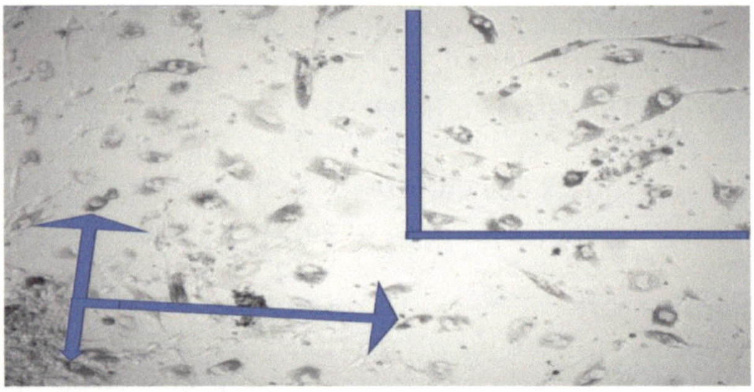

Figure 1.
In vitro *staining of IGF-1 biomarker human in human glioma cell culture. The tissue and cells are stained for IGF-1 using anti-IGF-1 antibodies applied in immunoperoxidase technique. Nine days of culture established from human glioblastoma biopsy. (left down) Note the cells (head arrows) proliferating from compact tissue of biopsy (left down corner) (200×); (right up) Note the cluster of cells showing dark cytoplasm of staining (400×).*

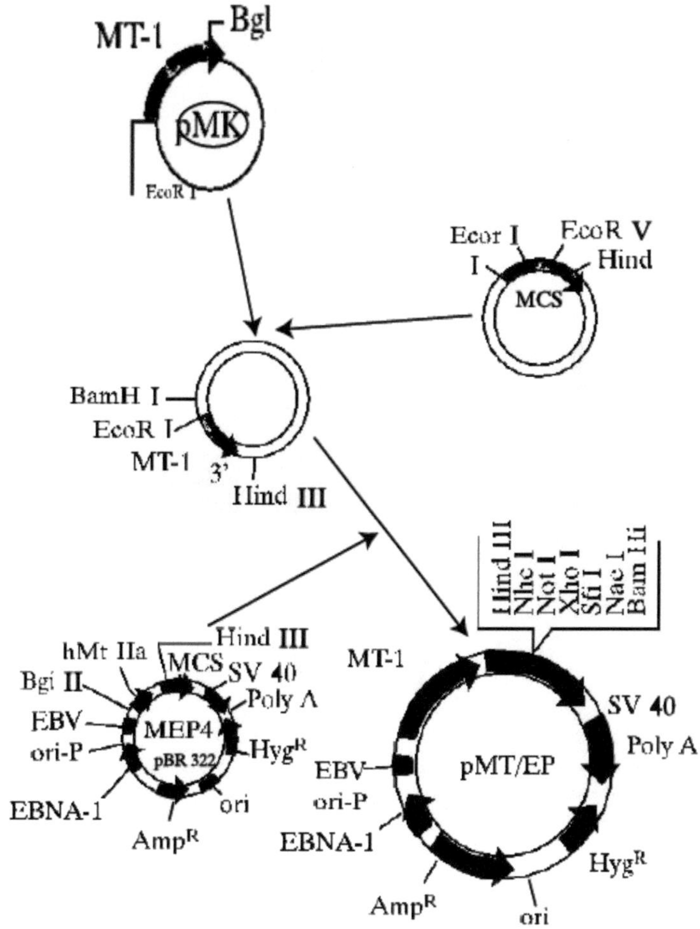

Figure 2.
Diagrammatic representation of steps employed to construct the episomal vector pMT/EP used for preparation of IGF-I antisense and triple helix expression vectors.

only an abundant 1.0 kb band. The transfected cultures were positively stained either for both MHC-I and B7 antigens (in 60% of cloned lines) or for MHC-I (only in 40% of cloned lines). The data show that transfection with "antisense" and "triple helix" vectors induced a significant increase in the expression of MHC-I and B7 (**Table 1**). The "triple helix" rat and human cells as compared to "antisense" cells showed slightly higher expression of MHC-I or B7. As to apoptosis, it was detected in approximately 70% of the IGF-I antisense and triple helix transfected cells. As expected, the hybridomas of IGF-I triple helix or IGF-I antisense cells fused to activated dendritic cells, IGF-I TH//DC or IGF-I AS//DC, were negative for IGF-I. The most important observations concerned the increased level of MHC-I and MHC-II, and especially the presence of B7 in IGF-I TH//DC and IGF-I AS//DC hybridomas (**Table 1**). No tumors were observed in animals injected subcutaneously with CNS-1 cells transfected with IGF-I "triple helix" vector, expressing both MHC-I and B7.

The simultaneous increase in the presence and role of B7 and MHC-I antigens in the induction of T-cell immunity against tumors has been extensively investigated [33, 93, 94]. The injection of IGF-I antisense and triple helix transfected cells presenting both MHC-I and B7 molecules stopped effectively the established rat glioma tumors. This was not the case for cells expressing MHC-I only (**Table 1**). Injection of cell hybridomas composed of IGF-I antisense cells and activated dendritic cells (IGF-I AS//DC) into tumor-bearing animals suppressed the established glioma

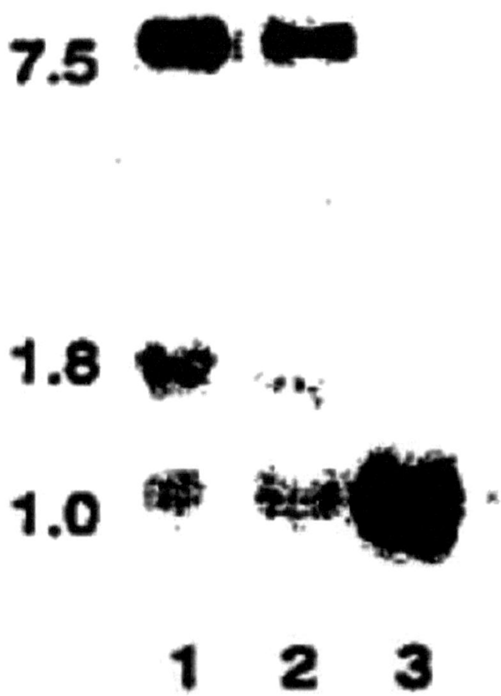

Figure 3.
Antisense transcripts in cultured C6 glioma cells. Molecular sizes of IGF-I transcripts are shown in kilobases. Lane 1, parental nontransfected C6 glial cells exposed to serum-free medium. Lanes 2 and 3, transfected C6 glioma cells incubated in serum-free medium in the absence (lane 2) or presence (lane 3) of ZnSO4. For lanes 2 and 3, nick-translated rat IGF-I cDNA was used.

tumors in 4/6 cases of Lewis rats. The experience was repeated using cell hybridomas composed of IGF-I triple helix cells and activated dendritic cells (IGF-I TH// DC). In this case, the subcutaneous injection of the hybridomas into glioma-bearing animals completely suppressed tumors in a ratio 6/6.

MHC-I molecules were in general not sufficient to stimulate T-cell response. In the absence of B7 molecule, MHC-peptide complexes could selectively inactivate T cells [105]. B7 molecules bound to the counter-receptor CD28 and/or CTLA4 expressed on the T cells [9, 106, 107]; enhancement in B7 costimulation through a cAMP mechanism linked to tyrosine kinase of the CD28 receptor has been previously reported [108]. The mechanism of signaling (tyrosine kinase activates IRS-1, and then IRS-1 activates PI3K [109, 110]) could be considered in the cytokine induced B7-1 expression demonstrated in fetal human microglia in culture [111].

Using CNS-1 glioma, we have confirmed the relation between the immunogenicity and apoptosis found in IGF-I transfected cells [96]. The phenotypic modifications due to apoptosis may explain the recognition of the transfected cells by the immune system like tumor-specific immunity mediated by CD8+ T described earlier by us [40, 98]. Apoptotic cells, in the context of MHC-I, are recognized by dendritic cells activating lymphocytes T-CD8 [112, 113]. B7 molecules can be included in this mechanism, because both MHC-I and B7 molecules are necessary for T-cell activation [4, 55, 79, 93, 114–116]. Considering the role of dendritic cells, the presented results may be useful in introducing IGF-I TH//DC "vaccines" into cellular therapy of human gliomas. Moreover, the obtained results of tumor suppression are in agreement with the immunogenic character of used "vaccines"—the efficiency of "vaccines" being related to the expression level of MHC-I, -II, and B7 (**Table 1**) [97, 117–119].

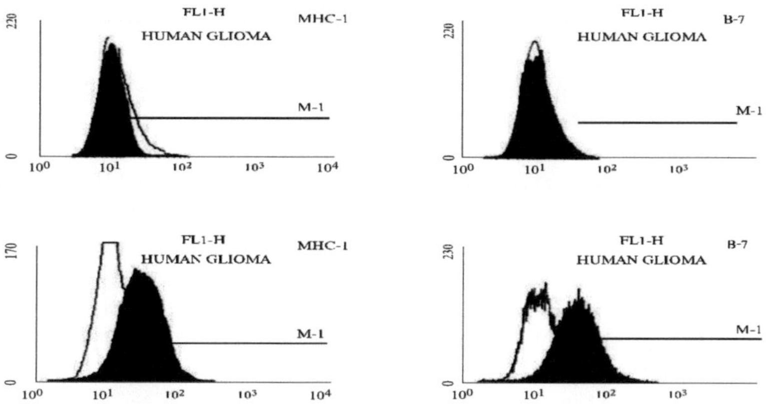

Figure 4.
Flow cytometry analysis (FACScan Becton Dickinson). Expression of MHC-I (left) and B7 (right) in primary human glioblastoma cell line. Upper panels: non transfected cells; lower panels: transfected cells (upregulation of MHC-I and B7).

Cells	Rat glioma CNS-1 cells		
	MHC-I	MHC-II	B7
NT	<0.5	<0.5	<0.5
IGF-I AS	12.3	<0.5	18.1
IGF-I TH	14.6	<0.5	19.6
IGF-I AS/IGF-I TH	12.8	<0.5	18.4
IGF-I AS/MHC-I AS/B7 AS	1.0	<0.5	1.0
IGF-I TH/MHC-I AS/B7 AS	1.0	<0.5	1.0
IGF-I AS//DC	14.7	3.8	19.3
IGF-ITH//DC	16.9	4.2	21.9

NT: parental nontransfected cells; pMT-EP: cells transfected with "empty vector"; IGF-I AS or IGF-II AS: cells transfected with IGF-I or IGF-II antisense expression vector; IGF-I TH: cells transfected with IGF-I triple helix expression vector; IGF-I AS/IGF-I TH: cotransfection with antisense and triple helix vectors; IGF-I AS/MHC-I AS/B7 AS, and IGF-I TH/MHC-I AS/B7 AS: triple cotransfection with IGF-I antisense or triple helix, MHC-I antisense and B7 antisense expression vectors; IGF-I TH//DC or IGF-I AS//DC: cells transfected with IGF-I antisense or triple helix expression vectors, and fused to dendritic cells.
**The data of flow cytometry (the average of three experiments) are presented as percent change in value of fluorescence relative to fluorescence in control nontransfected cells (CC). The increase in MHC-I, -II, and B7 is significant at the $P < 0.01$ level (Wilcoxon's signed rank test).*

Table 1.
*Expression of MHC-I, MHC-II, and B7 in the cells of rat glioma.**

5. Clinical gene therapy

5.1 Methodology

Using radiotherapy and chemotherapy, the mortality of glioblastoma remains close to 100% and the median survival, using conventional therapy, is 9–14 months. Current pharmacology increases the survival to 15 and rarely to 18 months [120]. The etiology of glioma is still being investigated using molecular biology techniques [64]. New or proposed therapies are based either on immune treatment or on immuno-gene strategies [121]. The AS and TH technologies [84–87] have permitted us to establish new and successful immuno-gene therapy strategies targeting glioma's growth factors [40, 122]. Other technologies include those of potentially useful siRNA [123, 124] and miRNA (microRNA) [125]. The role of 21–23mer double-stranded RNA (siRNA) in the silencing of genes is strongly similar to that of the TH DNA mechanism, which also involves 23mer RNA [85]. Whether or not siRNA technology or miRNA knockdown will supplant the AS oligodeoxynucleotide approaches remains in question at this time [124, 126, 127]. The AS oligodeoxynucleotides reinforced by association with polycations (polyethyleneimine), polylysine, or cationic lipids (DOTMA, DOTAP) were also used for transfection of cells with plasmids encoding antisense RNA [128].

As to growth factors, historically, first IGF-I and its receptor and then TGF-beta were targeted in experimental preclinical studies [40, 57, 122, 129, 130] and then glycogen synthase, GS [51]. The absence of IGF-I, TGF-beta, and GS synthesis in "AS" transfected cells leads to a compensated increase in IGF-I-receptor [51] (relation between the signal transduction pathway of tyrosine kinase (IGF-I-R) and the induction of B7 [131]). Other growth factors such as EGF and VEGF, and their receptors, have also been investigated by AS technology in preclinical studies. The *in vitro* and *in vivo* results were similar to the results obtained with AS IGF-I technology [51, 130]. Thus IGF-I via IGF-I-R not only increases cell proliferation but also "supervises" mitogenic action of other growth factors (EGF, PDGF, etc.) by its autocrine-paracrine stimulation, becoming some kind of growth factor director. In clinical IGF-I antisense/triple helix immunotherapy, the cells used for "vaccination" were downregulated in IGF-I and presented both MHC-I and B7.1 molecules (**Figure 4**).

5.2 Results and discussion

The first clinical assay for human GBM using AS IGF-I approach was performed by Anthony et al. and by Trojan et al. [96, 100, 114]. After each of three AS IGF-I vaccinations, there was an increase in the percentage of CD8+ T cells in peripheral blood lymphocytes with a characteristic phenotype—switch

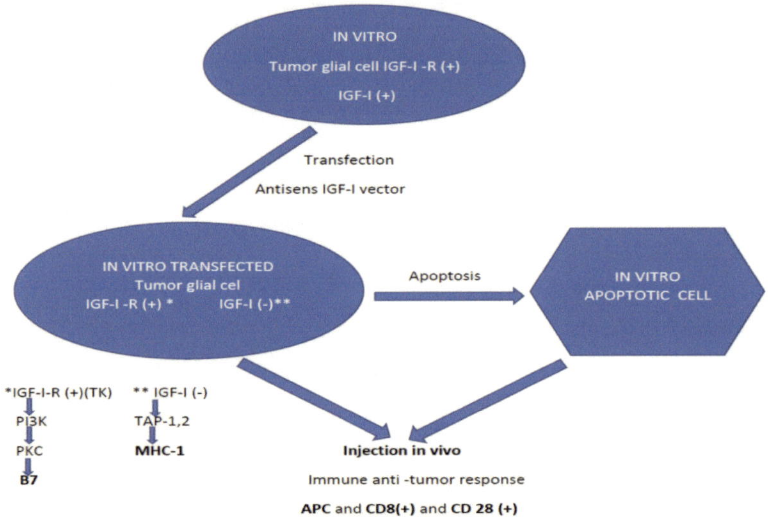

Figure 5.
Antisense immunotherapy. Example of antisense anti-IGF-I treatment of glial malignant tumor—glioblastoma. The schema of therapy shows transfected in vitro *brain tumor glial cells using a vector containing cDNA of IGF-I in antisense orientation. After transfection, the cells express IGF-I RNA antisense stopping the IGF-I synthesis characteristic for tumor cells. They become MHC-I [+] and B7 [+], and partially apoptotic. The transfected cells, together with apoptotic cells and APC cells induced* in vivo, *activate T lymphocytes (CTL CD8+CD28+). Abbreviations used in signal transduction pathway: TK (tyrosine kinase of growth factors receptor); PI3K (phosphatidylinositol 3 kinase); PKC (protein kinase C); TAP 1,2 (transporter associated with antigen processing antigen); APC (antigen presenting cell).*

CD8+CD11b+/CD8+CD11b– (**Figure 5**). In patients with GBM treated in Bromberg (NATO Science Programme—U.S.A./France/Poland), life from time of diagnosis to time of demise was 19 and 24 months.

Histopathologic examination of resected tumors showed peritumor necrosis and infiltration by lymphocytes CD8+ T and CD4+ T cells [100]. Moreover, we can underline, as described in our previous studies [51], that using anti-IGF-I approach without chemotherapy, median survival in GBM-treated patients has reached 19 months and has increased to more than 21 months (NATO Programme) when applied in combination with chemotherapy (temozolomide). The individualized therapy using IGF-I antigene treatment and pharmacology (temozolomide) has been applied in phase I/II trials [132].

In 2001, simultaneously with the first assay with AS IGF-I, Andrews et al. [133] treated 12 patients with recurrent glioblastoma and anaplastic astrocytoma using an antisense to IGF-I receptor, AS IGF-I-R, strategy. Histological analysis of tumors resected from patients with disease progression revealed lymphocytic infiltration and necrosis [133]. As new experimental therapies and efficient viral vectors expressing AS IGF-I-R are being developed, clinical trials using this approach will increase [66, 133, 134].

The approach of AS TGF-beta using an AS oligodeoxynucleotide, compound AP 12009, has given satisfactory results [135–137]. In another clinical AS TGF-beta study, a phase I clinical trial in grade IV astrocytoma (GBM) was performed using autologous tumor cells modified by an AS TGF-beta2 vector. There were indications of humoral and cellular immunity induced by the vaccine [138].

6. Conclusions

The clinical strategies of glioma treatment, using either inhibitors (i.e., imatinib and gefitinib) or antibodies (i.e., Avastin) targeting growth factors and their receptors [139–143], are currently focusing on antisense technology combined with pharmacological treatment.

The neuro-oncology research on glial cells focuses on the PI3K/AKT pathway becoming a potential target in antisense/triple helix strategy for the treatment of glioblastoma patients [59, 69]. The arrest of at least two links either IGF-I or TGF-beta or VEGF and GS of the pathway TK/PI3K/AKT/GSK3/GS [64] seems to be in line for a future clinical gene therapy trial strategy for treatment of GBM. The final result of this signal transduction pathway element inhibition is an immune response mediated *in vivo* by lymphocytes T CD8 and APC cells (**Figure 5**). But the near future in treating this group of disorders belongs to a combination of treatment [4, 42, 70, 79, 115, 130, 144–150]: classical surgery; radiotherapy with immunotherapy, including the use of dendritic cells pharmacologic therapy; growth factor inhibitors; and the use of the antisense/triple helix gene blockade approach targeting signal transduction pathway elements of cancer processes.

Conflict of interest

No conflict of interest.

Author details

Annabelle Trojan[1,2*], Heliodor Kasprzak[2,3], Oscar Gutierrez[4], Pedro Penagos[2,5], Ignacio Briceno[2,6], Heber O. Siachoque[7], Donald D. Anthony[8], Alvaro Alvarez[1] and Jerzy Trojan[2,9]

1 Faculty of Medicine, University of Cartagena, Cartagena de Indias, Colombia

2 ICGT—International Cancer Gene Therapy, Bogota, Colombia

3 Collegium Medicum, Department of Neurosurgery, UMK University, Bydgoszcz, Poland

4 Department of Neurosurgery, Kennedy Hospital, Bogota, Colombia

5 Department of Neurosurgery, INC—National Institute of Cancerology, Bogota, Colombia

6 Institute of Human Genetics, PUJ University, Bogota, Colombia

7 INS – National Institute of Health, Bogota, Colombia

8 School of Medicine, CWRU, Cleveland, OH, USA

9 INSERM, Cancer Centre, Villejuif, France

*Address all correspondence to: genetherapy@hotmail.fr

References

[1] Gaillard J, Caillaud JM, Maunoury R, et al. Expression of neuro-ectoblast in murine teratocarcinomas: Electron-microscopic and immunocytochemical studies, applications in embryology and in tumor pathology of central nervous system. (in French. Bulletin Institut Pasteur. 1984;**82**:335-385

[2] Trojan J, Gaillard J, Vedrenne C, et al. Localization of H blood group antigen in ectoblastic derivatives of murine teratocarcinoma. Tumour Biology. 1987;**8**:9-18

[3] Trojan J, Naval X, Johnson T, et al. Expression of serum albumin and of alphafetoprotein in murine normal and neoplastic primitive embryonic structures of teratocarcinoma. Molecular Reproduction and Development. 1995;**42**(4):369-378

[4] Castillo T, Trojan A, Noguera MC, et al. Epistemiologic experience in elaboration of molecular biology technology for immunogene therapy (in Spanish). Revista Cientifica. 2016;**2**(25). DOI: 10.14483/udistrital.jour.RC.2016.25.a6

[5] Trojan A, Aristizabal B, Jay LM, et al. Testing of IGF-I biomarker in an ethical context. Advances of Modern Oncology Research. 2016;**2**(4). DOI: 10.18282/amor:v2:i4.58

[6] Trojan J, Uriel J, Deugnier MA, Gaillard J. Immunocytochemical quantitative study of alphafetoprotein in normal and neoplastic neural development. Developmental Neuroscience. 1984;**6**:251-259

[7] François JC, Duc HT, Upegui-Gonzalez LC, et al. Alterations in tumorigenicity of embryonal carcinoma cells by IGF-I triple-helix induced changes in immunogenicity and apoptosis. Life Science. 2001;**68**(3):307-319

[8] Trojan J, Kasprzak H, Anthony D. How to stop glial neoplastic brain development: Antisense strategy. In: Bezerra MF, Alves CR, editors. Glioblastoma: Risk Factors, Diagnosis and Treatment Options. NY: Nova Science Publishers, Inc; 2012. pp. 1-14. ch. 6

[9] Harding BN, Golden JA. Developmental Neuropathology. Basel, Suiss: International Society of Neuropathology; 2004

[10] Dambska M, Wisniewski K. Normal and Pathologic Development of the Human Brain and Spinal Cord. London: Ed. John Libbey & Comp; 1999

[11] Stevens LC. Studies on transplantable testicular teratoma of strain 129 mice. Journal of National Cancer Institut. 1958;**20**:1257-1276

[12] Willis RA. Nervous tissue in teratomas. In: Minckler J, editor. Pathology of the Nervous System. Vol. 2. Hamburg: McGraw-Hill. pp. 1971, 1937-1943

[13] Damjanow I, Solter D, Serman D. Teratocarcinoma with the capacity for differentiation restricted to neuro-ectodermal tissue. Virchows Archives B: Zell Pathology. 1973;**13**:179-185

[14] Gaillard JA. Differentiation and organization in teratomas. In: Sherbert GV, editor. Neoplasia and Cell Differentiation. Basel: Karger. p. 1974

[15] Stevens LC, Varnum DS. The development of teratomas from part thenogenetically activated ovarian mouse eggs. Developmental Biology. 1974;**37**:369-380

[16] Gaillard JA. Experimental teratocarcinoma. Localisation of embryonal bodies inoculated into syngeneic mouse abdominal

cavity (in French). Bulletin Cancer. 1976;**63**:341-352

[17] De Armond SJ, Vandenberg SR, Herman MH. Neural differentiation in the OTT 60-50 mouse teratoma: Effects of intracerebral environment on the neural differentiation of embryoid bodies. Virchows Archives B: Zell Pathology. 1981;**393**:39-52

[18] Nogales FF Jr, Aguilar D. Neural tissues in human teratomas. In: Damjanov I, Knowles BB, Solter D, editors. The Human Teratomas. Clifton: Humana Press; 1983

[19] Trojan J, Gaillard JA, Uriel J. Localisation of alphafetoprotein in neuroepithelial derivatives of mouse teratocarcinoma (in French). Annales of Pathology. 1983;**3**:137-145

[20] Haugen OA, Taylor CR. Immunohistochemical studies of ovarian and testicular teratomas with antiserum to glial fibrillary acid protein. Acta Pathologica Microbiologica Scandinavia (Sect A). 1984;**92**:9-14

[21] Love S, Arie Perry A, Ironside J, Budka H. Greenfield's Neuropathology. 9th ed. NY: CRC Press; 2015

[22] Kleihues P, Luis DN, Scheithauer BW, et al. The WHO classification of tumors of the nervous system. Journal of Neuropathology & Experimental Neurology. 2002;**3**(61):215-225. DOI: 10.1093/jnen/61.3.215

[23] Benedetti E, Galzio R, D'Angelo B, et al. PPARs in human neuroepithelial tumors: PPAR ligands as anticancer therapies for the most common human neuroepithelial tumors. PPAR Research. 2010:401-427. DOI: 10.1155/2010/427401

[24] Walther W, Stein US. Gene Therapy of Cancer. Methods and Protocols. NY: Human Press; 2009

[25] Templeton NS. Gene and Cell Therapies. FL: CRC Press; 2009

[26] You Y. Targets in Gene Therapy. Vienna, Riyeka: InTech; 2011

[27] Lichtor T. Evolution of the Molecular Biology of Brain Tumors and The Therapeutic Implications. Vienna, Riyeka: InTech; 2013

[28] Daughaday WH, Hall K, Raben MS, et al. Somatomedin: Proposed designation for sulphation factor. Nature. 1972;**235**:107

[29] Froesch ER, Schmid C, Schwander J, Zapf J. Actions of insulin-like growth factors. Annual Review of Physiology. 1985;**47**:443-467

[30] Han VKM, Hill DJ. In: Shofield PN, editor. The Insulin-Like Growth Factors: Structure and Biological Functions. Oxford, England: Oxford University Press; 1992. pp. 178-121

[31] Baserga R, Sell C, Porcu P, Rubini M. The role of the IGF-I receptor in the growth and transformation of mammalian cells. Cell Proliferation. 1994;**27**:63-71

[32] Baserga R. Oncogenes and the strategy of growth factors. Cell. 1994;**79**:927-930

[33] Trojan J, Blossey BK, Johnson T, et al. Loss of tumorogenicity of rat glioblastoma directed by episome-based antisense cDNA transcription of insulin-like growth factor I. Proceedings of the National Academy of Sciences of the United States of America. 1992;**89**(11):4874-4878

[34] Trojan J, Johnson TR, Rudin SD, et al. Gene therapy of murine teratocarcinoma: Separate functions for insulin-like growth factors I and II in immunogenicity and differentiation. Proceedings of the National Academy of Sciences of the United States of America. 1994:6088-6092

[35] Sturm MA, Conover CA, Pham H, Rosenfeld RG. Insulin like growth factor receptors and binding proteins in rat neuroblastoma. Endocrinology. 1989;**124**:388-396

[36] Werther GA, Abate M, Hogg A, et al. Localisation of insulin like growth factor mRNA in rat brain by in situ hybridization—Relation to IGF-I receptor. Molecular Endocrinology. 1990;**4**:773-778

[37] Antoniades HN, Galanopoulis T, Nevile-Golden J, Maxwell M. Expression of insulin like growth factor I and II and their receptor mRNAs in primary human astrocytomas and meningiomas: In vivo studies using in situ hybridization and immunocytochemistry. International Journal of Cancer. 1992;**50**:215-222

[38] Zumkeller W, Westphal M. The IGF/IGFBP system in CNS malignancy. Molecular Pathology. 2001;**54**:227-229

[39] Baserga R. The insulin-like growth factor-I receptor as a target for cancer therapy. Expert Opinion on Therapeutic Targets. 2005;**9**:753-768

[40] Trojan J, Johnson T, Rudin S, et al. Treatment and prevention of rat glioblastoma by immugenic C6 cells expressing antisense insulin-like growth factor I RNA. Science. 1994;**259**:94-97

[41] Casper JT, Borella L, Sen L. Reactivity of human brain antiserum with neuroblastoma cells and nonreactivity with thymocytes and lymphoblasts. Cancer Research. 1977;**37**:1750-1758

[42] Trojan J, Pan YX, Wei MX, et al. Methodology for anti-gene anti-IGF-I therapy of malignant tumours. Chemotherapy Research and Practice. 2012. DOI: 10.1155/2012/721873

[43] Sandberg AC, Engberg C, Lake M, et al. The expression of insulin-like growth factor I and insulin-like growth factor II genes in the human fetal and adult brain and in glioma. Neuroscience Letters. 1988;**93**(1):114-119. DOI: 10.1016/0304-3940(88)90022-5

[44] Kiess W, Lee L, Graham DE, et al. Rat C6 glial cells synthesize insulin-like growth factor I (IGF-I) and express IGF-I receptors and IGF-II/mannose 6-phosphate receptors. Endocrinology. 1989;**124**(4):1727-1736. DOI: 10.1210/endo-124-4-1727

[45] Trojan J, Uriel J. Localisation of alphafeprotein (AFP) in murine teratocarcinoma. Biomedicine. 1981;**34**(3):140-146

[46] Guha A, Mukherjee J. Advances in the biology of astrocytomas. Current Opinion in Neurology. 2004;**17**(6):655-662. DOI: 10.1097/00019052-200412000-00004

[47] Ohgaki H, Dessen P, Jourde B, et al. Genetic pathways to glioblastoma: A population-based study. Cancer Research. 2004;**64**(19):6892-6899. DOI: 10.1158/0008-5472.CAN-04-1337

[48] Wrensch M, Rice T, Miike R, et al. Diagnostic, treatment, and demographic factors influencing survival in a population-based study of adult glioma patients in the San Francisco Bay Area. Neuro Oncology. 2006;**8**(1):12-26. DOI: 10.1215/S1522851705000268

[49] Hajeri-Germond M, Naval J, Trojan J. The uptake of alpha-foetoprotein by C-1300 mouse neuroblastoma cells. British Journal of Cancer. 1985;**51**: 791-797. DOI: 10.1038/bjc.1985.123

[50] Ostos H, Astaiza G, Garcia F, et al. Decreased incidence of defects of neural tube closure at the University Hospital of Neiva: Possible effect promotion of folic acid (in Spanish). Biomédica. 2000;**20**(1):18-24. DOI: 10.7705/biomedica.v20i1.1043

[51] Trojan J, Cloix JF, Ardourel MY, et al. Insulin-like growth factor type I biology and targeting in malignant gliomas. Neuroscience. 2007;**145**(3):795-811. DOI: 10.1016/j.neuroscience.2007.01.021

[52] Le Roith D, Bondy C, Yakar S, et al. The somatomedin hypothesis. Endocrinology Review. 2011;**22**(1): 53-74. DOI: 10.1210/edrv.22.1.0419

[53] Le Roith D. The insulin-like growth factor system. Experimental Diabesity Research. 2003;**4**(4):205-212. DOI: 10.1155/EDR.2003.205

[54] Adhami VM, Afaq F, Mukhtar H. Insulin-like growth factor-I axis as a pathway for cancer chemoprevention. Clinical Cancer Research. 2006;**12**(19):5611-5614. DOI: 10.1158/1078-0432.CCR-06-1564

[55] Chen H, Mester T, Raychaudhuri N, et al. Teprotumumab, an IGF-1R blocking monoclonal antibody inhibits TSH and IGF-1 action in fibrocytes. Journal of Clinical Endocrinology and Metabolism. 2014;**99**(9):E1635-E1640. DOI: 10.1210/jc.2014-1580

[56] Kooijman R. Regulation of apoptosis by insulin-like growth factor (IGF)-I. Cytokine Growth Factor Review. 2006;**17**(4):305-323. DOI: 10.1016/j.cytogfr.2006.02.002

[57] Pollak MN, Schernhammer ES, Hankinson SE. Insulin-like growth factors and neoplasia. Nature Review Cancer. 2004;**4**:505-518. DOI: 10.1038/nrc1387

[58] Kurmasheva RT, Houghton PJ. IGF-I mediated survival pathways in normal and malignant cells. Biochimica et Biophysica Acta. 2006;**1766**(1):1-22. DOI: 10.1016/j.bbcan.2006.05.003

[59] Beckner ME, Gobbel GT, Abounader R, et al. Glycolytic glioma cells with active glycogen synthase are sensitive to PTEN and inhibitors of PI3K and gluconeogenesis. Laboratory Investigation. 2005;**85**(12):1457-1470. DOI: 10.1038/labinvest.3700355

[60] Vignot S, Faivre S, Aguirre D, Raymond E. mTOR-targeted therapy of cancer with rapamycin derivatives. Annales Oncology. 2005;**16**(4):525-537. DOI: 10.1093/annonc/mdi113

[61] Schlingensiepen KH, Jaschinski F, Lang SA, et al. Transforming growth factor-beta 2 gene silencing with trabedersen (AP 12009) in pancreatic cancer. Cancer Science. 2011;**102**(6):1193-1200. DOI: 10.1111/j.1349-7006.2011.01917.x

[62] Trojan J, Anthony DD. Antisense strategies in therapy of gliomas. Current Signal Transduction Therapy. 2011;**6**(3):411-423. DOI: 10.2174/157436211797483895

[63] Patel S, Doble B, Woodgett JR. Glycogen synthase kinase-3 in insulin and Wnt signalling: A double-edged sword? Biochemical Society Transactions. 2004;**32**(5):803-808. DOI: 10.1042/BST0320803

[64] Jiang R, Mircean C, Shmulevich I, et al. Pathway alterations during glioma progression revealed by reverse phase protein lysate arrays. Proteomics. 2006;**6**(10):2964-2971. DOI: 10.1002/pmic.200500555

[65] Hutterer M, Gunsilius E, Stockhammer G. Molecular therapies for malignant glioma. Wiener Medizinische Wochenschrift. 2006;**156**(11):351-363. DOI: 10.1007/s10354-006-0308-3

[66] Sachdev D, Yee D. Disrupting insulin-like growth factor signaling as a potential cancer therapy. Molecular Cancer Therapy. 2007;**6**(1):1-12. DOI: 10.1158/1535-7163.MCT-06-0080

[67] Ardourel M, Blin M, Moret JL, et al. A new putative target for antisense gene

therapy of glioma: Glycogen synthetase. Cancer Biology and Therapy. 2007;**6**(5):719-723. DOI: 10.4161/cbt.6.5.4232

[68] Zhou X, Ren Y, Moore L, et al. Downregulation of miR-21 inhibits EGFR pathway and suppresses the growth of human glioblastoma cells independent of PTEN status. Laboratory Investigation. 2010;**90**: 144-155. DOI: 10.1038/labinvest. 2009.126

[69] Premkumar DR, Arnold B, Jane EP, Pollack IF. Synergistic interaction between 17-AAG and phosphatidylinositol 3-kinase inhibition in human malignant glioma cells. Molecular Carcinogenesis. 2006;**45**(1):47-59. DOI: 10.1002/mc.20152

[70] Sanson M, Laigle-Donadey F, Benouaich-Amiel A. Molecular changes in brain tumours: Prognostic and therapeutic impact. Current Opinion in Oncology. 2006;**18**(6):623-630. DOI: 10.1097/01.cco.0000245322.11787.72

[71] Esiri M, Perl D. Oppenheimer's Diagnostic Neuropathology. 3rd ed. FL: CRC Press; 2006

[72] Glick RP, Lichtor T, Unterman TG. Insulin-like growth factors in central nervous system tumors. Journal of Neuro-Oncology. 1997;**35**(3):315-325

[73] Johnson TR, Trojan J, Rudin SD, et al. Effects of actinomycin D and cycloheximide on transcript levels of IGF-I, actin, and albumin in hepatocyte primary cultures treated with growth hormone and insulin. Molecular Reproduction and Development. 1991;**30**(2):95-99. DOI: 10.1002/mrd.1080300204

[74] Obrepalska-Steplowska A, Kedzia A, Trojan J, Goździcka-Józefiak A. Analysis of coding and promoter sequences of the IGF-I gene in children with growth disorders presenting with normal level of growth hormone. Journal of Pediatric Endocrinology and Metabolism. 2003;**16**(9):1267-1275

[75] Zumkeller W. IGFs and IGF-binding proteins as diagnostic markers and biological modulators in brain tumors. Expert Review of Molecular Diagnostics. 2002;**2**(5):473-477. DOI: 10.1586/14737159.2.5.473

[76] Hu B, Niu X, Cheng L, et al. Discovering cancer biomarkers from clinical samples by protein microarrays. Proteomics Clinical Application. 2015;**9**(1-2):98-110. DOI: 10.1002/prca.201400094

[77] Ertl DA, Gleiss A, Sagmeister S, Haeusler G. Determining the normal range for IGF-I, IGFBP-3, and ALS: New reference data based on current internal standards. Wien Medicina Wochenschr. 2014;**164**(17-18):343-352. DOI: 10.1007/sl 0354-014-0299-4

[78] Gu F, Schumacher FR, Canzian F, et al. Eighteen insulin-like growth factor pathway genes, circulating levels of IGF-I and its binding protein, and risk of prostate and breast cancer. Cancer Epidemiology Biomarkers Prevention. 2010;**19**(11):2877-2887. DOI: 10.1158/1055-9965.EPI-10-0507

[79] Trojan A, Jay LM, Kasprzak H, et al. Immunotherapy of malignant tumors using antisense anti-IGF-I approach: Case of glioblastoma. Journal of Cancer Therapy. 2014;**5**:685-705

[80] Rodriguez-Tarduchy G, Collins MKL, Garcia I, Lopez-Rivas A. Insulin-like growth factor-I inhibits apoptosis in IL-3-dependent hemopoietic cells. European Journal of Immunology. 1992;**149**:535-540

[81] Upegui-Gonzalez LC, Duc HT, Buisson Y, et al. Use of the IGF-I antisense strategy in the treatment of the hepatocarcinoma. Advances in

Experimental Medicine and Biology. 1998;**451**:35-42

[82] Shevelev A, Burfeind P, Schulze E, et al. Potential triple helix mediated inhibition of IGF-I gene expression significantly reduces tumorigenicity of glioblastoma in an animal model. Cancer Gene Therapy. 1997;**4**:105-112

[83] Upegui-Gonzalez LC, Ly A, Sierzega M, et al. IGF-I triple helix strategy in hepatoma treatment. Hepato/Gastroenterology. 2001;**48**:660-666

[84] Derwan P. Reagents for the site-specific cleavage of mega-base DNA. Nature. 1992;**359**:87-88

[85] Helene C. Control of oncogene expression by antisense nucleic acids. European Journal of Cancer. 1994;**30**:1721-1726

[86] Rubinstein JL, Nicolas JF, Jacob F. L'ARN non sens (nsARN): Un outil pour inactiver spécifiquement l'expression d'un gène donné in vivo. Comptes Rendus Académie des Sciences Paris. 1984;**299**:271-274

[87] Weintraub H, Izant G, Harland RM. Anti-sense RNA as a molecular tool for genetic analysis. Trends in Genetics. 1985;**1**:23-25

[88] Green PJ, Pines O, Inouye M. The role of antisense RNA in gene regulation. Annual Review of Biochemistry. 1986;**55**:569-597

[89] Kim SK, Wold BJ. Stable reduction of thymidine kinase activity in cells expressing high levels of anti-sense RNA. Cell. 1985;**42**:129-138

[90] Whitesell L, Rosolen S, Neckers LM. Episome-generated N- myc antisense RNA restricts the differentiation potential of primi-tive neuroectodermal cell lines. Molecular Cell Biology. 1991;**11**:1360-1371

[91] Blanchet O, Bourge JF, Zinszner H, et al. Altered binding of regulatory factors to HLA class I enhancer sequence in human tumor cell lines lacking class I antigen expression. Proceedings of National Academy of Sciences of the United States of America. 1992;**89**:3488-3492

[92] Plautz GE, Yang ZY, Wu BY, et al. Immunotherapy of malignancy by in vivo gene transfer into tumors. Proceedings of National Academy of Sciences of the United States of America. 1993;**90**:4645-4649

[93] Townsend SE, Allison JA. Tumor rejection after direct costimulation of CD8+ T cell transfected melanoma cells. Science. 1993;**259**:368-370

[94] Guo Y, Wu M, Chen H, et al. Effective tumor vaccine generated by fusion of hepatoma cells with lymphocytes B cells. Science. 1994;**263**:518-520

[95] Trojan J, Duc H, Upegui-Gonzalez L, et al. Presence of MHC-I and B-7 molecules in rat and human glioma cells expressing antisense IGF-I mRNA. Neuroscience Letters. 1996;**212**:9-12

[96] Ly A, Duc HT, Kalamarides M, et al. Human glioma cells transformed by IGF-I triple-helix technology show immune and apoptotic characteristics determining cell selection for gene therapy of glioblastoma. Journal of Clinical Pathology. 2001;**54**:230-239

[97] Trojan LA, Ly A, Kopinski P, et al. Antisense and triple helix anti IGF-I tumour vaccines: Gene therapy of gliomas. International Journal of Cancer Prevention. 2007;**2**(4):227-243

[98] Lafarge-Frayssinet C, Sarasin A, Duc HT, et al. Gene therapy for hepatocarcinoma: Antisense IGF-I transfer into a rat hepatoma cell line

inhibits tumorigenesis into syngeneic animal. Cancer Gene Therapy. 1997;**4**:276-285

[99] Rininsland F, Johnson T, Chernicky C, et al. Suppression of insulin-like growth factor type-I receptor by a triple-helix strategy inhibits IGF-I transcription and tumorigenic potential of rat C6 glioblastoma cells. Proceedings of the National Academy of Sciences of the United States of America. 1997;**94**:5854-5859

[100] Wongkajornslip A, Ouyprasertkul M, Sangruchi T, et al. The analysis of peri-tumor necrosis following the subcutaneous implantation of autologous tumor cells transfected with an episome transcribing an antisense insulin-like growth factor I RNA in a glioblastoma multiforme subject. Journal of Medical Association of Thailand. 2001;**4**:740-747

[101] Siena S, Di Nicola M, Bregni M, et al. Massive ex vivo generation of functional dendritic cells from mobilized CD34+ blood progenitors for anticancer therapy. Experimental Hematology. 1995;**23**:1465-1473

[102] Pickl WF, Majdic O, Kohl P, et al. Molecular and functional characteristics of dendritic cells generated from highly purified CD14+ peripheral blood monocytes. Journal of Immunology. 1996;**157**(9):3850-3859

[103] Guo Y, Wu M, Chen H, et al. Effective tumor vaccine generated fusion of hepatoma cells with lymphocytes B cells. Science. 1994;**263**:518-520

[104] Robin A. Immunochemistry in Practice. NY: Blackwell; 1988

[105] Steiman RM, Turkey S, Mellman I, Inaba K. The induction of tolerance by dendritic cells that have captured apoptotic cells. Journal of Experimental Medicine. 2000;**191**:411-416

[106] Linsley PS, Clark EA, Ledbetter JA. T-cell antigen CD28 mediates adhesion with B cells by interacting with activation antigen B7/13. Proceedings of the National Academy of Sciences of the United States of America. 1990;**87**:5031-5035

[107] Freeman GB, Gray GS, Gimmi CD, et al. Structure, expression and T cell costimulatory activity of murine homologue of the human B lymphocyte activation antigen B7. Journal of Experimental Medicine. 1991;**174**:625-631

[108] Schwartz RH. Costimulation of T lymphocytes: The role of CD28, CTLA-4 and B7/BBI in interleukin-2 production and immunotherapy. Cell. 1992;**71**:1065-1068

[109] D'Ambrosio C, Ferber A, Resnicoff M, Baserga R. A soluble insulin-like growth factor receptor that induces apoptosis of tumor cells in vivo and inhibits tumorigenesis. Cancer Research. 1996;**56**:4013-4020

[110] Dudek H, Datta SR, Franke TS, et al. Regulation of neuronal survival by the serine-threonine protein kinase Akt. Science. 1997;**275**:661-665

[111] Satoh J, Lee YB, Kim SU. T-cell costimulatory molecules B7-1 (CD80) and B7-2 (CD86) are expressed in human microglia but not in astrocytes in culture. Brain Research. 1995;**704**:95-96

[112] Sotomayor E, Fu Y, Lopez-Cepero M, et al. Role of tumor derived cytokines on the immune system of mice bearing a mammary adenocarcinoma. Journal of Immunology. 1991;**147**:2816-2823

[113] Matthew L, Saiter B, Bhardwag N. Dendritic cells acquire antigen from apoptotic cells and induce class I restricted CTL. Nature. 1998;**392**:86-89

[114] Anthony D, Pan Y, Wu S, et al. Ex vivo and in vivo IGF-I antisense RNA strategies for treatment of cancer in humans. Advances in Experimental Medicine and Biology. 1998;**451**:27-34

[115] Pan Y, Trojan J, Guo Y, Anthony D. Rescue of MHC-1 antigen processing machinery by down-regulation in expression of IGF-I in human glioblastoma cells. PLoS One. 2013;**8**(3):e58428. DOI: 10.1371/0058428

[116] Zhu C, Trabado S, Fan Y, et al. Characterization of effector components from the humoral and cellular immune response stimulated by melanoma cells exhibiting modified IGF-1 expression. Biomedicine & Pharmacotherapy. 2015;**70**:53-57. DOI: 10.1016/j.biopha.2015.01.002

[117] Trojan J. From unsolved mysteries of neoplastic brain development to market of gene therapyof brain tumors—glioblastoma. In: BIT's 5th Annual World Congress of NeuroTalk 2014, Session: Frontier of Neurosystem Matters; Nanjing, China; 19 May. 2014

[118] Trojan J. Cellular therapy of malignant tumours: Anti-gene anti IGF-I approach. In: BIT'S 7th Annual World Congress – WCC 2014; Session: Cancer Immunology and Cancer Metabolism; Nanjing, 22 May. 2014

[119] Trojan J. Cell immunogene therapy of cancers using anti-gene anti IGF-I vaccines. In: 3rd International Conference Vaccines R&D, Session Therapeutic Vaccination; Washington, USA. November 2017

[120] Stupp R, Hegi ME, van den Bent MJ, et al. Changing paradigms—An update on the multidisciplinary management of malignant glioma. The Oncologist. 2006;**11**:165-180

[121] Kjaergaard J, Wang L, Kuriyama H, et al. Active immunotherapy for advanced intracranial murine tumors by using dendritic cell-tumor cell fusion vaccines. Journal of Neurosurgery. 2005;**103**:156-164

[122] Fakhrai H, Dorigo O, Shawler DL, et al. Eradication of established intracranial rat gliomas by transforming growth factor beta antisense gene therapy. Proceedings of the National Academy of Sciences of the United States of America. 1996;**93**(7):2909-2914

[123] Boado RJ. RNA interference and nonviral targeted gene therapy of experimental brain cancer. NeuroRx. 2005;**2**(1):139-150

[124] Pai SI, Lin YY, Macaes B, et al. Prospects of RNA interference therapy for cancer. Gene Therapy. 2006;**13**(6):464-477

[125] Berezikov E, Thuemmler F, van Laake LW, et al. Diversity of microRNAs in human and chimpanzee brain. Nature Genetics. 2006;**38**(12):1375-1377

[126] Corsten MF, Miranda R, Kasmieh R, et al. MicroRNA-21 knockdown disrupts glioma growth in vivo and displays synergistic cytotoxicity with neural precursor cell delivered S-TRAIL in human gliomas. Cancer Research. 2007;**67**(19):8994-9000

[127] Dias N, Stein CA. Basic concepts and antisense oligonucleotides mechanisms. Molecular Cancer Therapeutics. 2002;**1**:347-355

[128] Galderisi U, Cascino A, Goirdano A. Antisense oligonucleotides as therapeutic agents. Journal of Cell Physics. 1999;**181**:251-257

[129] Resnicoff M, Li W, Basak S, et al. Inhibition of rat C6 glioblastoma tumor growth by expression of insulin-like growth factor I receptor antisense mRNA. Cancer Immunology and Immunotherapy. 1996;**42**(1):64-68

[130] Trojan J. Anti-gene anti IGF-I technology applied for cancer immunotherapy. World Journal of Research Review. 2016;**1**(3):67-75

[131] Schwartz RH. Costimulation of T lymphocytes: The role of CD28, CTLA-4, and B7/BB1 in interleukin-2 production and immunotherapy. Cell. 1992;**71**:1065-1068

[132] Kasprzak HA, Trojan J, Bierwagen M, et al. Usefulness of the antisense and triplex anti-IGF-1 techniques for postoperative cellular gene therapy of malignant gliomas expressing IGF-1. Neurology Neurochirurgy. 2006;**40**(6):509-515

[133] Andrews DW, Resnicoff M, Flanders A, et al. Results of a pilot study involving the use of an antisense oligodeoxynucleotide directed against the insulin-like growth factor type I receptor in malignant astrocytomas. Journal of Clinical Oncology. 2001;**19**:2189-2200

[134] Samani AA, Fallavollita L, Jaalouk DE, et al. Inhibition of carcinoma cell growth and metastasis by a vesicular stomatitis virus G-pseudotyped retrovector expressing type 1 insulin-like growth factor receptor antisense. Human Gene Therapy. 2001;**12**:1969-1977

[135] Schlingensiepen R, Goldbrunner M, Szyrach MNI, et al. Intracerebral and intrathecal infusion of the TGF-beta2-specific antisense phosphorothioate oligonucleotide AP 12009 in rabbits and primates: Toxicology and safety. Oligonucleotides. 2005;**15**(2):94-104

[136] Schlingensiepen KH, Schlingensiepen R, Steinbrecher A, et al. Targeted tumor therapy with the TGF-beta2 antisense compound AP 12009. Cytokine & Growth Factor Reviews. 2006;**17**:129-139

[137] Hau P, Jachimczak P, Schlingensiepen R, et al. Inhibition of TGF-beta2 with AP 12009 in recurrent malignant gliomas: From preclinical to phase I/II studies. Oligonucleotides. 2007;**17**(2):201-212

[138] Fakhrai H, Mantil JC, Liu L, et al. Phase I clinical trial of a TGF-beta antisense-modified tumor cell vaccine in patients with advanced glioma. Cancer Gene Therapy. 2006;**13**(12):1052-1060

[139] Goudar RK, Shi Q, Hjelmeland MD, et al. Combination therapy of inhibitors of epidermal growth factor receptor/vascular endothelial growth factor receptor 2 (AEE788) and the mammalian target of rapamycin (RAD001) offers improved glioblastoma tumor growth inhibition. Molecular Cancer Therapy. 2005;**4**:101-112

[140] Lamszus K, Brockman MA, Eckerich C, et al. Inhibition of glioblastoma angiogenesis and invasion by combined treatments directed against vascular endothelial growth factor receptor-2, epidermal growth factor receptor, and vascular endothelial-cadherin. Clinical Cancer Research. 2005;**11**:4934-4940

[141] Reardon DA, Quinn JA, Vredenburgh JJ, et al. Phase 1 trial of gefitinib plus sirolimus in adults with recurrent malignant glioma. Clinical Cancer Research. 2006;**12**:860-868

[142] Halatsch ME, Schmidt U, Behnke-Mursch L, et al. Epidermal growth factor inhibition for the treatment of glioblastoma multiforme and other malignant brain tumours. Cancer Treatment Review. 2006;**32**:74-89

[143] Wen PY, Yung WK, Lamborn KR, et al. Phase I/II study of imatinib mesylate for recurrent malignant gliomas: Norty American Brain Tumour

Consortium Study 99-08. Clinical Cancer Research. 2006;**12**:4899-4907

[144] Schlingensiepen KH, Fischer-Blass B, Schmaus S, Ludwig S. Antisense therapeutics for tumor treatment: The TGF-beta2 inhibitor AP 12009 in clinical development against malignant tumors. Recent Results in Cancer Research. 2008;**177**:137-150

[145] Trojan LA, Ly A, Upegui-Gonzalez LC, et al. Antisense anti IGF-I therapy of primary hepatic cancer. Journal of African Cancer. 2009;**1**:1-10

[146] Biroccio A, Leonett C, Zupi G. The future of antisense therapy: Combination with anticancer treatment. Oncogene. 2003;**22**:6579-6588

[147] Meng Y, Carpentier AF, Chen L, et al. Successful combination of local CpG-ODN and radiotherapy in malignant glioma. International Journal of Cancerology. 2005;**116**:992-997

[148] Gonzalez J, Gilbert MR. Treatment of astrocytomas. Current Opinion in Neurology. 2005;**18**:632-638

[149] Jane EP, Premkumar DR, Pollack IF. Coadministration of sorafenib with rottlerin potently inhibits cell proliferation and migration in human malignant glioma cells. Journal of Pharmacology and Experimental Therapy. 2006;**319**:1070-1080

[150] Vega EA, Graner MW, Sampson JH. Combating immunosuppression in glioma. Future Oncology. 2008;**4**(3):433-442

Chapter 12

Advances in the Systemic Treatment of Melanoma Brain Metastases

Philip Friedlander

Abstract

It is estimated that up to 40% of patients with distantly metastatic melanoma develop clinically detectable brain metastases. The prognosis for these patients is very poor with an historical median overall survival of approximately 4 months. Targeted surgical and radiotherapy-based approaches can improve outcomes in certain patients. Over the past decade, the efficacy of systemic treatments for metastatic melanoma has improved with the development of anti-CTLA-4 and anti-PD-1-based immunotherapies (checkpoint inhibitors) that provide survival benefit. In patients whose melanoma expresses a V600 BRAF mutation which activates the MAPK signaling pathway, the targeted inhibition of BRAF and MEK also confers survival benefit. These immunomodulatory and molecular-targeted approaches have recently been studied in patients with melanoma brain metastases to determine efficacy of these approaches in treating the brain metastases. Advances in use of chemotherapy, immune checkpoint inhibitors, and BRAF plus MEK inhibitors to treat melanoma brain metastases are discussed.

Keywords: melanoma, brain, metastases, immunotherapy, PD-1, BRAF, targeted therapy

1. Introduction

Melanoma arises through the accumulation of genetic aberrations in melanocytes which lead to uncontrolled cellular proliferation, resistance to apoptosis, and escape from immune surveillance. Melanoma has the potential to metastasize distantly through hematologic and lymphatic channels. When distant spread is present, the melanoma is classified as stage IV. The American Joint Committee on Cancer (AJCC) eighth edition subcategorizes stage IV melanoma into four prognostic subgroups with the worst prognostic group (stage IV M1d) defined by the presence of brain metastases [1]. Melanoma is the third most common type of cancer to metastasize to the brain following breast and lung cancer. It is estimated that 10–40% of patients with stage IV melanoma eventually develop clinically detectable brain metastases [2]. In autopsy series, a high incidence of subclinical metastasis is noted as over 50% of patients have brain metastases [2].

2. Management of melanoma brain metastases

Brain metastases can lead to morbidity with the development of seizures, cerebral edema, and neurologic symptoms reflective of the part of the brain involved. However, several retrospective analyses have shown that the majority of patients with brain metastases are asymptomatic [2]. While metastases can develop in any part of the brain, the incidence is not evenly distributed. A study evaluating the location of 115 brain metastases showed that 43.5% were located in the frontal lobe with only 8.6% in the cerebellum and less than 1% in the hippocampus [3]. Similarly, a retrospective single center analysis of 6064 brain metastases in 632 cancer patients revealed that fewer than 1% of the metastases develop in the hippocampus, while the distribution is highest in the frontal lobe (31.6%) [4].

The prognosis for patients with melanoma metastatic to the brain is very poor with an historical median overall survival of approximately 4 months [5]. However, prognosis is heterogeneous with a small subset of patients demonstrating greater than 3-year survival despite the development of brain metastases. A retrospective review of 702 patients with melanoma-related brain metastases identified a small subset of patients who survived greater than 3 years. These patients were largely categorized by the presence of an isolated brain metastasis that was treated surgically [5].

Several retrospective studies have attempted to associate clinical and pathological characteristics with the development of brain metastases and with the outcome following the development of brain metastasis. A review of clinical features and survival outcome in melanoma patients who enrolled in any of 12 clinical trials at a single cancer center identified factors prognostic for overall survival [6]. About 44% of 743 chemotherapy naive melanoma patients developed brain metastases with the median overall survival following diagnosis of brain metastases being only 4.3 months. Age at the time of diagnosis of brain metastases did not predict for survival outcome. However, the year of diagnosis was prognostic as patients diagnosed prior to 1996, the midpoint for inclusion of these patients, had worse survival than patients diagnosed after the start of 1996 (4.14 months vs. 5.92 months, $p = 0.01$). While prognosis has improved over time, survival outcomes remain very poor. Other prognostic factors included the number of brain metastases with a median survival for patients with one to three metastases of 5.92 months as opposed to 3.52 months for those with more than three brain metastases (HR 1.57, $p = 0.001$). The presence of leptomeningeal involvement conferred an even worse prognosis with a median overall survival of only 1.2 months. The development of brain metastases after receiving systemic therapy for extracranial metastases conferred worse overall survival compared to developing the brain metastases before or synchronous to extracranial metastases (HR 1.78, $p < 0.0001$). Therefore, in multivariate analysis, the year of diagnosis, number of parenchymal brain metastases, and timing of metastases relative to extracranial metastases were significantly associated with overall survival. Another retrospective analysis of 49 patients with melanoma metastatic to the brain identified as part of a melanoma database collected from 1998 to 2012 associated survival to the presence or absence of symptoms, number of parenchymal brain lesions (one vs. two or more), and response to chemotherapy [2]. A multivariate analysis of 89 melanoma patients from a single institution who developed brain metastases and who were part of a larger prospectively accrued cohort of 900 melanoma patients revealed that the presence of neurologic symptoms and extracranial metastases predicted for worsened survival [7].

The modality used to treat brain metastases may reflect prognosis. The median survival of 686 patients with melanoma and cerebral metastases treated at the Sydney Melanoma Unit between 1985 and 2000 was 8.9, 8.7, 3.4, and 2.1 months, respectively, in patients treated with surgery plus postoperative radiotherapy, surgery alone, radiotherapy alone, and supportive care alone [8]. While outcomes differed in patients receiving surgery and/or radiotherapy compared to best supportive care, the differences may reflect patient selection based on performance status, extent of extracranial metastases, comorbidities, and number, size, and location of brain metastases. These features impact the decision to recommend surgery or radiation therapy. Furthermore, the size, location, and number of metastases impact the ability to perform stereotactic radiosurgery as opposed to whole brain radiation therapy.

Overall survival of stage IV melanoma patients also is determined by the effectiveness of systemic therapy. Systemic treatment options have improved over the past decade through the development of efficacious immunotherapies and molecularly targeted approaches translating into improvements in survival. Prior to 2011, the only two systemic therapies Food and Drug Administration (FDA) approved for the treatment of stage IV melanoma were the cytotoxic chemotherapy dacarbazine (DTIC) and the cytokine immunotherapy high-dose interleukin-2 (HD-IL2). DTIC is an intravenously administered alkylating agent that confers responses in 5–20% of stage IV melanoma patients but the responses are largely partial and not durable [9]. Treatment with HD-IL2 confers a 16% response rate with 5% of patients developing complete durable responses [10]. The potential for HD-IL2 to cause capillary leak syndrome and cerebral edema limits the ability to use this treatment in patients with brain metastases. Neither HD-IL2 nor DTIC have been shown in randomized studies to confer overall survival benefit.

Temozolomide is an oral alkylating agent that is metabolized to MTIC the same active agent that dacarbazine is metabolized to. Treatment of stage IV melanoma patients randomized to treatment with dacarbazine or temozolomide showed equivalency in terms of response rate and survival [11]. Temozolomide has better penetrance of the central nervous system. A retrospective analysis comparing CNS relapse rate in patients who responded to treatment with temozolomide versus dacarbazine showed that temozolomide-treated patients had significantly fewer CNS relapses [12]. This suggests that temozolomide may prevent development of brain metastases in melanoma patients. To assess efficacy of temozolomide in treating brain metastases in melanoma patients where the metastases did not require immediate radiation therapy, a phase II study was performed treating 151 patients with temozolomide at dose of 150 milligrams per meter squared (mg/m^2) per day for 5 days in row every 28 days. Among the 117 patients who did not receive prior systemic therapy, the response rate was 7%, while 29% had stabilization of the brain metastases. Of the 34 patients who received prior systemic therapy, only 1 patient responded and 6 patients developed stable disease in the brain [13]. Therefore, while temozolomide demonstrates efficacy in treating melanoma brain metastases, the benefit is limited and seen only in a small subset of patients.

An improved mechanistic understanding of the positive and negative regulation of the immune system through multiple immune-mediated checkpoints has led to the development of more efficacious treatment for stage IV melanoma patients. Since 2011, the FDA has approved for treatment of stage IV melanoma an inhibitor of the negative regular cytotoxic T-lymphocyte-associated protein 4 (CTLA-4), ipilimumab, and two inhibitors of the negative regulator programmed death-1 (PD-1), nivolumab and pembrolizumab. Ipilimumab is administered intravenously at a dose of 3 milligrams per kilogram (mg/kg) every 3 weeks for a total of four doses. Nivolumab is administered intravenously at a flat dose of 240 mg intravenously every 2 weeks or 480 mg every 4 weeks. Pembrolizumab is administered at a dose of 200 mg every 3 weeks.

T-cell activation requires binding of the T-cell receptor to an antigen-derived amino acid sequence complexed to MHC molecules on antigen presenting cells. For T-cell activation, costimulatory interactions are necessary with binding of CD28 on the T-cell to B7 on the antigen presenting cell. CTLA-4 is expressed on T-cells and binds to B7 with higher affinity that CD28 leading to disruption of CD28-B7 interaction thereby dampening the immune response. Ipilimumab is a fully human IgG1 monoclonal antibody that binds to CTLA-4 in an inhibitory fashion enhancing T-cell priming and decreasing suppressor T-cell activity [14]. A phase III study that randomized previously treated stage IV melanoma patients to treatment with ipilimumab alone at a dose of 3 mg/kg intravenously every 3 weeks for four treatments, a peptide vaccine GP-100 alone, or the combination of ipilimumab plus the vaccine demonstrated a statistically significant improvement in overall survival following ipilimumab treatment [14]. The median overall survival was 10.1 months in the ipilimumab group as opposed to 6.4 months in the gp100 vaccine group (hazard ratio for death of 0.68; p-value < 0.001). A pooled analysis of long-term data from 12 phase II and phase III studies encompassing 1861 melanoma patients treated with ipilimumab showed a mean overall survival of 11.4 months with a survival rate at 3 years of 22% [15].

Nivolumab and pembrolizumab are monoclonal antibodies which inhibit the activity of PD-1 leading to increased T-cell activity in the tumor microenvironment [16, 17]. PD-1 is expressed on the surface of tumor infiltrating T-cells and binds to PD-L1 which is aberrantly expressed on tumor cells leading to functional inhibition of the T-cells. Both of the PD-1 inhibitors confer 35–40% response rates and lead to significantly improved survival when compared to outcomes following ipilimumab treatment [18, 19]. The Keynote-006 phase III study randomized 834 melanoma patients to treatment with pembrolizumab or ipilimumab. Median overall survival with a median follow-up of 22.9 months was not reached in the pembrolizumab-treated patients as opposed to 16 months in the ipilimumab-treated patients ($p = 0.0009$). Twenty-four-month overall survival was 55 and 43% in the pembrolizumab and ipilimumab groups, respectively ($p = 0.0009$) [18].

CTLA-4 and PD-1 inhibitors modulate different parts of the immune system, and preclinical murine models demonstrate synergistic activity following concurrent CTLA-4 and PD-1 blockade [20]. The CheckMate 067 study randomized 945 advanced melanoma patients to placebo-controlled treatment with ipilimumab monotherapy, nivolumab monotherapy, or the combination of ipilimumab plus nivolumab [21]. Ipilimumab-treated patients received ipilimumab at dose of 3 mg/kg every 3 weeks for a total of four treatments. Nivolumab-treated patients were treated with 3 mg/kg nivolumab every 2 weeks. Patients receiving combination therapy were treated with ipilimumab at a dose of 3 mg/kg plus nivolumab 1 mg/kg every 3 weeks for a total of four doses and then nivolumab alone every 2 weeks at a dose of 3 mg/kg. Objective responses were noted in 58, 45, and 19% of combination therapy, nivolumab monotherapy- and ipilimumab monotherapy-treated patients, respectively. With a minimum 4 year follow-up, the median overall survival was not reached in the combination group, was 36.9 months in the nivolumab group, and was 19.9 months in the ipilimumab group.

Inhibition individually or in combination of the CTLA-4 and PD-1 checkpoints leads to survival benefit for stage IV melanoma patients. However, the initial clinical trials excluded patients with untreated brain metastases. To determine the antimelanoma efficacy of these immune modulatory approaches in patients with untreated brain metastases, clinical trials were developed specifically enrolling melanoma patients with untreated brain metastases.

A phase II study of patients with melanoma and untreated brain metastases treated with ipilimumab showed intracranial responses in 8 of 51 (16%) of asymptomatic patients who did not need steroids and 1/21 (5%) of patients requiring steroids because of perimetastasis edema or neurologic symptoms related to the metastases. Median overall survival remained poor being 7 months for patients not needing steroids and 3.7 months for patients requiring steroids [22]. The overall survival assessment also reflects the time period when the study was conducted prior to availability of anti-PD-1 immunotherapies.

A single center phase II study treated 18 stage IV melanoma patients with at least 1 untreated or progressive brain metastasis between 5 and 20 mm in diameter and without associated neurologic symptoms to treatment with pembolizumab at a dose of 10 mg/kg every 2 weeks. Four of the patients (22%) developed a partial response in the brain. The responses were durable lasting at least 4 months, and at the time of data, cutoff was ongoing in all responders [23].

To determine the intracranial efficacy of combined CTLA-4 and PD-1 blockade, a phase II multicenter study, CheckMate 204, treated melanoma patients who had at least one measurable nonirradiated brain metastasis with a diameter between 0.5 and 3 cm and with no associated neurologic symptoms to combined treatment with nivolumab and ipilimumab [24]. The primary endpoint was intracranial clinical benefit defined as complete or partial response or stable disease at 6 months. Brain metastases were felt to not need immediate resection or radiosurgery and patients did not receive steroid treatment for at least 10 days prior to treatment initiation. The nivolumab was administered at dose of 1 mg/kg and ipilimumab 3 mg/kg every 3 weeks for four doses followed by single agent nivolumab at dose of 3 mg/kg every 2 weeks until disease progression or prohibitive toxicity. With a median of 14 month follow-up, the rate of intracranial benefit in the 94 patients who were followed for at least 6 months was 56% with a 26% complete response rate and 30% partial response rate. About 2% of patients had intracranial stable disease that lasted greater than 6 months. About 64% of patients did not experience intracranial progression of brain metastases 6 months after treatment initiation. The extracranial clinical benefit rate was 56% similar to the intracranial rate. As expected, the combination immunotherapy treatment led to a 55% rate of high-grade toxicity felt related to the immunotherapy. Treatment-related adverse events involving the central nervous system were seen in 36% of patients and high-grade CNS toxicity developed in 7% of the patients. The most common treatment-related nervous system toxicity of any severity was headache affecting 22% of patients with 3% having severe headaches.

Additional evidence that anti-PD-1 immunotherapy has efficacy in treating active brain metastases comes from the results of a phase II study conducted at four sites in Australia. Melanoma patients with asymptomatic brain metastases that did not receive prior localized treatment were randomized to systemic therapy with nivolumab or combined nivolumab plus ipilimumab blockade. Efficacy was appreciated in both cohorts with intracranial response rates of 20 and 46% seen in nivolumab alone versus combination therapy-treated patients, respectively [25].

Treatment of stage IV melanoma has improved not only through the use of immunotherapy but also through the use of molecular-targeted therapies. Approximately, 40% of melanomas select for an activating mutation in the protein BRAF which is a component of the mitogen-activated protein kinase (MAPK) signaling pathway. The MAPK signaling pathway is a cascade initiated by extracellular signals binding to cell membrane receptors activating RAS which then activated CRAF and BRAF leading to downstream activation of MEK and ERK. Greater than 90% of BRAF mutations in melanoma are activating hotspot mutations present at position 600 with the most common being a V600E mutation. Activation of BRAF leads to melanoma proliferation and survival due to enhanced signaling through the MAPK pathway. Three different combinations of BRAF plus MEK inhibitors (the BRAF inhibitors dabrafenib, vemurafenib, and encorafenib combined with the MEK inhibitors trametinib, cobimetinib, and binimetinib, respectively) are FDA approved for the treatment of unresectable melanoma expressing a V600E BRAF mutation [26–28]. Randomizing 947 previously untreated patients with unresectable melanoma to treatment with dabrafenib plus placebo or dabrafenib plus trametinib as part of an international phase III study demonstrated overall survival benefit favoring the dual inhibitor approach [29]. Treatment with dabrafenib monotherapy conferred a 53% response rate, while dabrafenib plus trametinib treatment led to a 69% response rate. Efficacy is limited by the development of resistance with median progression free survival being 8.8 and 11 months for patients treated with dabrafenib monotherapy or combination therapy, respectively. Two-year overall survival was 42% for patients treated with BRAF inhibition alone and improved to 51% for patients treated with concurrent BRAF and MEK inhibition [29]. Eligibility requirements for the trial required definitive treatment of any preexisting brain metastases with confirmed stability of at least 12 weeks. Patients with untreated or unstable brain metastases were excluded from enrollment.

To determine the ability of combined BRAF and MEK inhibition to treat progressive brain metastases in patients with melanoma expressing a V600 BRAF mutation, a multicenter international phase II (COMBI-MB) study was performed which treated four cohorts with dabrafenib plus trametinib [30]. The four cohorts were: A. Patients with melanoma expressing a V600E BRAF mutation and with asymptomatic brain metastases, no prior localized therapy to the brain metastases, and an ECOG performance status 0 or 1. B. Patients with melanoma expressing a V600E BRAF mutation and asymptomatic brain metastases and an ECOG performance status 0 or 1 but who received prior localized therapy to the brain metastases. C. Patients with melanoma expressing a V600 D/K/R mutation and asymptomatic brain metastases and ECOG performance status of 0–1 with or without prior localized treatment of the brain metastases. D. Patients with melanoma expressing a V600 D.E/K/R BRAF mutation and with symptomatic brain metastasis and an ECOG performance status of 0, 1, or 2. The primary endpoint was investigator-assessed intracranial response in the first patient cohort. Intracranial response in the other three cohorts was a secondary endpoint. With a median follow-up of 8.5 months, the intracranial response rate in the 76 patients enrolled in cohort A was 58%. The intracranial response rates in the 16 patients enrolled in cohort B, 16 patients enrolled in cohort C, and 17 patients enrolled in cohort D were 56, 44, and 59%, respectively. Therefore, clinical benefit intracranially was appreciated in all four cohorts even in patients with worsened performance status (ECOG 2) and symptomatic brain metastases. Longer follow-up is needed to determine effects on survival and long-term intracranial metastases control rates.

While systemic therapies can lead to intracranial efficacy in a subset of metastatic melanoma patients, multimodality approaches may lead to further improvement in clinical outcome. A meta-analysis performed in April 2017 identified six retrospective studies which compared treatment with stereotactic radiotherapy alone to radiotherapy plus ipilimumab [31]. Of the 411 patients identified, 128 were treated with a combined radiotherapy and immunotherapy approach, while 283 received radiotherapy alone. Combination therapy significantly improved survival (HR 0.74, p = 0.04) without significantly increasing the incidence of adverse events. The authors conclude that combining stereotactic radiosurgery (SRS) is safe and effective treatment option.

Given the survival benefits of initial immunotherapy treatment with a PD-1 inhibitor as opposed to ipilimumab in patients with melanoma who have brain metastases, one may expect that SRS plus a PD-1 inhibitor may incrementally improve intracranial response and survival compared to treatment with SRS plus ipilimumab. A study of patients who received SRS plus a PD-1 inhibitor had a median overall survival of 20.4 months as opposed to 7.5 months in patients treated with SRS plus CTLA-4 blockade [32]. A single institution retrospective study assessed the intracranial metastasis control rate in patients treated with SRS for melanoma brain metastases within 3 months of receiving treatment with anti-PD-1 immunotherapy, anti-CTLA-4 immunotherapy, BRAF plus MEK inhibitor targeted therapy, anti-BRAF monotherapy, or cytotoxic chemotherapy [33]. The 12-month distant melanoma metastasis control rates were 38, 21, 20, 8, and 5%, respectively. Local melanoma brain metastasis control rates were similar among the groups. Combining systemic therapy with SRS was overall well tolerated without significant increase in neurotoxicity. Multivariate analysis showed improved overall survival in patients treated with immunotherapy or BRAF targeted therapy when compared to those treated with cytotoxic chemotherapy.

3. Conclusions

Treatment of patients with melanoma brain metastases should be based upon a personalized treatment plan that may include multimodality approaches utilizing systemic therapy, surgery, and radiation therapy. The treatment approach will be impacted by multiple factors including but not limited to comorbidities, performance status, number, size, and location of brain metastases, CNS metastasis-related symptoms, steroid needs, prior therapy, the presence or absence of a BRAF mutation, and patient preference. Recent advances identifying immunomodulatory and BRAF-targeted therapies with intracranial efficacy have led to outcomes that are better than historically expected through the use of anti-PD-1 monotherapy, combined anti-CTLA-4 plus anti-PD-1 blockade, and if patients with a V600 BRAF mutation combined BRAF and MEK inhibition.

Conflict of interest

Advisory Board Member for Seattle Genetics, Regeneron, Array Biopharma, EMD Serono, and Castle Biosciences. Consultant for Aspyrian Therapeutics.

Author details

Philip Friedlander
Division of Hematology and Medical Oncology, Icahn School of Medicine, Mount Sinai Hospital, Tisch Cancer Institute, New York, NY, USA

*Address all correspondence to: philip.friedlander@mssm.edu

References

[1] Gershenwald JE et al. Melanoma staging: Evidence-based changes in the American joint committee on cancer eighth edition cancer staging manual. CA: A Cancer Journal for Clinicians. 2017;**67**(6):472-492

[2] Bottoni U et al. Predictors and survival in patients with melanoma brain metastases. Medical Oncology. 2013;**30**(1):466

[3] Hong AM et al. Low incidence of melanoma brain metastasis in the hippocampus. Radiotherapy and Oncology. 2014;**111**(1):59-62

[4] Wu SG et al. Distribution of metastatic disease in the brain in relation to the hippocampus: A retrospective single-center analysis of 6064 metastases in 632 patients. Oncotarget. 2015;**6**(41):44030-44036

[5] Sampson JH et al. Demographics, prognosis, and therapy in 702 patients with brain metastases from malignant melanoma. Journal of Neurosurgery. 1998;**88**(1):11-20

[6] Davies MA et al. Prognostic factors for survival in melanoma patients with brain metastases. Cancer. 2011;**117**(8):1687-1696

[7] Zakrzewski J et al. Clinical variables and primary tumor characteristics predictive of the development of melanoma brain metastases and post-brain metastases survival. Cancer. 2011;**117**(8):1711-1720

[8] Fife KM et al. Determinants of outcome in melanoma patients with cerebral metastases. Journal of Clinical Oncology. 2004;**22**(7):1293-1300

[9] Chapman PB et al. Phase III multicenter randomized trial of the Dartmouth regimen versus dacarbazine in patients with metastatic melanoma. Journal of Clinical Oncology. 1999;**17**(9):2745-2751

[10] Atkins MB et al. High-dose recombinant interleukin-2 therapy in patients with metastatic melanoma: Long-term survival update. The Cancer Journal from Scientific American. 2000;**6**(Suppl 1):S11-S14

[11] Middleton MR et al. Randomized phase III study of temozolomide versus dacarbazine in the treatment of patients with advanced metastatic malignant melanoma. Journal of Clinical Oncology. 2000;**18**(1):158-166

[12] Paul MJ et al. Effect of temozolomide on central nervous system relapse in patients with advanced melanoma. Melanoma Research. 2002;**12**(2):175-178

[13] Agarwala SS et al. Temozolomide for the treatment of brain metastases associated with metastatic melanoma: A phase II study. Journal of Clinical Oncology. 2004;**22**(11):2101-2107

[14] Hodi FS et al. Improved survival with ipilimumab in patients with metastatic melanoma. The New England Journal of Medicine. 2010;**363**(8):711-723

[15] Schadendorf D et al. Pooled analysis of long-term survival data from phase II and phase III trials of ipilimumab in unresectable or metastatic melanoma. Journal of Clinical Oncology. 2015;**33**(17):1889-1894

[16] Robert C et al. Pembrolizumab versus ipilimumab in advanced melanoma. The New England Journal of Medicine. 2015;**372**(26):2521-2532

[17] Weber JS et al. Nivolumab versus chemotherapy in patients with advanced melanoma who progressed after anti-CTLA-4 treatment (CheckMate 037):

A randomised, controlled, open-label, phase 3 trial. The Lancet Oncology. 2015;**16**(4):375-384

[18] Schachter J et al. Pembrolizumab versus ipilimumab for advanced melanoma: Final overall survival results of a multicentre, randomised, open-label phase 3 study (KEYNOTE-006). Lancet. 2017;**390**(10105):1853-1862

[19] Hodi FS, Chiarion-Sileni V, Gonzalez R. Nivolumab plus ipilimumab or nivolumab alone versus ipilimumab alone in advanced melanoma (CheckMate 067): 4-year outcomes of a multicentre, randomised, phase 3 trial (vol 19, pg 1480, 2018). Lancet Oncology. 2018;**19**(12):E668-E668

[20] Selby MJ et al. Preclinical development of ipilimumab and nivolumab combination immunotherapy: Mouse tumor models, in vitro functional studies, and cynomolgus macaque toxicology. PLoS One. 2016;**11**(9):e0161779

[21] Hodi FS et al. Nivolumab plus ipilimumab or nivolumab alone versus ipilimumab alone in advanced melanoma (CheckMate 067): 4-year outcomes of a multicentre, randomised, phase 3 trial. The Lancet Oncology. 2018;**19**(11):1480-1492

[22] Margolin K et al. Ipilimumab in patients with melanoma and brain metastases: An open-label, phase 2 trial. The Lancet Oncology. 2012;**13**(5):459-465

[23] Goldberg SB et al. Pembrolizumab for patients with melanoma or non-small-cell lung cancer and untreated brain metastases: Early analysis of a non-randomised, open-label, phase 2 trial. The Lancet Oncology. 2016;**17**(7):976-983

[24] Tawbi HA et al. Combined nivolumab and ipilimumab in melanoma metastatic to the brain. The New England Journal of Medicine. 2018;**379**(8):722-730

[25] Long GV et al. Combination nivolumab and ipilimumab or nivolumab alone in melanoma brain metastases: A multicentre randomised phase 2 study. The Lancet Oncology. 2018;**19**(5):672-681

[26] Ascierto PA et al. Cobimetinib combined with vemurafenib in advanced BRAF(V600)-mutant melanoma (coBRIM): Updated efficacy results from a randomised, double-blind, phase 3 trial. The Lancet Oncology. 2016;**17**(9):1248-1260

[27] Dummer R et al. Overall survival in patients with BRAF-mutant melanoma receiving encorafenib plus binimetinib versus vemurafenib or encorafenib (COLUMBUS): A multicentre, open-label, randomised, phase 3 trial. The Lancet Oncology. 2018;**19**(10):1315-1327

[28] Long GV et al. Long-term outcomes in patients with BRAF V600-mutant metastatic melanoma who received dabrafenib combined with trametinib. Journal of Clinical Oncology. 2018;**36**(7):667-673

[29] Long GV et al. Dabrafenib and trametinib versus dabrafenib and placebo for Val600 BRAF-mutant melanoma: A multicentre, double-blind, phase 3 randomised controlled trial. Lancet. 2015;**386**(9992):444-451

[30] Davies MA et al. Dabrafenib plus trametinib in patients with BRAF(V600)-mutant melanoma brain metastases (COMBI-MB): A multicentre, multicohort, open-label, phase 2 trial. The Lancet Oncology. 2017;**18**(7):863-873

[31] Khan M et al. SRS in combination with ipilimumab: A promising new dimension for treating melanoma brain metastases. Technology in Cancer Research & Treatment. 2018;**17**:1533033818798792

[32] Choong ES et al. Survival of patients with melanoma brain metastasis treated with stereotactic radiosurgery and active systemic drug therapies. European Journal of Cancer. 2017;**75**:169-178

[33] Ahmed KA et al. Clinical outcomes of melanoma brain metastases treated with stereotactic radiosurgery and anti-PD-1 therapy, anti-CTLA-4 therapy, BRAF/MEK inhibitors, BRAF inhibitor, or conventional chemotherapy. Annals of Oncology. 2016;**27**(12):2288-2294

Chapter 13

Angiogenesis in Malignant Gliomas and Bevacizumab Resistance

Scott G. Turner

Abstract

Standard therapy for malignant gliomas includes maximal resection followed by radiotherapy and temozolomide. The increase in neovascularization in high-grade gliomas serves the increased metabolic demands of these fast-growing tumors and the main pathway mediating this process involves vascular endothelial growth factor (VEGF) and its receptor. This pathway is targeted by bevacizumab (BEV), an anti-VEGF monoclonal antibody. Though preclinical trials with BEV were promising, clinical trials failed to show improvement in overall survival, and ultimately GBM become resistant to BEV. By better understanding the molecular mechanisms involved in angiogenesis, new targets may be identified and by elucidating the mechanism behind BEV resistance, new treatment modalities may be developed to treat these aggressive tumors.

Keywords: angiogenesis, bevacizumab, vascular endothelial growth factor, glioma, glioblastoma

1. Introduction

Glioblastoma multiforme (GBM) is the most common primary adult brain tumor with 9000 predicted new cases in the US each year [1]. Prognosis remains poor and standard therapy includes maximal safe resection followed by radiotherapy and temozolomide chemotherapy [2]. Because of their high metabolic demand, GBM tend to outgrow their blood supply, leading to a hypoxic, necrotic core [3]. One of the hallmarks of these aggressive tumors, therefore, is their ability to signal new blood vessels to grow into the tumor mass to counteract this effect. This chapter will examine the current state of our understanding of these pro-angiogenic pathways involving VEGF, integrins, angiopoietins, platelet-derived growth factor (PDGF), protein kinase C and mTOR [4–6]. The primary pathway involves VEGF [6] and is targeted by bevacizumab (BEV), a monoclonal antibody to VEGF [7]. BEV resistance, thought to be due, in part, to redundant angiogenic pathways, remains a serious concern, as few subsequent treatment options exist. Other mechanisms of BEV resistance will be discussed, including vessel co-option, vascular intussusception, vascular mimicry, and recruitment of bone-marrow-derived cells.

IntechOpen

2. Angiogenesis

Normal endothelial cells form a monolayer interconnected by tight and adherens junctions made up of molecules such as occludin, claudin, and junction adhesion molecule proteins. These structures form the basis of the blood brain barrier. Endothelial cells are surrounded by pericytes, which regulate cell proliferation and a vascular basement membrane is formed by the endothelial cells and pericytes [8].

Sprouting is the process by which new blood vessels are produced from existing blood vessels and this serves to supply the increased metabolic demands of rapidly growing tumors [10]. This is achieved by increasing the production of proangiogenic factors, of which, VEGF is one of the most important players [6]. Often, hypoxia is the trigger for signaling the expression of proangiogenic factors via the expression of hypoxia-induced factor (HIF1α) [11], although other hypoxia-independent pathways exist involving the mitogen-activated protein kinase (MAPK) and phosphoinositide 3-kinase PI3K) pathways [4]. A balance of proangiogenic and antiangiogenic signals within the tumor microenvironment determine whether angiogenesis will occur, the so-called "angiogenic switch" [9]. When the proangiogenic signal predominates, pericytes secrete matrix metalloproteases and detach from the basement membrane. Endothelial cells loosen theist tight and adherens junctions. Plasma proteins leak out of the blood vessel and supply a scaffold for the new blood vessel. Endothelial cells migrate into this extracellular matrix in response to integrin signaling. A single endothelial serves as the "tip cell" to direct the nascent blood vessel toward the proangiogenic signal. The trailing "stalk cells" form the lining of the new lumen. Signaling by Ang-2, VEGF, Notch, PDGF, neuropilins and others are involved in this process. These new blood vessels, however, tend to be tortuous and lack an intact blood-brain barrier, making them leaky, leading to vasogenic edema in the vicinity of the tumor [12]. Hypoxic tumors also tend to be more resistant to standard chemotherapy regimens. Agents targeting angiogenic pathways, therefore, could reduce peritumoral edema, reduce hypoxia, and improve the delivery of cytotoxic agents [13].

The VEGF family consists of VEGF-A, B, C, D and placental growth factors (PlGF1–4) and their receptors—VEGFR-1, 2, 3, neuropilin (NRP)-1, and NRP-2 [5, 14–17]. This family has been shown to be important in normal and pathologic angiogenesis, maintenance of blood vessels, migration of endothelial cells, and vascular permeability. The most important of these is VEGF-A (VEGF) [18] that forms disulfide-linked homodimers that then bind to VEGFR-1 and VEGF-2. These are both receptor tyrosine kinases that in turn signal through the PI3K/MAPK pathway as well as the AKT1 signaling pathway [19]. Most of the proangiogenic signaling is effected by VEGF-A binding to VEGF-2, which has strong tyrosine kinase activity [20]. VEGFR-1 binding tis thought to modulate VEGFR-2 signaling by sequestering VEGF-A, which binds to VEGFR-1 with higher affinity than it does to VEGFR-2 [21].

3. Bevacizumab

Standard of care for high-grade gliomas starts with maximal surgical resection [22] followed by Temozolomide chemotherapy [2]. Because of the FDA approval of BEV with Irinotecan (IRI) in colorectal cancer, two single-arm Phase II prospective studies for patients with recurrent malignant gliomas were undertaken in 2007.

The BRAIN trial started with two cohorts of 35 patients with GBM who progressed after standard therapy. Twenty-three patients received both BEV and IRI every 14 days and once this was deemed safe, a second cohort of 12 patients was treated with IRI for 4 doses in 6 weeks and BEV every 3 weeks. The results seemed promising with a 6 month progression-free survival (PFS-6) of 46% (vs. 15% in historic controls) and median overall survival (OS) of 42 weeks, vs. 21 months in historic controls). However, complications included thromboembolism, grade 2–3 proteinuria, and intracranial hemorrhage [23]. A second trial involved 9 Grade III and 23 Grade IV glioma patients who had progressed on standard therapy treated with BEV and IRI every 2 weeks of a 6-week cycle. PFS-6 was 38% and the median overall survival was 40 weeks in Grade IV patients. Though no intracranial hemorrhages occurred, three patients developed deep venous thromboses or pulmonary emboli, and one patient had an arterial ischemic stroke [24]. As a result of these studies, BEV was FDA approved for use as a combination with IRI or alone in recurrent high-grade glioma in 2009. In 2014, the BELOB trial, a randomized Phase II trial randomized 148 patients to receive BEV 10 mg/kg every 2 weeks, lomustine 110 mg/m^2 every 6 weeks or combination of both. The primary endpoint was OS at 9 months and was found to be 38% in the BEV arm, 43% in the lomustine arm, and 59% in the BEV/lomustine arm [25]. The EORTC-2601 trial compared lomustine monotherapy to BEV plus lomustine combination therapy and though PFS was improved (4.2 vs. 1.5 months), no significant difference in OS (9.1 vs. 8.6 months) was noted [26].

Because BEV looked promising in the recurrent setting, three trials were commenced to determine its efficacy in newly diagnosed GBM. The first of these was a single-arm, multicenter Phase II trial of 70 patients with newly diagnosed GBM comparing combined RT, TMZ and BEV (concurrent administration of daily TMZ and biweekly BEV with RT followed by TMZ for 5 days every 4 weeks and continued biweekly BEV) with a control arm in which patients received RT/TMZ followed by TMZ for 5 days every 4 weeks and BEV at recurrence. Though addition of BEV improved PFS (13.6 vs. 7.6 months), no significant improvement in OS was seen (19.6 vs. 21.1 months). Importantly, the BEV cohort showed increased incidence of cerebrovascular ischemia, wound infections, GI perforations, GI bleeds, and CNS hemorrhage [27]. RTOG 0825 was a large randomized, placebo-controlled, double-blinded trial of 637 patients in which patients received Stupp protocol with either BEV or placebo from week 4 of RT continued for 12 weeks. Though there was an improvement in PFS was slightly improved (10.7 vs. 7.3 months) no significant survival benefit was seen in the BEV group (15.7 vs. 16.1 months). There was an increased incidence of hypertension, thromboembolism, wound dehiscence, visceral perforation, serious hemorrhage, and serious neutropenia in the BEV group [28]. Finally, in a similar design, the AVAglio study randomized 921 patients to receive Stupp protocol with BEV or placebo every 2 weeks starting during RT and continuing until the disease progressed or unacceptable toxic effects developed. The median PFS was improved (10.6 vs. 6.2 months) but no improvement in overall survival (16.8 vs. 16.7 months) was seen. BEV did, however, appear to decrease dependence on steroids and prolong cognitive function in this study, though the rate of adverse events was higher with bevacizumab than with placebo [29].

Other chemotherapy agents such as carboplatin, irinotecan, erlotinib, and etoposide have shown no improvement in survival when added to Bevacizumab [30–33]. Aflibercept (VEGF Trap), is a recombinant fusion protein of the

Extracellular domains of VEGF fused to the Fc portion of immunoglobulin G1; it binds with high affinity to both VEGF and placental growth factor (PlGF) and thus scavenges both VEGF and PlGF. A Phase II study of patients with recurrent high glioma demonstrated no survival benefit and moderate toxicities including hypertension, lymphopenia, and wound healing complications [34]. Other antiangiogenic agents such as sunitinib, cediranib, and vandetanib, which are tyrosine-kinase inhibitors that target VEGF, have likewise failed to show survival benefit [35–37].

4. Pseudoprogression and pseudoresponse

Pseudoprogression is an inflammatory treatment-related effect seen on MRI that can occur weeks to months after the end of therapy. Therefore, new gadolinium enhancement and T2 signal in the vicinity of the resection cavity may not necessarily represent recurrent tumor as pseudoprogression is thought to occur occurs in about 30% of cases [38]. Furthermore, only surgery can definitively distinguish between pseudoprogression and true progression, though spectroscopy, PET scan, functional MRI, and magnetic resonance perfusion have been employed, but with sensitivities of less than 80% [39]. Pseudoprogression has been treated with corticosteroids, hyperbaric oxygen, pentoxifylline, and vitamin E. Bevacizumab has also been used to treat pseudoprogression as it stabilizes the blood-brain barrier [40].

Confounding the picture further is the phenomenon of pseudoresponse. Because bevacizumab normalizes tumor vasculature, restoring the blood-brain barrier and reducing peritumoral edema [41, 42], MRI tend to show reduced T2 signal and gadolinium enhancement, making it difficult to visualize the underlying tumor. Bevacizumab may, however, increase perfusion, reduce hypoxia, and improve delivery of cytotoxic agents to the tumor [43, 44]. These tend to be a transient effect, however.

5. Bevacizumab resistance

Though it seems to improve PFS and reduce steroid dependence, bevacizumab does not confer a survival benefit. Ultimately, malignant gliomas overcome the antiangiogenic effect of BEV and tumor progression occurs. There are many mechanisms by which tumor cells can achieve resistance to bevacizumab [8]. In a process called vessel co-option, tumor cells migrate along and grow around existing blood vessels. Intussusception is the process by which existing blood vessels are enlarged and bifurcated. Tumor cells may incorporate into the endothelium of native blood vessels in a process called vascular mimicry that is associated with invasion, rapid tumor growth, and resistance to radiotherapy. Endothelial progenitor cells may be recruited, and cancer-like stem cells may differentiate into endothelial cells or pericytes to supply new blood vessels [45].

As antiangiogenic agents like BEV cause vessel regression and hypoxia, tumor cells switch from a proliferative to a migratory phenotype [42]. This type of migratory cell expresses mesenchymal markers and matrix metalloproteases used to degrade the extracellular matrix and allow for cell migration [46]. The c-MET tyrosine kinase and its ligand, hepatocyte growth factor (HGF) are both strongly up-regulated in hypoxic environments as well as in patients with BEV resistance. Its downstream targets are likewise phosphorylated, including focal adhesion kinase (FAK) and STAT3, which are involved in promoting cell migration [47]. Targeting members of this signaling pathway could lead to improvements in survival and may help to overcome BEV resistance [48] and rilotumumab, a monoclonal antibody to HGF is currently under investigation [49].

BEV-induced hypoxia may also alter the metabolism of tumor cells toward aerobic glycolysis to increase glucose uptake and promoting proliferation and migration. Hypoxic microenvironments cause increased levels of hexokinase-2 [50, 51] known to promote proliferation and drug resistance, and pyruvate dehydrogenase kinase-1 ultimately blocking pyruvate from entering the Krebs cycle [52]. The phosphinositol-3-kinase (PI3K)/Akt pathway and Myc also are involved in this metabolic shift [53, 54].

Finally, BEV treatment may lead to the adoption of other proangiogenic pathways involving fibroblast growth factor, platelet-derived growth factor, transforming growth factor-α, Ang-2, and Tie-2 [55]. The integrin family of cell-adhesion molecules is attractive targets for antiangiogenic therapy as hypoxia induces overexpression of αvβ3 and αvβ5 in GBM and correlate with tumor aggressiveness [56, 57]. α5 integrin is upregulated and β1 and α5 integrin were downregulated in tumor cells resistant to BEV.

6. Conclusion

GBM remains an incurable and difficult to treat malignancy. Due to its aggressive nature, the tendency for tumor cells to invade into normal brain along blood vessels and white matter tracks, and its ability to supply its metabolic needs via a number of complimentary proangiogenic mechanisms, new targets and therapies are needed. Targeting multiple angiogenic pathways simultaneously with monoclonal antibodies and receptor tyrosine kinase inhibitors may help mitigate the problem of targeting angiogenesis and bevacizumab resistance.

Acknowledgements

I would like to thank Brandon Bowman for assistance with the manuscript and the members of the Department of Neuro-Oncology at the Marion Bloch Neuroscience Institute at Saint Luke's Hospital, Kansas City, MO.

Conflict of interest

I have no conflicts of interest to declare.

Author details

Scott G. Turner
Saint Luke's Medical Center, Kansas City, MO, USA

*Address all correspondence to: sgturner@saint-lukes.org

References

[1] Ostrom QT, Gittleman H, Stetson L, Virk SM, Barnholtz-Sloan JS. Epidemiology of gliomas. Cancer Treatment and Research. 2015;**163**:1-14

[2] Stupp R, Mason WP, van den Bent MJ, Weller M, Fisher B, Taphoorn MJ, et al. Radiotherapy plus concomitant and adjuvant temozolomide for glioblastoma. The New England Journal of Medicine. 2005;**352**:987-996

[3] Louis DN. Molecular biology of malignant gliomas. Annual Review of Pathology. 2006;**1**:97-117

[4] Maity A, Pore N, Lee J, Solomon D, O'Rourke DM. Epidermal growth factor receptor transcriptionally up-regulates vascular endothelial growth factor expression in human glioblastoma cells via a pathway involving phosphatidylinositol 3-kinase and distinct from that induced by hypoxia. Cancer Research. 2000;**60**(20):5879-5886

[5] Schmidt NO, Westphal M, Hagel C, Ergün S, Stavrou D, Rosen EM, et al. Levels of vascular endothelial growth factor, hepatocyte growth factor/ scatter factor and basic fibroblast growth factor in human gliomas and their relation to angiogenesis. International Journal of Cancer. 1999;**84**(1):10-18

[6] Huang H, Held-Feindt J, Buhl R, Mehdorn HM, Mentlein R. Expression of VEGF and its receptors in different brain tumors. Neurological Research. 2005;**27**:371-377

[7] Ferrara N, Hillan KJ, Gerber HP, Novotny W. Discovery and development of bevacizumab, an anti-VEGF antibody for treating cancer. Nature Reviews. Drug Discovery. 2004;**3**:391-400

[8] Carmeliet P, Jai RK. Molecular mechanisms and clinical applications of angiogenesis. Nature. 2011;**473**(7347):298-307

[9] Baeriswyl V, Christofori G. The angiogenic switch in carcinogenesis. Seminars in Cancer Biology. 2009;**19**(5):329-337

[10] Hanahan D, Weinberg RA. The hallmarks of cancer. Cell. 2000;**100**(1):57-70

[11] Kaur B, Khwaja FW, Severson EA, Matheny SL, Brat DJ, Van Meir EG. Hypoxia and the hypoxia-inducible-factor pathway in glioma growth and angiogenesis. Neuro-Oncology. 2005;**7**:134-153

[12] Jain RK, Booth MF. What brings pericytes to tumor vessels? The Journal of Clinical Investigation. 2003;**112**(8):1134-1136

[13] Jain RK. Normalization of tumor vasculature: An emerging concept in antiangiogenic therapy. Science. 2005;**307**(5706):58-62

[14] Ferrara N, Gerber HP, LeCouter J. The biology of VEGF and its receptors. Nature Medicine. 2003;**9**(6):669-676

[15] Staton CA, Kumar I, Reed MW, Brown NJ. Neuropilins in physiological and pathological angiogenesis. The Journal of Pathology. 2007;**212**(3):237-248

[16] Hattori K, Heissig B, Wu Y, Dias S, Tejada R, Ferris B, et al. Placental growth factor reconstitutes hematopoiesis by recruiting VEGFR1(+) stem cells from bone-marrow microenvironment. Nature Medicine. 2002;**8**(8):841-849

[17] Zhou YH, Tan F, Hess KR, Yung WK. The expression of PAX6, PTEN, vascular endothelial growth factor, and epidermal growth factor receptor in

gliomas: Relationship to tumor grade and survival. Clinical Cancer Research. 2003;**9**(9):3369-3375

[18] Leung DW, Cachianes G, Kuang WJ, et al. Vascular endothelial growth factor is a secreted angiogenic mitogen. Science. 1989;**246**:1306-1309

[19] Petrova TV, Makinen T, Alitalo K. Signaling via vascular endothelial growth factor receptors. Experimental Cell Research. 1999;**253**(1):117-130

[20] Holmes K, Roberts OL, Thomas AM, Cross MJ. Vascular endothelial growth factor receptor-2: Structure, function, intracellular signalling and therapeutic inhibition. Cellular Signalling. 2007;**19**(10):2003-2012

[21] Zygmunt T, Gay CM, Blondelle J, Singh MK, Flaherty KM, Means PC, et al. Semaphorin-plexinD1 signaling limits angiogenic potential via the VEGF decoy receptor sFlt1. Developmental Cell. 2007;**21**(2):301-314

[22] Lacroix M, Toms SA. Maximum safe resection of glioblastoma multiforme. Journal of Clinical Oncology. 2016;**32**(8):727-728

[23] Vredenburgh JJ, Desjardins A, Herndon JE 2nd, Marcello J, Reardon DA, Quinn JA, et al. Bevacizumab plus irinotecan in recurrent glioblastoma multiforme. Journal of Clinical Oncology. 2007;**25**:4722-4729

[24] Vredenburgh JJ, Desjardins A, Herndon JE 2nd, Dowell JM, Reardon DA, Quinn JA, et al. Phase II trial of bevacizumab and irinotecan in recurrent malignant glioma. Clinical Cancer Research. 2007;**13**:1253-1259

[25] Taal W, Oosterkamp HM, Walenkamp AME, Dubbink HJ, Beerepoot LV, Hanse M, et al. Final analysis of the BELOB trial (A randomized phase II study on bevacizumab versus bevacizumab plus lomustine single agent in recurrent glioblastoma). Neuro-Oncology. 2014;**16**:v20-v21

[26] Wick W, Brandes AA, Gorlia T, Bendszus M, Sahm F, Taal W, et al. EORTC 26101 phase III trial exploring the combination of bevacizumab and lomustine in patients with first progression of a glioblastoma. Journal of Clinical Oncology. 2016;**34**(15_suppl):2001-2010

[27] Lai A, Tran A, Nghiemphu PL, Pope WB, Solis OE, Selch M, et al. Phase II study of bevacizumab plus temozolomide during and after radiation therapy for patients with newly diagnosed glioblastoma multiforme. Journal of Clinical Oncology. 2011;**29**:142-148

[28] Gilbert MR, Dignam JJ, Armstrong TS, Wefel JS, Blumenthal DT, Vogelbaum MA, et al. A randomized trial of bevacizumab for newly diagnosed glioblastoma. The New England Journal of Medicine. 2014;**370**:699-708

[29] Cinot OL, Wick W, Mason W, Henriksson R, Saran F, Nishikawa R, et al. Bevacizumab plus radiotherapy-temozolomide for newly diagnosed glioblastoma. The New England Journal of Medicine. 2014;**370**:709-722

[30] Field KM, Simes J, Nowak AK, et al. Randomized phase 2 study of carboplatin and bevacizumab in recurrent glioblastoma. Neuro-Oncology. 2015;**l17**:1504-1513

[31] Friedman HS, Prados MD, Wen PY, et al. Bevacizumab alone and in combination with irinotecan in recurrent glioblastoma. Journal of Clinical Oncology. 2009;**27**:4733-4740

[32] Sathornsumetee S, Desjardins A, Vredenburgh JJ, et al. Phase II trial of bevacizumab and erlotinib in patients with recurrent malignant glioma. Neuro-Oncology. 2010;**12**:1300-1310

[33] Arakaw Y, Mizowaki T, Murata D, Fujimoto K, Kikuchi T, Kunieda T, et al. Retrospective analysis of bevacizumab in combination with ifosfamide, carboplatin, and etoposidein patients with second recurrence of glioblastoma. Neurologia Medico-Chirurgica (Tokyo). 2013;**53**(11):779-785

[34] de Groot JF, Lamborn KR, Chang SM, et al. Phase II study of aflibercept in recurrent malignant glioma: A North American brain tumor consortium study. Journal of Clinical Oncology. 2011;**29**(19):2689-2695

[35] Duerinck J, Du Four S, Sander W, Van Binst AM, Everaert H, Michotte A, et al. Sunitinib malate plus lomustine for patients with temozolomide-refractory recurrent anaplastic or low-grade glioma. Anticancer Research. 2015;**35**(10):5551-5557

[36] Batchelor TT, Mulholland P, Neyns B, et al. Phase III randomized trial comparing the efficacy of cediranib as monotherapy, and in combination with lomustine, versus lomustine alone in patients with recurrent glioblastoma. Journal of Clinical Oncology. 2013;**31**(26):3212-3218

[37] Kreisl TN, McNeill KA, Sul J, Iwamoto FM, Shih J, Fine HA. A phase I/II trial of vandetanib for patients with recurrent malignant glioma. Neuro-Oncology. 2012;**14**(12):1519-1526

[38] Knudsen-Baas KM, Moen G, Fluge O, Storstein A. Pseudoprogression in high grade glioma. Acta neurologica Scandinavica. Supplementum. 2013;**196**:31-37

[39] O'Brien BJ, Colen RR. Post-treatment imaging changes in primary brain tumors. Current Oncology Reports. 2014;**16**:397

[40] Miyata K, Hori T, Shimomura Y, Joko M, Takayasu M, Okumura A. Pseudoprogression successfully treated with bevacizumab in a child with spinal pilocytic astrocytoma. Child's Nervous System. 2018;**34**(11):2305-2308

[41] Gonzalez J, Kumar AJ, Conrad CA, Levin VA. Effect of bevacizumab on radiation necrosis of the brain. International Journal of Radiation Oncology, Biology, Physics. 2007;**67**:323-326

[42] Jain RK. Antiangiogenesis strategies revisited: From starving tumors to alleviating hypoxia. Cancer Cell. 2014;**26**:605-622

[43] Winkler F, Kozin SV, Tong RT, et al. Kinetics of vascular normalization by VEGFR2 blockade governs brain tumor response to radiation: Role of oxygenation, angiopoietin-1, and matrix metalloproteinases. Cancer Cell. 2004;**6**:553-563

[44] Batchelor TT, Sorensen AG, di Tomaso E, et al. AZD2171, a pan-VEGF receptor tyrosine kinase inhibitor, normalizes tumor vasculature and alleviates edema in glioblastoma patients. Cancer Cell. 2007;**11**:83-95

[45] Ricci-Vitiani L, Pallini R, Biffoni M, et al. Tumour vascularization via endothelial differentiation of glioblastoma stem-like cells. Nature. 2010;**468**:824-828

[46] Chen Q, Jin M, Yang F, Zhu J, Xiao Q, Zhang L. Matrix metalloproteinases: Inflammatory regulators of cell behaviors in vascular formation and remodeling. Mediators of Inflammation. 2013;**2013**:928315-928329

[47] Abounader R, Laterra J. Scatter factor/hepatocyte growth factor in brain tumor growth and angiogenesis. Neuro-Oncology. 2005;7:436-451

[48] Sierra JR, Tsao MS. c-MET as a potential therapeutic target and biomarker in cancer. Therapeutic

Advances in Medical Oncology. 2011; **3**(1 Suppl):S21-S35

[49] Wen PY, Schiff D, Cloughesy TF, Raizer JJ, Laterra J, Smitt M, et al. A phase II study evaluating the efficacy and safety of AMG 102 (rilotumumab) in patients with recurrent glioblastoma. Neuro-Oncology. 2011;**13**:437-446

[50] Mathupala SP, Ko YH, Pedersen PL. Hexokinase II: Cancer's doubleedged sword acting as both facilitator and gatekeeper of malignancy when bound to mitochondria. Oncogene. 2006;**25**:4777-4786

[51] Xu RH, Pelicano H, Zhou Y, Carew JS, Feng L, Bhalla KN, et al. Inhibition of glycolysis in cancer cells: A novel strategy to overcome drug resistance associated with mitochondrial respiratory defect and hypoxia. Cancer Research. 2005;**65**:613-621

[52] Semenza GL. HIF-1 mediates metabolic responses to intratumoral hypoxia and oncogenic mutations. The Journal of Clinical Investigation. 2013;**123**(9):3664-3671

[53] Marie SK, Shinjo SM. Metabolism and brain cancer. Clinics (São Paulo, Brazil). 2011;**66**(Suppl 1):33-43

[54] Ward PS, Thompson CB. Metabolic reprogramming: A cancer hallmark even warburg did not anticipate. Cancer Cell. 2012;**21**:297-308

[55] Oltrock ZK, Mahfouz RA, Makarem JA, Shamseddine AI. Understanding the biology of angiogenesis: Review of the most important molecular mechanisms. Blood Cells, Molecules & Diseases. 2007;**39**:212-220

[56] Bello L, Francolini M, Marthyn P, Zhang J, Carroll RS, Nikas DC, et al. Alpha(v)beta3 and alpha(v)beta5 integrin expression in glioma periphery. Neurosurgery. 2001;**49**:380-389

[57] DeLay M, Jahangiri A, Carbonell WS, Hu YL, Tsao S, Tom MW, et al. Microarray analysis verifies two distinct phenotypes of glioblastomas resistant to antiangiogenic therapy. Clinical Cancer Research. 2012;**18**(10):2930-2942

Chapter 14

Innovations in Metastatic Brain Tumor Treatment

Caleb Stewart, Brody Stewart and Marcus L. Ware

Abstract

Metastatic brain tumors (MBTs) are the most common intracranial tumor and occur in up to 40% of patients with certain cancer diagnoses. The most common and frequent primary locations are cancers originating from the lung, breast, kidney, gastrointestinal tract or skin, and also may arising from any part of the body. Treatment for brain metastasis management includes surgery, whole brain radiotherapy (WBRT), stereotactic radiosurgery (SRS), and chemotherapy. Standard treatment for MBTs includes surgery and SRS which offer the best outcomes, while the WBRT is still an important treatment option for patients who cannot tolerate surgery and SRS or patients with multiple brain metastases. Newer approaches such as immunotherapy and molecularly targeted therapy (e.g., small molecules and monoclonal antibodies) are currently being evaluated for the treatment of MBTs. In this chapter, we will review current available treatments for MBTs and discuss treatments that are undergoing active investigation.

Keywords: brain metastasis, chemotherapy, radiotherapy, targeted-therapy, neuroimaging

1. Introduction: epidemiology and pathophysiology

Metastatic brain tumors (MBTs) are the most common central nervous system tumors in the United States [1, 2]. Patients are living longer with cancer with the advent of imaging modalities leading to earlier detection and improved systemic therapies. As a result, the probability of patients developing brain metastases (BM) over time has increased [2]. A number of studies support the expected trend of rising MBT incidence. A cohort study in Sweden found the incidence for brain metastases doubled from 1987 to 2006 [3]. Another study from the Swedish National Cancer Registry reported that patients diagnosed with breast cancer from 2004 to 2006 had a 44% increase in risk in brain metastasis as compared to patients in 1998 and 2000 [4]. A forecast for greater frequency of metastatic brain cancer (MBC) emphasizes the need for continued innovation in MBT treatment.

Roughly 200,000 patients are newly diagnosed with MBC annually in the United States [5, 6]. The incidence rate for primary central nervous tumors was estimated at 6.4 per 100,000, while the incidence for metastatic brain tumors has been estimated between 8.3 and 11.3 per 100,000 [2, 7]. More recent studies suggest that MBTs may occur as much as 10 times more frequently than primary tumors [2, 8, 9]. For cancer patients, an estimated 8.5–9.6% will be diagnosed with brain metastasis [2]. In adults, the most common sources of brain metastases are lung, breast, melanoma, renal and colorectal cancer [10–13]. Another study of patients in Detroit from 1973 to 2001 found the incidence for brain metastases for melanoma (6.9%) and renal carcinoma (6.5%) superseded breast cancer (5.1%) as the second and third most common sources [5]. A 2002 study examined patients from 1986 to 1995 and found renal carcinoma was the second most common MBC followed by melanoma and breast cancer [14]. In contrast, MBC in children has the lowest incidence and has previously estimated at 1.5 per 100,000 between the ages of 0 and 14 years [15]. A study following children diagnosed with cancer at MD Anderson Cancer Center found 1.4% of individuals had a BM, which most commonly originated from sarcomas and melanomas [16]. Previous studies reported incidence as high as 4 and 4.9% among children diagnosed with solid tumors [17, 18]. For adults, melanoma, testicular and renal carcinomas have the greatest tendency to metastasize to the brain, but their relative scarcity translates to lower frequencies compared to other types of metastatic brain cancers [13] Whereas metastases in children most frequently emanated from neuroblastoma, sarcomas, and germ cell tumors [18–20].

Barnholtz-Sloan et al. reported that race, gender and age impact the incidence of brain metastasis. Shifts in these demographic features of MBC can be explained by the rising incidence of lung cancer among women compared to men [5, 21]. Investigation by Barnholtz-Sloan found that men had higher incidence percentage (IP%) of BM for each type of systemic cancer with the exception of breast and lung cancers. In patients with lung cancer, the cumulative incidence for BM in women was 21.8 and 18.9% for men [5]. There is a higher cumulative incidence of BMs in African Americans as compared to Caucasians for lung, melanoma, and breast cancers [5]. Renal cancers displayed a higher IP% among Caucasian patients compared to African American patients. Lastly, the IP% for colorectal cancer was similar between the two populations [5]. The frequency of BM increases with age for most cancer types. Primary cancers presenting with BM increases proportionally with age with a peak around 60 years old [22]. A 1996 study estimated incidence rates for MBTs by age and found the highest incidence was in the age bracket of 65–74 years at 53.7 per 100,000 [15].

1.1 Clinical presentation

MBTs might present with a number of different signs and symptoms. The most common clinical sign is headache, which occurs in as many as 50% of cases [23]. Headaches that are ≤10 weeks in duration have been suggested to be more predictive of BM [24]. These headaches usually can be generalized or localized. They can persist for hours and reoccur at various intervals. Tension headaches, migraines and even cluster type headaches are not uncommon. Lateralization of the headaches to the ipsilateral side only happened in the minority of cases [25]. The headaches have been suggested to be due to increase intracranial pressure due to mass effect and a resulting hydrocephalus. An even smaller number of patients (~20%) have a resulting papilledema due to increase intracranial pressure. Another common presenting symptom is nausea and vomiting. This has been suggested to occur in as many as 54% of cases to as few as 12% of cases [26, 27].

Focal neurological deficits are a common clinical manifestation of MBTs. They occur in approximately 40% of cases [28]. The deficits that patients suffer depends on a number of factors including number of BMs, areas of the brain affected, and more tumor specific factors such as growth, associated swelling or recent hemorrhage. These deficits can progress as the tumor increases in size. These symptoms can present acutely in a stroke-like manner due to hemorrhage or as a slow ominous progression. Weakness has been the primary presenting complaint in between 20 and 40% of BMs. Sensory deficits have been reported to be slightly less common than weakness.

Other frequently encountered symptoms included altered mental status, seizures, ataxia, and dysphagia. The actual rates of occurrence are not clear. These variations are largely predicated on the fact that MBTs unpredictably seed the central nervous system. Most frequently BMs seed the frontal lobe (32%). The parietal (18%), occipital (13%), and temporal (12%) lobes each make up a significant portion. Cerebellar metastases make up approximately 18% of BM. The least common area is the brainstem [26, 29, 30]. Studies have suggested that the sites of BMs vary based on the primary site of origin and cerebral blood flow. There are data that suggest that the differences in surface characteristics make specifics sites more conducive to invasion by circulating cancer cells. The exact mechanisms or characteristics have not been elicited [31].

1.2 Genomics

Metastatic tumors may have very different rates of occurrence and different responses to treatment. There are a number of studies that suggest that these can be explained by genetic and/or epigenetic differences. Research on BM models has shown idiosyncratic expressions of genes that mediate metastasis [32, 33]. Several chromosomal translocations are associated with the development of brain metastases. Lee et al. identified that regions 5q53, 10q23, and 17q23-24 were correlated with development of BM within 3 months of primary tumor diagnosis [34]. Specific genes have also been associated with development of BM in lung cancer such as PLGF, VEGFR1, c-MET, and CXCR4 [35–37]. Other genes suggest a greater risk for brain relapse [38–42]. Metastatic pathophysiology is not limited to protein-coding regions, since non-coding RNA regions are associated with many cancer types [43]. Studies documenting unique mutations in MBTs compared to the source tumor indicate lesions evolve in character and underscore the need for genomic evaluation for best-fit therapies [44]. Although the molecular mechanisms leading to early brain metastasis are poorly understood, these insights provide potential targets for therapy.

1.3 Microenvironment

A growing focus among researchers is understanding the dynamic interactions of cancer cells with astrocytes that may provide several novel therapeutic options. Following extravasation, individual cancer cells are surrounded by reactive astrocytes [45, 46]. Astrocytes serve as the first line of protection in the central nervous system (CNS) [45, 47, 48]. With regard to brain metastasis (BM), astrocytes reduce the number of potential metastatic cells by activating plasmin [45]. Adaptive cancer cells can evade these defense systems by expressing serpins [45]. Serpins represent a target for future therapies.

Neoplastic cells surviving this phase usually seed in the perivascular niche [49, 50], adjacent to neural stem cells and nearby nutrient and oxygen supplies [51–53]. Proliferation in perivascular niches establishes micrometastases where only a fraction of sites reach detectable volumes [54]. Recent research suggests the natural selection of micrometastases is regulated by reactive astrocytes in the microenvironment [55, 56]. Astrocytic-neoplastic interactions depend upon the presence of protocadherin 7 (PCDH7) which mediates contact between the cell groups [56]. Following interaction, gap junctions form and cell-cell communication occurs that increase cancer cell growth and resistance to chemotherapeutic apoptosis [57]. Born out of the pro-metastatic astrocytes research, silibinin represents a targeted therapy attacking the microenvironment with promising results [58]. Meclofenamate and tonabersat are another promising set of medications that target carcinoma-astrocyte gap junctions that suppressed brain metastasis in mice models [56].

2. Metastatic brain tumor diagnosis

Magnetic resonance imaging (MRI) is the current gold standard for brain mass evaluation. MRI provides a wide array of benefits including lesion detection and characterization as well guiding treatment by establishing differential diagnoses, guiding invasive procedures, and monitoring patients for changes over time. Within the past decade we have witnessed imaging transition from indirect diagnosis of lesions using cerebral angiography to precise lesion diagnosis by implementing multi-planar CT and MRI. Modern tumor imaging can be categorized as anatomic, metabolic, and functional (physiological) in nature. This section reviews conventional and advanced imaging techniques provided by CT, MRI, PET, and biomarkers as it relates to the management of metastatic brain cancer.

2.1 Computer tomography

Computed tomography images are obtained by transmitting precisely collimated beams of radiation through specimens at multiple angles. Detectors opposite the radiation source record absorbed and scattering of beams whereby computer algorithms derive attenuation at each location. Currently, multislice CT scanners (MSCT) implement a multilayered matrix system of detectors to generate registration simultaneously for several helical trajectories [59]. The chief advantage of MSCT is higher resolution and faster scan times. Metastases appear as isodense lesions or lower density relative to the density of normal brain matter in native CT scans. Tumor boundaries can be distinguished adjacent to edematous regions. Nonenhanced CT is capable of detecting neurosurgical emergencies such as hydrocephalus, hemorrhage, and mass effect. In cases where patients have implants that are not compatible with MRI, we still rely heavily on CT for diagnosis and to evaluate response to treatment. Another advantage of CT is its ability to detect the extent of bony destruction from calvarial metastases [60]. Sensitivity and ionizing-radiation exposure are the two main limitations when imaging for tumors with CT. Visibility of metastases can be enhanced with contrast-based injections typically with iodine-based injections [61].

Three-dimensional (3D) imaging technology has improved the standards of neurosurgical diagnostics and planning in general [62, 63]. 3D renderings convey greater information (e.g., the scope of bony involvement and destruction) and improves localization of abnormal lesions in relation to surrounding tissues. Combining 3D technology with CT angiography (CTA) helps elucidate tumor blood supply and their orientation with cerebral arteries. Visualizing vasculature information permits better planning for surgical access and the extent of tumor resection. CTA provides higher spatial resolution than MR angiography (MRA), but poorer contrast between arteries and surrounding tissues. One of the more useful CT technological advances in the treatment of brain tumors is perfusion CT. Perfusion CT (PCT) administers an intravenous bolus of contrast agent to evaluate changes in density characteristics of tissue. Quantitative estimates of hemodynamic perfusion cerebral blood volume (CBV), cerebral blood flow (CBF), mean transit time (MTT), microvascular permeability (PS) can be acquired for monitoring the effectiveness of cancer treatment. This technique opens up the possibility for measuring the hemodynamics in brain tissue, tumors, and proximate regions. Perfusion methods estimate and quantify blood flow feeding brain regions through specialized workstations calculating CBF, CBV, MTT, and PS parameters for each voxel [64, 65] Initially, CT perfusion was utilized to evaluate the extent of ischemic brain damage by visualizing brain hypoperfusion within minutes of an ischemic attack [66, 67]. More recently, PCT has been implemented for brain tumor diagnosis and differentiation from adjacent lesions based on hemodynamic characteristics [68, 69]. Visual perfusion analysis reconstructs parametric color maps that are proportional to the selected perfusion parameter. Maps codify the quantitative data into a visual system, which allows medical specialists to examine the vasculature supplying structures of interest [70]. It also allows greater appreciation of solid components and distinguishing the regions of viable neoplastic tissue. Parametric maps for CBF and MTT have been used to generate mean values for different metastatic tumor types, which may serve to predict the sources of tumors. A comparative assessment of perfusion parameters performed on varying lesion sizes found CBF values were higher than in smaller lesions. However, MTT values were not affected significantly with regard to lesion size. Presently, CTP is implemented for primary diagnosis of MBTs and assessing post-radiation changes. Changes in the perfusion parameters proved more effective for monitoring radiation therapy at earlier stages (2 months post-treatment) when compared to CT and MRI methods [71]. Lastly, positron emission imaging hybridized with CT image data (PET-CT) can serve to localize brain abnormalities with useful anatomical landmarks while correcting photon attenuation.

2.2 Magnetic resonance imaging (MRI)

MR imaging utilizes electromagnetic waves in radiofrequency ranges to generate incident energy and contrast between tissues. Advantages of MRI compared with CT include superior contrast in soft tissues, greater selection of contrasts between tissues, versatility of advanced imaging techniques, and lack of ionizing radiation [72]. Pulse sequences are different patterns of incident radiofrequency waves that generate multiple types of contrast between tissues. After a radiofrequency wave emitted by the scanner perturbs nuclei of the body, the body transmits a signal to MRI receivers. The returning waveform varies based on the rate of relaxation of the excited nuclei towards its initial state. Two types of relaxation are measured, i.e., longitudinal and transverse. T1 sequence is the time it takes longitudinal magnetization to return to 63% of its equilibrium value after excitation. While, T2 sequence is the same percent value for transverse magnetization. Each sequence has specific functions with particular advantages and disadvantages relative to others.

Typically, tumors have greater water content than brain parenchyma and thus exhibit hypoattenuation on T1-weighted images relative to parenchyma. This pattern is regularly altered with the presence of necrosis, fat, proteinaceous fluid, hemorrhage, and calcifications. MBTs, in particular, are roughly spherical, highly vascularized and tend to hemorrhage more than primary brain tumors. The effects of hemorrhage oftentimes obscure tumors and hematomas and require follow-up imaging, imaging with contrast or perfusion-based imaging to reveal an underlying image. Metastases develop in parenchyma and wide range of nonparenchymal regions including calvarium, diploic space, meninges, choroid plexus, and pituitary gland. Typically, contrast-enhanced MRI is the preferred imaging modality for evaluating metastases in these regions for its superior contrast, resolution, and multitude of sequences [73].

MR has higher sensitivity for recognizing small metastases compared to CT and CT/PET [74, 75]. Knowledge of the size, location, and number of metastases are essential in treating patients with MBs. The ability to detect very small tumors is essential in treatment. Multiple gadolinium-based contrast agents (GBCA) are available to enhance the sensitivity of MRI scans. These agents vary in biophysical properties but generally increase T1 relaxivity resulting in greater signal-to-noise ratios [76, 77]. Increasing GBCA leads to increased sensitivity, particularly for lesions smaller than 5 mm, but at the expense of increasing false-positive results [78]. In the same vein, stronger magnets (1.5–3.0 T) increase MRI field strengths and improves metastatic detection. Theoretical predictions suggest signal-to-noise ratios (SNR) should improve linearly as field strength increases [79]. Altering these two variables has profoundly improved sensitivity for detection of suspected metastatic lesions [80, 81]. The emergence of 7 T MRI machines may allow for better lesion detection while reducing the contrast dose and scan time [82]. In light of the association between GBCA and nephrogenic fibrosis, higher doses may be avoided without compromising scan quality. Magnets have been manufactured for 8 and 9.4 T systems are currently being used on humans [83]. We expect image quality and tumor elucidation to continue to improve into the near future. Another option for enhancing detection is to increase time delay between contrast administration and T1 acquisition [84]. The development of machine learning and automated detection of brain lesions with human interpretation could generate greater sensitivity and accuracy of lesion characterization [85, 86].

The hallmark of malignancy is uncontrolled cell proliferation and an increase in blood supply once the tumor reaches 2–4 mm^3 [87]. Tumor growth leads to focal hypoxia and hypoglycemia which stimulates angiogenesis. Tumor-derived blood vessels differ from normal brain vessels in vascular consistency, fragility, permeability, trajectory underlie the differences observed in hemodynamic parameters measured in MRI perfusion [88–90]. MRI perfusion technique administers a bolus of contrast agent and calculates the intensity of the MR signal during its transit [91–93]. CBF, CBV, and MTT maps assess tumor vascularity similar to PCT, but perfusion MRI avoids several pitfalls, e.g., radiation exposure and iodine-based contrast agents. MR perfusion has several common techniques including dynamic susceptibility contrast (DSC), arterial spin labeling (ASL), and dynamic contrast-enhanced (DCE) which have different tradeoffs. Ktrans is a DCE derived perfusion-based metric that describes leakiness of blood vessels [94]. ASL can be acquired without GBCA by labeling blood water protons to generate an endogenous tracer [95]. MRI perfusion also maintains its superior anatomical characterization of tumors along with hemodynamic measurements [96, 97]. While perfusion MRI has existed for over 20 years, it has not been used as much as other techniques and has not become standard of care for brain tumor patients [98, 99]. Reasons for underutilization include an unclear reimbursement scheme, lack of approved GBCA for perfusion MRI, insufficient methodological standardization, and limited evidence supporting a significant advantage for patients than current practices [99]. Despite these limitations, perfusion MRI is an intriguing candidate for determining tumor grade, prognosis and therapeutic efficacy.

2.3 Metabolic imaging: PET

Positron emission tomography (PET) is an imaging technique that depicts the metabolism of brain metastases and other brain lesions [100]. A wide range of PET tracers are labeled with a positron-emitting radionuclide to promote decay by positron emission. Collisions with nearby electrons produces two gamma-rays with a fixed energy separated by 180°. Detectors absorb the photon energy and reemit the energy as visible light. Visible light is converted into electrical current, which is proportional to the incident photon energy and reconstructed into a 3D image [101–103]. Common positrons employed with tracers consist of ^{18}F (110-minute half-life) and ^{11}C (20-minute half-life). While the most common tracer is FDG, a glucose analog taken up by insulin-dependent GLUT 1 transporters. Phosphorylation of the tracer inside the cell prevents further metabolism resulting in greater uptake in cells that are metabolically active. Image registration is exceedingly important to accurately correlate PET metabolic findings with MRI abnormalities.

There are several limitations for FDG tracers within the brain. One important problem is the high background activity present in the cortex and basal ganglia as a result of these tissues elevated glucose consumption. High background activity sizeably degrades the SNR and reduces image sensitivity, which is critical for distinguishing small lesions from cortical regions [104]. Resolution is another hindrance (5 mm compared to sub 2 mm for MRI) stemming from multiple technical factors. As a consequence, both sensitivity and specificity for FDG PET are reduced for the detection of brain metastases when compared to MRI [75, 105, 106]. Therefore, FDG uptake is not specific for solely brain tumors, but may also indicate nontumorous lesions such as inflammatory lesions, focal epilepsy, and recent ischemic infarcts.

Despite the aforementioned limitations for diagnosing lesions, PET is particularly adept at differentiating between recurrent or residual tumor and necrotic tissue post-radiation therapy [107]. One study found that sensitivity of FDG-PET for detecting recurrent tumors versus radiation-induced necrosis was 75% and the specificity was 81% [108]. However, significant variation has been observed for low-grade, high-grade tumors, inflammatory and other brain lesions [109]. Another utility of PET is discerning responders from nonresponders in its earliest stages during chemotherapy treatment. Identification of nonresponders has practical implications in avoiding essential bone marrow reserves, patient quality of life, and unnecessary expenses on ineffective treatment [110].

Constraints posed by FDG tracer has researchers focused on developing alternative tracers to capture greater metabolic information and produce favorable imaging outcomes. Tracers reflecting amino acid metabolism help to characterize metastatic brain tumors. Amino-acid tracers take advantage of the L-amino acid transporter type 1 system to avoid the inefficient process of blood-brain barrier (BBB) breakdown for uptake. Alternative uptake for amino acid tracers greatly reduces brain background activity and correlates with a variety of malignant activities, e.g., cell proliferation and angiogenesis. Amino acid tracers appear to perform better than FDG tracer in differentiating postradiation changes from recurrent tumors. Even in brain lesions without increased uptake for FDG-PET, sensitivity and specificity for tumors (89 and 100%) were obtained [111].

2.4 Proton magnetic resonance spectroscopy

Magnetic resonance spectroscopy (MRS) is a noninvasive MRI technique that produces metabolic spectra rather than producing anatomic images. Several nuclei (proton, carbon, sodium, fluorine) can be used but proton is the most common because of its high sensitivity. MRS can be used to measure the metabolite concentrations or the chemical composition of tissues. Commonly measured metabolites include N-acetyl aspartate (NAA) and choline (Cho) that are markers for neuronal integrity and membrane turnover in gliomas. Lactate, lipids, amino acids, and myoinositol can also be detected by MRS [112, 113]. MRS imaging of peri-enhancing brain regions may be useful for distinguishing solitary metastases from primary brain tumors. Gliomas often show elevated Cho in surrounding tissue, whereas MBTs are generally encapsulated and do not exhibit elevated Cho signals [114, 115]. Elevated Cho and lipid signals on MRSI make glioblastomas more likely than MBC [116]. MRSI may also have a role in evaluating prognosis based upon metabolite ratios [117–119]. However, MR spectroscopy was not adept at differentiating metastatic brain tumors of disparate etiologies. For that reason, its utility in MBT diagnostics is unproven [59].

2.5 Functional imaging

A unique feature of MRI is the ability to visualize thermal or Brownian motion of water molecules in the brain tissues. Diffusion properties of water in an isotropic medium is represented by Fick's law relating molecular flow vectors to concentration gradient [120]. Water molecules in solutions above absolute zero exhibit Brownian motion, which in pure water behaves randomly and isotropically. The higher the diffusion coefficient value, the greater the distance molecules can move within the same time period. Apparent diffusion coefficient (ADC) acts as a surrogate for this motion and can be calculated by MRI techniques. B values are parameters of DWI pulse sequence and represent the diffusion weighting. DWI acquisition with a minimum of two distinct b values enables derivation of diffusivity for each individual voxel. Multiple images with varying b values generate ADC maps. Molecular water movement occurs within individual cells (restricted diffusion) and extracellular spaces amongst structures that constrain the motion of molecules (free and hindered diffusion). Generally, the magnitude of diffusion coefficient is dependent on microstructural organization and its respective chemical composition. Abnormal areas of reduced diffusion appear bright on DWI. The first diffusion-weighted image (DWI) was procured in 1985, but DWI did not reach clinical practice until the third generation of MR scanners emerged [121, 122].

On diffusion-weighted MR imaging, MBTs are characterized by heterogeneous changes on DWI and ADC maps. Homogenous MRI signals on DWI usually originated from solid lesions. A variety of biophysical conditions of tissue can result in reduction of diffusion. For instance, edema and increased cellularity can inhibit the motion of water molecules. DWI is considered the standard imaging technique for early diagnosis of cerebral ischemia, as it visualizes impaired diffusion following cytotoxic edema and microstructural damage to cells. In addition to this clinical application, DWI is highly sensitive to cerebral abscesses, epidermoid cysts, traumatic shearing injuries, encephalitis, and postoperative brain injury. One major drawback to DWI is the sensitivity to lesions containing high concentrations of magnetic materials, e.g., blood products, calcium, metal, bone or air. This is particularly true for postoperative DWI imaging.

2.6 Diffusion tensor imaging

Within certain brain tissues, barriers restricting water diffusion are isotropically distributed meaning water diffuses in all directions. At other sites in the brain, barriers will be distributed anisotropically leading to directional diffusion perpendicular to the barriers. In white matter, diffusion runs parallel to axonal projections and myelin fibers and restricted perpendicularly by biological membranes. Diffusion tensor imaging applies diffusion gradients in three orthogonal directions. When the three directions are compared, important differences become visible. The corpus callosum exhibits these differences with the greatest intensity. When diffusion gradients are applied in the z direction, diffusion is greatly restricted and has low signal intensity. When the gradient is applied in the x direction, diffusion is unrestricted in the right-to-left orientation and parallel to the corpus callosum fibers. This region of the brain displays anisotropy with the greatest intensity. Tensor models help quantify diffusion anisotropy by measuring ADC in three perpendicular directions x, y, and z and all combinations of the selected directions. Diagonal elements are transformed to coincide with the principle axis of diffusion for each voxel. New diagonal elements correspond to three eigenvectors and three eigenvalues codifying the main directions of diffusion and associated diffusivities (radial, axial, median). Fractional anisotropy (FA) measures the mean anisotropic diffusion. Color-coded maps can then be developed corresponding to directionality of water movement along axons.

DTI-tractography is a post-processing method for selecting white matter pathways in the brain. Fiber bundles in the brain correspond to the color maps. Diffusion tensor MRI is the means for evaluating the brain with attention to the anatomic microstructure or brain white matter. These white matter maps can then be used to infer functional pathways. This knowledge allows neurosurgeons to plan surgical resections with a better margin of safety. Before the onset of modern brain mapping, complications rates for brain tumor resections were as high as 26% [123–126]. DTI and presurgical brain mapping have made a tremendous impact on surgical risk-benefit analysis and outcomes following surgery [127]. Tractography provides the qualitative information for assessing nerve bundle status, whether there is mass effect, tumor infiltration, edema, or functional reorganization [128]. Mass effect often leads to deviation in nerve tracts. Infiltration refers to any section of the tract with lower anisotropy but preserved morphology. Degeneration of tracts can be visualized with reduced fiber size or lower anisotropic values. Finally, fibers may appear interrupted or discontinuous indicating organizational alteration lesions. Appreciation of these features by surgeons allows for preoperative planning for maximal resection, targeting specific regions for biopsy, and avoiding functional tissue. DTI is a promising imaging technique for examining microscopic differences in tumors. In combination with intraoperative localization techniques, neurosurgeons can tailor presurgical mapping data to reduce operation times by testing language and motor functions while dissecting along tumor borders. Electrical stimulation is one method implemented for testing the white matter function [129, 130]. Transient speech or language deficit during dissection means imminent white matter injury is within millimeters beyond the dissection plane. Importation of DTI mapping data into neuronavigation systems allow real-time interaction with spatial relationships between lesions and functional nerve pathways.

2.7 Advanced diffusion imaging

High angular diffusion imaging (HARDI) method detects diffusion greater directions than DTI. HARDI implements 55 to over 100 gradient directions as compared to the standard 6 gradient directions in DTI [130]. The HARDI model estimates fiber orientations (orientation distribution function) that minimizes scan acquisition time compared to other methods (diffusion spectrum imaging). By changing from an ellipsoid model to orientation distribution function, HARDI appreciates multiple fibers in a single voxel. Scan acquisition time for DTI is roughly 3–10 minutes, whereas HARDI requires a minimum of 12 minutes. HARDI scan times are more reasonable for research and clinical use as opposed to other novel techniques [130].

By propagating fiber trajectories in multiple alternative directions, HARDI is more sensitive in picking up fibers displaced by brain lesions. White matter critical for speech, language, and motor functions better delineated by HARDI in cases where lesion-induced deviation or interruption may occur. Corticospinal tracts (CST) near the centrum semiovale run against crossing white matter tracts from the corpus callosum and superior longitudinal fasciculus [131]. Identifying motor fibers represented by CST is critical for presurgical brain mapping in tumor resection cases.

Neurite orientation dispersion and density imaging (NODDI) is a recent diffusion MRI technique detecting microstructural features of brain tissue with higher resolution than DTI [132, 133]. NODDI maps both gray and white matter microstructure. Detection of diffusion for both dendrites and axons constitutes the term neurite. Neurite density (intracellular volume fraction) and orientation dispersion are calculated using 17 b values and 153 gradient directions, making it tedious for clinical translation [134]. Quantifying neurite morphology in terms of density and orientation provides alternative information for the structural basis of brain disorders. Branching complexity can be computed in terms of dendritic density. Areas with less complex dendritic structures tend to engage in early information processing, while regions with greater complexity participate in the end stages of information processing [135]. Changes in neurite morphology is associated with development as humans age [136], numerous neurological disorders including multiple sclerosis [137], amyotrophic lateral sclerosis [138, 139], and Alzheimer's disease [140].

Prior to the advent of NODDI, changes in the brain microstructure from brain disorders were studied using scarce postmortem tissue samples. There is growing evidence that neurite morphology from NODDI methods is comparable to independent measures derived from histology [141]. NODDI provides a promising tool for differentiating glioblastomas from solitary brain metastases and assessing tumor malignancy grades [142–144].

3. Metastatic brain tumor therapeutics

3.1 Surgery

Despite advances in other technologies, surgical resection of BMs remains a mainstay of treatment. Surgical resection provides a number of immediate benefits to patients including symptomatic relief from BMs through resolution of mass effect and reducing edema [145]. Often this is for emergent situations in which complications, like increased intracranial pressure, become life threatening. Surgical resection of the tumor can also be a non-pharmacological solution to seizures. The epileptic medications can have significant interactions with chemotherapy due to inhibition of the cytochrome p450. Another valuable product of surgical resection is histological evaluation of the tumor. This gives pathologist a change to determine the source of metastatic tumors in the event of undiagnosed primary disease, and also the opportunity to evaluate the genetic variations to help guide further clinical decision making.

Aggressive surgical resection of BMs of solitary tumors has gained greater popularity in the last few decades. This type of management gained more traction in the 90s and early 2000s when studies began to show benefits for surgical resection over radiation therapies. Studies demonstrated a reduction in local recurrence, increase life expectancy, and improved quality of life [146–148]. The difficulties in assessing the indications for surgical resection over other treatment modalities have led to the development of nonograms like recursive partitioning analysis (RPA) that classify MBT patients into three classes. Class I patients have a Karnofsky Performance Status (KPS) ≥ 70, are younger than 60 years of age, have a well-controlled primary tumor and metastatic disease that is limited to the brain [149]. These patients have been shown to be the best surgical candidates of the RPA classes. This has demonstrated that subgroups of this patient population will benefit from more aggressive treatment. Various nonograms have been developed in more recent years to help define this population of patients more clearly. This has been somewhat of a moving target as surgical advancements have been made which can improve outcomes through reduced surgical complication and more accurate resection of tumors and tumor margins.

3.2 Augmented reality

A number of technological advancements over the last couple of decades have culminated to allow for new developments in the realm of augmented reality (AR) use in surgery. Modeling of patient-specific anatomy and pathology has become easier to produce and more accurate. With this and other advancements like smaller, less bulky AR hardware, intraoperative use of AR more feasible. One of the most difficult obstacles AR is facing is determining the best method for image alignment and maintaining this alignment during tissue movement [150]. Several studies have demonstrated that some of these techniques have an accuracy that meets the clinical requirement of under 2 mm [151, 152]. One study even demonstrated an accuracy of 0.8 ± 0.25 mm for projecting images on the skull and brain [153]. This can allow the surgeon direct visualization of the tumor and has the potential to increase the accuracy of resection. It has been demonstrated that AR has shown to be beneficial of a 2D approach in rates of correct localization and in efficiency [154]. It has also been demonstrated that there may be no difference in terms of error between operators [155].

AR technology requires much more work before being used routinely in the operative setting. Larger scale studies are needed to compare AR in tumor resection to other techniques like fluorescence guided surgery. These studies need to determine whether AR improves clinical outcomes, such as reducing morbidity, mortality, and local tumor recurrence. Headset technology and computing platform limitations with regard to field of view, positional tracking and coregistration with moving tissue need further development. The larger hope for developers is integrating artificial intelligence, robotics and AR technology to merge machine-learning with pre-programmed trajectories and spatial parameters from the overlay [156].

3.3 Whole brain radiotherapy

Whole-brain radiotherapy had long been the standard of care for the management of patients with brain metastases (BM). Toxicities associated with whole-brain radiotherapy has led to greater selectivity for its use. Multiple Radiation Therapy Oncology Group (RTOG, now NRG) have examined optimal WBRT dose regimen [157–160]. Typical WBRT fractionation schedule consisted of 20 Gy in five fractions, 30 Gy in 10 fractions, or 37.5 Gy in 15 fractions to produce noticeable effects on imaging [161]. Multiple randomized trials have shown WBRT is an effective treatment for controlling intracranial metastases and preventing new occurrences [162–165]. Studies have also reported that WBRT is associated with both stabilized or improvements in neurological signs and symptoms [166–168]. Despite the benefits of tumor control and neurological improvements, routine use of WBRT for all patients is still controversial. The QUARTZ trial examined patients with nonsmall cell lung cancer (NCLC) patients with BM [168]. Over 500 patients were evaluated comparing patients receiving WBRT with supportive care. The trial reported no difference in survival, quality-adjusted life years, or steroid use. This study suggests that WBRT provides little to no benefit for patients unsuitable for surgical resection.

Routine use of WBRT as an adjuvant for patients with BM following resection remains controversial [162]. A randomized trial in 1998 examined WBRT after surgery and found WBRT was associated with lower rates of recurrence and less neurologic death, however, no improvement in overall survival was reported. A phase III randomized trial evaluating adjuvant WBRT after surgery versus solely stereotactic radiosurgery (SRS) or surgical resection in patients with one to three MBTs found greater control by WBRT than the alternatives [164]. In 2016, another phase III trial compared postoperative SRS with post-resection WBRT and found 6-month cognitive deterioration was worse in the WBRT group [169]. Although cognitive deterioration was worse following WBRT, intracranial control was still better in the WBRT group than the SRS group. No overall survival benefit was reported for WBRT and quality of life was worse.

In an effort to prevent new metastases WBRT has been combined with SRS in multiple randomized control trials (RCTs). Despite increased tumor control, multiple trials have shown no survival benefit by adding WBRT [163, 164, 170]. Furthermore, patients with WBRT following SRS had worse memory, verbal fluency and quality of life outcomes [170]. Novel WBRT techniques have been developed to preserve neurocognitive and quality-of-life by avoiding the hippocampus during treatment. RTOG studied the effect of hippocampal avoidance and found much lower declines in Hopkins Verbal Learning Test—Revised compared to traditional WBRT [171]. Pharmacologic therapy has provided another method for greater neuroprotection after WBRT. Memantine and donepezil have shown some potential in reducing the rate of cognitive decline and memory loss in patients [172]. Limitations in these studies necessitate more RCTs to validate these protective therapies [173].

3.4 Stereotactic radiosurgery

SRS is a treatment for MBTs that converges multiple, well-collimated beams of ionizing radiation to tumors, while reducing toxic exposure to surrounding brain tissues. In many cases, SRS can be performed as a direct alternative to surgical resection. SRS is often preferred over surgical resection for tumor located within or near eloquent brain structure for in areas that may be challenging to access such as the brainstem, thalamus, and basal ganglia [174, 175]. In addition SRS, may be used as an adjuvant following resection. Several retrospective studies and one incomplete RCT have compared SRS + WBRT versus resection + WBRT and SRS versus resection + WBRT. Generally, these studies show no significant difference in outcomes between treatment groups for median survival, neurologic death, or functional outcome [176–180]. Since survival outcomes are the same for surgical resection and SRS, many institutions perform resection in cases with unclear histology, significant mass effect or patients with neurological deficits. Radiosurgery is the primary option for tumors smaller than 3 cm in diameter. Overall, SRS provides high local tumor control rates, low toxicity, and reduced risk of hemorrhage, infection, and tumor seeding [181, 182].

More recently, MBC is managed with SRS in combination with targeted agents and immunotherapies. SRS and BRAF inhibitors have been safely combined for cases of melanoma brain metastases with no resulting toxicity [183, 184]. Several studies demonstrated greater median survival for patients treated with SRS and targeted therapies in melanoma and nonsmall cell lung cancer brain metastases [185–187]. However, some studies have not shown a benefit when combining SRS with targeted agents [188, 189]. Concurrent delivery of SRS and immunotherapy may enhance the effectiveness of SRS. Several studies have reported better outcomes after treating metastatic brain melanoma with combination radiosurgery and immunotherapy [221, 222]. One downside to this treatment is the inflammatory response may be overactive resulting in elevated peritumoral edema and more severe neurologic symptoms [190, 191]. Efficacy and safety of concurrent SRS and immunotherapy needs further investigation.

3.5 Chemotherapy

Cytotoxic chemotherapy for metastatic brain cancer is currently considered when surgical resection and radiation therapies are not adequate or sufficient for treatment. This is often the case for patients with lower prognostic factors such as patients in RPS class II or III. Patient who have no targetable genetic factors and for which immunotherapeutic agents are inappropriate or contraindicated are considered for cytotoxic chemotherapeutic agents. The agent(s) change based on the primary tumor. A number of phase II and III trials have evaluated the role of chemotherapy for NSCLC MBTs. Patients were treated with six cycles of cisplatin and pemetrexed followed by WBRT in one trial and recorded a response rate of 34.9% [192]. Median survival in the same study was 7.4 months. A more recent cisplatin/pemetrexed study examined patients with BM from lung adenocarcinoma. Overall response rates were comparable to the aforementioned study with median overall survival of 12 months [193].

A randomized phase III trial reversed the order of treatment in patients with NSCLC MBTs where WBRT was followed by chemotherapy [194]. In this study, patients received cisplatin and vinorelbine for six cycles. Intracranial response rates were similar for both the group receiving chemotherapy alone and those receiving WBRT early and concurrently [194]. Another study evaluated paclitaxel and cisplatin chemotherapy in MBTs from NSCLC. The response rate after completion of the course resulted in slightly higher response rates (38%) compared to previous trials. Multiple chemotherapeutic agents have been studied for the treatment of MBTs from breast cancer. Cisplatin, etoposide, cyclophosphamide, high dose methotrexate and 5-fluorouracil have achieved response rates over 50% [195, 196]. Innovation to systemic chemotherapy for brain metastases has been modest with regard to drug development. Modifications to drug delivery ranging from direct injection, convection-enhanced, and implantable seeds have been examined for efficacy [197–200].

3.6 Brachytherapy

Brachytherapy delivers high doses of radiation with small pieces of radioactive material placed within the resection cavity for treating residual tumor. Brachytherapy enables delivery of customizable doses for sparing of functional tissue. Brachytherapy seeds have been used in neurosurgery for over a half-century with mixed results [201–203]. Isotypes used in brachytherapy changed since the 1960s. More recently, cesium-131 and iodine-125 are now replacing gold and iridium-based isotypes. Modern brachytherapy has been studied for the treatment of meningiomas, gliomas, and metastases [204, 205]. Intraoperative brachytherapy may also be used as salvage treatment for recurrent cancers [206]. Recently, a randomized trial evaluated cesium-131 for the treatment of MBTs [207]. Twenty-four patients underwent total resection followed by intraoperative placement of cesium-131 with a planned dose of 80 Gy [207, 208]. The patients had no local recurrence, symptomatic radiation necrosis, and minimal surgical morbidity. Despite limitations in the study including small sample size, these promising results confirm the need for more robust trials.

3.7 Laser interstitial thermal therapy

MR-guided laser interstitial thermal therapy (LITT) builds upon previous thermal ablation technology with safer and more accurate results. LITT is performed by implanting a laser catheter into the tumor and heating it to temperatures monitored by MRI thermography. Patients often return home the day after treatment. Two studies have shown promising results for tumors failing to respond to radiotherapy. LITT is minimally invasive and requires only a 2-mm access port. Four patients with six tumors were treated with LITT without complications and no recurrence within 90-day follow up [209]. Another study demonstrated similar results using LITT for five metastases [210]. More recent studies have bolstered LITT in larger sample sizes as an alternative option for patients unresponsive to radiotherapy. Ahluwalia et al. reported LITT stabilized the Karnofsky Performance Scale (KPS) score, prolonged quality of life, reduced steroid usage with minimal complications [211]. With the advent of real-time monitoring and damage estimation, LITT has emerged as a valuable management modality for metastatic tumors. Larger scale trials need to standardize protocols and specify indications [212].

3.8 Checkpoint inhibitors

Immunotherapies are treatments that activate the immune system to destroy cancer and have been around for over a century. The brain has limited infiltration of leukocytes [213]. Following an injury or metastasis, infiltration of non-resident cell will take place. Metastatic brain infiltrate consists of a mixed array of immune cells, specifically, CD3+, CD4+, CD8+, FoxP3+, CD45RO+ lymphocytes, natural killer (NK) cells, and macrophages [214, 215]. Patient survival is correlated to the quantity of tumor-infiltrating leukocytes in peritumoral edema [214]. In the last decade, exciting advancements from a group of monoclonal antibody treatments called checkpoint inhibitors. Checkpoint inhibitors act to prevent lymphocyte suppression. Several clinical trials have studied immune checkpoint inhibitors efficacy on patients with MBC [216–218].

Programmed cell death proteins (PD-1) are immunomodulatory molecules expressed on the surfaces of immune cells to prevent T-cell overactivation [219]. There are two ligands for PD-1 (PD-L1 and PD-L2) found on the surface of tissue macrophages that regulate the immune response of T cells against pathogens and foreign cells [220]. Cancers are known to express PD-L1 and PD-L2 on their surface to suppress the cytotoxic T lymphocytes (CTLs) response. Nivolumab and pembrolizumab are both anti-PD-1 antibodies that selectively block PD-1 receptor interaction with ligands PD-L1 and PD-L2. These antibodies were approved by the FDA based on efficacy data from phase III trials for the treatment of melanoma, NSCLC, renal cell carcinoma, and head-neck cancer [221–228]. Three new PD-1 antibodies against PD-L1 (durvalumab, atezolizumab, and avelumab) are currently being investigated in phase III trials. Despite a large number of studies examining. Caponnetto et al. provide a timely overview of immunotherapy studies for the treatment of brain metastases [229]. PD-L1 antibodies have been studied on NSCLC brain metastases that resulted in the majority of participants discontinuing treatment from exacerbation of neurologic symptoms [230]. A study by Goldman et al., did not report high toxicity rates in the treatment of NSCLC BM with nivolumab and observed improved overall survival for patients [231]. Large prospective studies will be needed to confirm initial results.

Cytotoxic T lymphocyte-associated molecule-4 (CTLA-4) is another similar checkpoint molecule regulating CTL activity. CTLA-4 is on the surface of CTLs, which connect with CD28 and deactivate T cells [232]. Ipilimumab, an anti-CTLA-4 antibody, has demonstrated promising results in multiple trials in patients with metastatic melanoma [233, 234]. Another Phase III trial reported enhanced overall survival in patients with advanced melanoma and BM [233]. More tests will be required to determine if ipilimumab provides durable responses against melanoma, which is a limitation for BRAF inhibitors. Combination ipilimumab and nivolumab has shown promising results in several studies [228, 235, 236]. Unfortunately, there are no studies testing combination therapy on non-melanoma tumor types. Combination immunotherapy with radiotherapy is limited MBT studies, but radiation necrosis is an emerging concern [237]. Long-term effects of combination treatment and more robust studies to determine its efficacy.

3.9 Adoptive cellular therapy

Adoptive Cellular Therapy (ACT) for the treatment of BM extracts T cells from the patient, genetically modify and culture the cells in vitro before returning them to the same patient. Growth factors are usually added to the cells prior to reintroduction to stimulate survival and expansion in vivo [238]. There are three forms of ACT that use T cells including tumor-infiltrating lymphocyte (TIL) therapy, chimeric antigen receptor (CAR) T-cell therapy, and endogenous T-cell (ETC) therapy. Similar to the process described previously, TIL therapy removes T cell from the patient's tumor, expands them in vitro with an immune signaling molecule (Interleukin-2), before being infused back into the patient [239]. CAR T-cell therapy genetically engineer T cells to recognize specific tumor antigens. ETC neither requires a tumor source nor genetic engineering. Rather, ETC selects intrinsically tumor-reactive T cells in the peripheral blood and expands them. These cells are exceptionally rare and require intense processing methods. Several studies have reported successful treatment of melanoma brain metastases with ACT or combination therapy that includes ACT [240–243].

3.10 Targeted cancer therapy

Targeted cancer treatments are treatments that target specific proteins, processes, and pathways that have become pathological in cancer cells. Generally, targeted entities involve surface proteins on cancer cell membranes, faulty or overactive enzymes in cytoplasm, or faulty cell signaling pathway. The majority of these therapies can be classified under two categories, namely, monoclonal antibodies or kinase inhibitors. It is estimated that 18% of patients with MBTs are susceptible to targeted therapies [244]. Recent developments in the field of tumor biology have presented new therapeutic targets with greater BBB penetrance for a variety of metastatic brain cancers.

3.11 Breast cancer and brain metastases

MBTs occur in 10–15% of patients with breast cancer, although studies based on findings at autopsy suggest that the incidence is closer to 40% of cases [245]. Human epidermal growth factor receptor-2 (HER2) is overexpressed in approximately 15–20% of patients with breast cancer [246]. HER2-positive breast cancer is associated with higher rates of MBTs and prolonged survival than HER2-negative breast cancer [246]. Trastuzumab, a recombinant monoclonal antibody against HER2, improves tumor control and confers a survival benefit for HER2-positive patients [246]. However, the relative higher incidence of BM when treated with trastuzumab has prompted development of alternative therapies with enhanced blood-brain barrier (BBB) penetrance [247]. Lapatinib, a dual tyrosine kinase inhibitor (TKI) of epidermal growth factor receptor (EGFR) and HER2, has been used for treating patients with resistance to trastuzumab [248]. In contrast to trastuzumab, lapatinib can penetrate the BBB when combined with capecitabine. The intracranial response rate was 66% in a Phase II study of HER2-positive breast cancer patients with brain metastases [249–251]. By comparison, lapatinib as a single agent demonstrates only modest activity [249, 252]. Similar findings were observed with neratinib in combination with capecitabine [253, 254].

Triple-negative breast cancer (TNBC) does not express hormone receptors and presents a greater challenge identifying molecular targets. Approximately, 10–15% of breast cancers are TNBC, which have higher incidence and reduced survival [245, 255]. One potential target is poly adenosine diphosphate ribose polymerase (PARP) inhibitors that potentiate chemotherapy and radiotherapy [256]. PARP inhibitors can be effective as single agents for BRCA associated breast and ovarian cancers. Iniparib has begun Phase II trials and in combination with irinotecan yielded a modest benefit for treatment of TNBC [257]. Another potential candidate for TNBC are histone deacetylase (HDAC) inhibitors that prevent transcription of particular genes and expression of cellular activities [258, 259]. Vorinostat, an HDAC inhibitor, has prevented brain metastatic colonization by over 62% in mouse models [260]. Polo-like kinase 1 (Plk1) is another well-performing molecular target in BM from breast cancer. Inhibitors of Plk1 prevented the development of large BMs by 62% and prolonged survival by 17% in mouse models with breast cancer [261]. Plk1 inhibitors may be a new target for MBT prevention and treatment [262].

However, studies reported to date have not demonstrated improvements to overall survival with these treatments. An important factor for these findings may be the failure of targeted therapies to achieve complete responses in the brain [263]. To address these shortcomings, researchers are unraveling the mechanisms for therapeutic resistance, revising brain metastasis models, and developing more penetrative treatments. Specifically, these modifications include patient-derived xenografts, 3D bioprinted metastatic models, genetically-modified mouse models, and nanoparticles for enhanced drug delivery [264]. Vorinostat has undergone a Phase I clinical trial to study its use as a radiosensitizer for WBRT [265]. Treatment was well-tolerated by patients and is expected to enter a Phase II study.

3.12 Lung cancer and brain metastases

Approximately 40–50% of patients with lung cancer are diagnosed with MBC during their disease course [266]. Small cell lung cancer (SCLC) has a greater tendency to metastasize early in its development [267]. MBTs are more commonly encountered in this histological type than NSCLC. Overall, lung cancer patients commonly present with brain metastases at diagnosis [268]. As of today, no targeted therapies have been developed for BM in SCLC.

Roughly, 2–4% of lung cancer brain metastases originate from EGFR mutant [269]. Another 5% of lung cancer MBTs derive from ALK-translocated primary tumors (ibid). Gefitinib and Erlotinib are two first-generation EGFR TKIs approved for the management of EGFR mutant NSCLC [270]. Recent evidence has validated its effectiveness in decreasing the tumor burden by over 30% in over 80% of patients [271, 272]. The median time to progression was also extended for patients treated with erlotinib from 11.7 to 5.8 months [271]. Other studies have confirmed these findings with overall progression-free survival (PFS) of 15.2 months versus 4.4 months for patients without the mutation [273]. Gefitinib or erlotinib may be useful as prophylaxis since they were found to reduce the risk of progression in patients with NSCLC [274]. Similar findings have been observed for another EGFR inhibitor, osimertinib [275]. Osimertinib outperformed patients receiving chemotherapy in a Phase III trial with brain metastasis patients (ibid). Crizotinib is the first TKI approved for ALK-translocated lung cancer [276]. However, it exhibited suboptimal BBB penetration. Next-generation TKIs (e.g., brigatinib and alectinib) targeting translocated ALK have greater penetrance with greater intracranial responsiveness [277, 278].

3.13 Melanoma and brain metastases

Melanoma brain metastases have also benefited from targeted therapies. MBTs are found approximately in 10–20% of patients with melanoma, although autopsies suggest the incidence is as high as 70% in such patients [279]. Targeted therapies such as BRAF V600 TKI dabrafenib have exhibited 39% intracranial response in BMs that increased to 58% in studies combining dabrafenib and trametinib [280, 281]. Another BRAF inhibitor, vemurafenib, recorded a response rate of 18% in another trial [282]. In a previous study, vemurafenib resulted in complete or partial tumor regression and improved overall survival in patients positive for BRAF V600E metastatic melanoma [283]. The downside with BRAF inhibitors is that the majority of melanoma patients develop drug resistance and eventual relapse [284]. Combination therapies with targeted approaches will be necessary to counteract cancer resistance.

4. Experimental therapies

4.1 Nanooncology

Biotechnologies are increasingly used in cancer research [285]. The application of nanotechnology in cancer research is termed nanooncology and has generated promising solutions to address our current limitations in imaging and treatment of brain tumors [286]. Currently, two nanotechnology-based products are approved for the treatment of cancer, e.g., Doxil (liposomal doxorubicin) and Abraxane (nanoparticle formulated paclitaxel). Novel cancer therapeutics ranging from tiny carbon nanotubes and polymeric nanoparticles to large-scale thermal therapies such as magnetic nanoparticle-based hyperthermia [287, 288]. This field of research is growing rapidly with approximately 150 drugs currently in development that incorporate nanotechnology. The purpose of this section is to provide exposure to the field of nanooncology and highlight some promising materials.

4.2 Liposome-based nanoparticles

Liposomes are one of the most established nanomedicines in cancer therapy and theranostics. It is an effective delivery system with their flexibility, versatility, biocompatibility, and biodegradability [289]. Liposomes resemble biological membranes by adopting a lipid bilayer structure and house a wide range of cytotoxic drugs and imaging agents. The vesicle structure of liposomes permits encasement of a variety of lipophilic and hydrophilic cargos. The drug adopts the pharmacokinetic properties of the liposomal carrier until they are released [290]. This feature results in enhanced therapeutic index and reduction in systemic toxicity [291–293]. Additionally, hydrophilic polymers and ligands may be attached to the liposomes to modulate circulation time and targeting capabilities [294, 295]. Several studies have reported enhanced uptake and efficacy of ligand-targeted liposomes in diseased tissue versus non-targeted liposomes. Ligands are selected that have high affinity for highly-expressed receptor on cancer cells [296, 297].

Different strategies have been developed to promote the loading and release of therapeutics for cancer treatments. Liposomes act to protect encapsulated drugs from degradation, dilution and premature release [298]. As a consequence, therapeutic efficacy of anticancer drugs are increased since higher amounts reach the destination [299, 300]. Liposomal doxorubicin-cyclophosphamide for the treatment of breast cancer patients with MBTs demonstrated greater response rates and median survival time for both mouse models and human patients [299, 300]. One challenge for liposome-based nanoparticles is the encapsulation inefficiency (<30%) for passive loading of hydrophilic therapeutics [301]. In contrast, hydrophobic drugs tend to load with much higher efficiency because they readily dissolve inside the lipid bilayer.

4.3 Quantum dots

Quantum dots (QDs) are extremely small nanoparticles measuring a few nanometers in size. QDs emit light of specific frequencies modifiable by altering the size, shape, and material of the dots. QDs possess great potential for tumor fluorescence imaging and delivering therapies. Fluorescence imaging is a potent tool for cancer diagnosis and achieves more complete resections [302]. Biomolecules can be used to modify QDs which provides several improvements from other organic fluorophores, e.g., higher photoluminescence efficiency, greater photostability, and sharp emission profile. QD-based fluorescence also has good biocompatibility and low toxicity [303–307].

Visible fluorescence imaging uses light in the visible wavelength spectrum (400–700 nm) and is adept at cancer diagnosis and enhancing spatial resolution. For in vivo tumor fluorescence imaging, imaging agent delivery to brain tumors is challenging because the BBB restricts the passage of large molecules [308]. Thus, BBB prevents the transposition of many imaging agents and cancer therapeutics ergo attenuating their effect on tumor treatment and illumination. QDs provide a workaround for these physiological constraints due to their miniscule dimensions. Recent studies have developed QD nanoprobes that cross the BBB and target tumors specifically [309, 310]. These QDs cross the BBB and target cancer cells for in vivo imaging.

4.4 Gene therapy

Gene therapy of the nervous system is now a commonplace tool used around the world. Widely used to generate preclinical models, gene therapy is now demonstrating success in the clinic for both safety and efficacy for the treatment of congenital blindness and neurodegenerative disorders [311, 312]. A major component to gene therapeutics is the delivery system known as vectors. Vectors are commonly categorized as viral and non-viral vectors. Adenoviral vectors have proven valuable in the development of anticancer agents by selectively replicating within cancer cells [313]. Retroviral vectors are another useful delivery system for cancer treatment. Previous studies have demonstrated its ability to activate enzymes that convert 5-fluorocytosine (5FC) into toxic 5-fluorouracil (5FU) for treatment of gliomas [314, 315]. RRV with prodrug is currently being tested in randomized trials, however, this concept may be tested on MBTs in combination with immunotherapy [316]. Another rising technology is Clustered Regularly Interspaced Short Palindromic Repeats (CRISPR) that allows gene editing within organisms. Recently, CRISPR was used to engineer tumor cells to exhibit homing behavior [317]. After engineering, cells are released back into circulation and return back to the main tumor site. Cells were designed to secrete death receptor-targeting ligands that destroy the main tumor cells. Self-homing cells were also programmed with a drug-triggered cellular suicide system to eliminate them following tumor death. CRISPR has also been used to enhance therapeutic T cells in cancer immunotherapy [318]. These new capacities may expand into brain metastatic treatment in the near future.

5. Conclusion

In 1971, the National Cancer Act was signed to strengthen the National Care Institute with the objective to eliminate cancer as a leading cause of death in the United States [319]. This was expected to be achieved by funding research for understanding the mechanisms of cancer biology and developing effective treatments. Although cancer death rates have declined for the past 25 years in the United States, the results have overall been disappointing when considering total cancer deaths and mortality rate. Much of the progress against cancer can be attributed to the decline in tobacco use and the development of screening tools for earlier detection [320]. Since 1971, there has been expansion of knowledge in cancer biology and diversification of diagnostic tools and treatment options. With respect to brain metastases, the median survival has improved modestly [321] and innovative approaches to MBC management continue to emerge in the fields of imaging, biotechnology, and pharmaceuticals. Having said that, it is fair to question whether the rate of progress for cancer patient outcomes and innovation is decelerating and whether subsequent inventions will be as impactful as those previous [322, 323]. As Gordon has pointed out, successive Industrial Revolutions after the 1960s have made depreciating impacts on productivity and economic growth [322]. A similar trend is observed in pharmaceuticals with a noticeable decline in research and development (R&D) efficiency defined as the number of new drugs approved for every billion dollars spent on R&D [323]. Studies have haggled over the cost for one new drug approval with estimates between roughly $700 million and $2.5 billion dollars [324, 325]. This trend is referred to as Eroom's Law, which means drug discovery becomes slower and more expensive with time. Additionally, we have seen a decline in the state of competition and economic dynamism characterized by rising mergers and declining start-up rates [323, 326]. Even with newer treatments reaching market, we see evidence of diminishing returns for the treatment of cancer [327]. Despite these problematic economic and healthcare patterns, innovation in MBC management remains resilient producing robust tools for improving treatment safety and efficacy.

Author details

Caleb Stewart[1], Brody Stewart[2] and Marcus L. Ware[1,3]*

1 The University of Queensland School of Medicine, Ochsner Clinical School, New Orleans, LA, United States

2 Southern Illinois University School of Medicine, Springfield, IL, United States

3 Department of Neurological Surgery, Ochsner Clinic Foundation, New Orleans, LA, United States

*Address all correspondence to: mware@ochsner.org

References

[1] Alexandru D, Bota DA, Linskey ME. Epidemiology of central nervous system metastases. In: Current and Future Management of Brain Metastasis. Vol. 25. Basel, Switzerland: Karger Publishers; 2012. pp. 13-29

[2] Nayak L, Lee EQ, Wen PY. Epidemiology of brain metastases. Current Oncology Reports. 2012;**14**(1):48-54

[3] Smedby KE, Brandt L, Bäcklund ML, Blomqvist P. Brain metastases admissions in Sweden between 1987 and 2006. British Journal of Cancer. 2009;**101**(11):1919

[4] Bachmann C et al. CNS metastases in breast cancer patients: Prognostic implications of tumor subtype. Medical Oncology. 2015;**32**:400

[5] Barnholtz-Sloan JS, Sloan AE, Davis FG, Vigneau FD, Lai P, Sawaya RE. Incidence proportions of brain metastases in patients diagnosed (1973 to 2001) in the Metropolitan Detroit Cancer Surveillance System. Journal of Clinical Oncology. 2004;**22**(14):2865-2872

[6] Kohler BA, Ward E, McCarthy BJ, Schymura MJ, Ries LA, Eheman C, et al. Annual report to the nation on the status of cancer, 1975-2007, featuring tumors of the brain and other nervous system. Journal of the National Cancer Institute. 2011;**103**:714-736

[7] LAG R, Eisner MP, Kosary CL, Hankey BF, Miller BA, Clegg L, et al., editors. SEER Cancer Statistics Review, 1975-2000. Bethesda, MD: National Cancer Institute; 2003. Available from: https://seer.cancer.gov/csr/1975_2000/

[8] Feng W, Zhang P, Zheng X, Chen M, Mao WM. Incidence and treatment of brain metastasis in patients with esophageal carcinoma. World Journal of Gastroenterology—WJG. 2015;**21**(19):5805

[9] Villano JL, Durbin EB, Normandeau C, Thakkar JP, Moirangthem V, Davis FG. Incidence of brain metastasis at initial presentation of lung cancer. Neuro-Oncology. 2014;**17**(1):122-128

[10] Noone AM, Howlader N, Krapcho M, Miller D, Brest A, Yu M, et al., editors. SEER Cancer Statistics Review, 1975-2015. Bethesda, MD: National Cancer Institute. Available from: https://seer.cancer.gov/csr/1975_2015/, based on November 2017 SEER data submission, posted to the SEER web site, April 2018

[11] Nussbaum ES, Djalilian HR, Cho KH, Hall WA. Brain metastases: Histology, multiplicity, surgery, and survival. Cancer: Interdisciplinary International Journal of the American Cancer Society. 1996;**78**(8):1781-1788

[12] Sawaya R, Bindal RK, Lang FF, Abi-Said D. Metastatic brain tumors. In: El K, editor. Brain Tumors: An Encyclopedic Approach. 2nd ed. London: Churchill Livingstone; 2001

[13] Posner JB, Chernik NL. Intracranial metastases from systemic cancer. Advances in Neurology. 1978;**19**:579-592

[14] Schouten LJ, Rutten J, Huveneneers HA. Incidence of brain metastases in a cohort of patients with carcinoma of the breast, colon, kidney, and lung and melanoma. Cancer Institute. 2002;**105**:551-562

[15] Counsell CE, Collie DA, Grant R. Incidence of intracranial tumors in the Lothian region of Scotland 1989-90. Journal of Neurology, Neurosurgery, and Psychiatry. 1996;**61**:142-150

[16] Suki D, Khoury Abdulla R, Ding M, et al. Brain metastases in patients

diagnosed with a solid primary cancer during childhood: Experience from a single referral cancer center. Journal of Neurosurgery. Pediatrics. 2014;**14**:372-385

[17] Curless RG, Toledano SR, Ragheb J, Cleveland WW, Falcone S. Hematogenous brain metastasis in children. Pediatric Neurology. 2002;**26**:219-221

[18] Paulino AC, Nguyen TX, Barker JL Jr. Brain metastases in children with sarcoma, neuroblastoma, and Wilms' tumor. International Journal of Radiation Oncology, Biology, Physics. 2003;**57**:177-183

[19] Graus F, Walker RW, Allen JC. Brain metastases in children. The Journal of Pediatrics. 1983;**103**:558-561

[20] Kebudi R, Ayan I, Gorgun O, Agaoglu FY, Vural S, Darendeliler E. Brain metastasis in pediatric extracranial solid tumors: Survey and literature review. Journal of Neuro-Oncology. 2005;**71**:43-48

[21] Jemal A, Miller KD, Ma J, Siegel RL, Fedewa SA, Islami F, et al. Higher lung cancer incidence in young women than young men in the United States. New England Journal of Medicine. 2018;**378**:21

[22] Surveillance Epidemiology and End Results (SEER) Program. SEER*Stat Database: Incidence – SEER 18 Regs Research Data + Hurricane Katrina Impacted Louisiana Cases. Nov 2015 Sub (1973-2013 varying) – Linked To County Attributes – Total U.S., 1969-2014 Counties, National Cancer Institute, DCCPS, Surveillance Research Program, Surveillance Systems Branch, released April 2016, based on November 2015 submission; 2016

[23] Kaal EC, Taphoorn MJ, Vecht CJ. Symptomatic management and imaging of brain metastases. Journal of Neuro-Oncology. 2005;**75**(1):15-20

[24] Christiaans MH, Kelder JC, Arnoldus EP, Tijssen CC. Prediction of intracranial metastases in cancer patients with headache. Cancer. 2002;**94**(7):2063-2068

[25] Pfund Z, Szapary L, Jaszberenyi O, Nagy F, Czopf J. Headache in intracranial tumors. Cephalalgia. 1999;**19**(9):787-790

[26] Saha A, Ghosh SK, Roy C, Choudhury KB, Chakrabarty B, Sarkar R. Demographic and clinical profile of patients with brain metastases: A retrospective study. Asian Journal of Neurosurgery. 2013;**8**(3):157

[27] Wilne SH, Ferris RC, Nathwani A, Kennedy CR. The presenting features of brain tumours: A review of 200 cases. Archives of Disease in Childhood. 2006;**91**(6):502-506

[28] Soffietti R, Cornu P, Delattre JY, Grant R, Graus F, et al. Brain metastases. In: European Handbook of Neurological Management. Oxford, England, UK: Wiley-Blackwell; 2010. pp. 437-445

[29] Wu SG, Rao MY, Zhou J, et al. Distribution of metastatic disease in the brain in relation to the hippocampus: A retrospective single-center analysis of 6064 metastases in 632 patients. Oncotarget. 2015;**6**(41):44030-44036

[30] Wu SG, Sun JY, Tong Q, Li FY, He ZY. Clinical features of brain metastases in breast cancer: An implication for hippocampal-sparing whole-brain radiation therapy. Therapeutics and Clinical Risk Management. 2016;**12**:1849-1853

[31] Graf AH, Buchberger W, Langmayr H, Schmid KW. Site preference of metastatic tumours of the brain. Virchows Archiv A. 1988;**412**(5):493-498

[32] Nguyen DX et al. WNT/TCF signaling through LEF1 and HOXB9

mediates lung adenocarcinoma metastasis. Cell. 2009;**138**:51-62

[33] Bos PD et al. Genes that mediate breast cancer metastasis to the brain. Nature. 2009;**459**:1005-1009

[34] Lee HW, Seol HJ, Choi YL, Ju HJ, Joo KM, Ko YH, et al. Genomic copy number alterations associated with the early brain metastasis of non-small cell lung cancer. International Journal of Oncology. 2012;**41**:2013-2020

[35] Benedettini E, Sholl LM, Peyton M, Reilly J, Ware C, Davis L, et al. Met activation in non-small cell lung cancer is associated with de novo resistance to EGFR inhibitors and the development of brain metastasis. The American Journal of Pathology. 2010;**177**:415-423

[36] Chen G, Wang Z, Liu XY, Liu FY. High-level CXCR4 expression correlates with brain-specific metastasis of non-small cell lung cancer. World Journal of Surgery. 2011;**35**:56-61

[37] Li B, Wang C, Zhang Y, Zhao XY, Huang B, Wu PF, et al. Elevated PLGF contributes to small-cell lung cancer brain metastasis. Oncogene. 2013;**32**:2952-2962

[38] Martinez-Aranda A et al. FN14 and GRP94 expression are prognostic/predictive biomarkers of brain metastasis outcome that open up new therapeutic strategies. Oncotarget. 2015;**6**:44254-44273

[39] Li B et al. Elevated PLGF contributes to small-cell lung cancer brain metastasis. Oncogene. 2013;**32**:2952-2962

[40] Sevenich L et al. Analysis of tumour- and stroma-supplied proteolytic networks reveals a brain-metastasis-promoting role for cathepsin S. Nature Cell Biology. 2014;**16**:876-888

[41] Wrage M et al. Identification of HERC5 and its potential role in NSCLC progression. International Journal of Cancer. 2015;**136**:2264-2272

[42] Jilaveanu LB et al. PLEKHA5 as a biomarker and potential mediator of melanoma brain metastasis. Clinical Cancer Research. 2015;**21**:2138-2147

[43] Shen L, Chen L, Wang Y, Jiang X, Xia H, Zhuang Z. Long noncoding RNA MALAT1 promotes brain metastasis by inducing epithelial-mesenchymal transition in lung cancer. Journal of Neuroncology. 2015;**121**:101-108

[44] Dagogo-Jack I et al. Brain metastasis: Clinical implications of branched evolution. Trends in Cancer. 2016;**2**:332-337

[45] Valiente M et al. Serpins promote cancer cell survival and vascular co-option in brain metastasis. Cell. 2014;**156**:1002-1016

[46] Lorger M, Felding-Habermann B. Capturing changes in the brain microenvironment during initial steps of breast cancer brain metastasis. The American Journal of Pathology. 2010;**176**:2958-2971

[47] Wang X et al. Astrocytic Fas ligand expression is required to induce T-cell apoptosis and recovery from experimental autoimmune encephalomyelitis. European Journal of Immunology. 2013;**43**:115-124

[48] Wanner LB et al. Glial scar borders are formed by newly proliferated, elongated astrocytes that interact to corral inflammatory and fibrotic cells via STAT3-dependent mechanisms after spinal cord injury. The Journal of Neuroscience. 2013;**33**:12870-12886

[49] Kienast Y et al. Real-time imaging reveals the single steps of brain metastasis formation. Nature Medicine. 2010;**16**:116-122

[50] Carbonell WS et al. The vascular basement membrane as 'soil' in brain metastasis. PLoS One. 2009;**4**:e5857

[51] Rafi S et al. Angiocrine functions of organ-specific endothelial cells. Nature. 2016;**529**:316-325

[52] Loulier K et al. Beta1 integrin maintains integrity of the embryonic neocortical stem cell niche. PLoS Biology. 2009;**7**:e1000176

[53] Shen Q et al. Adult SVZ stem cells lie in a vascular niche: A quantitative analysis of niche cell-cell interactions. Cell Stem Cell. 2008;**3**:289-300

[54] Garcia MA et al. Discovery of additional brain metastases on the day of stereotactic radiosurgery: Risk factors and outcomes. Journal of Neurosurgery. 2017;**126**:1756-1763

[55] Xing F et al. Reactive astrocytes promote the metastatic growth of breast cancer stem-like cells by activating notch signaling in brain. EMBO Molecular Medicine. 2013;**5**:385-396

[56] Chen Q et al. Carcinoma-astrocyte gap junctions promote brain metastasis by cGAMP transfer. Nature. 2016;**533**:493-498

[57] Lin Q et al. Reactive astrocytes protect melanoma cells from chemotherapy by sequestering intracellular calcium through gap junction communication channels. Neoplasia. 2010;**12**:748-754

[58] Priego N et al. STAT3 labels a subpopulation of reactive astrocytes required for brain metastasis. Nature Medicine. 2018;**24**:1024-1035

[59] Dolgushin M, Kornienko VN, Pronin IN. Brain Metastases—Advance Neuroimaging. Cham, Switzerland: Springer International Publishing; 2018

[60] Maroldi R, Ambrosi C, Farina D. Metastatic disease of the brain: Extra-axial metastases (skull, dura, leptomeningeal) and tumour spread. European Radiology. 2005;**15**:617-626

[61] Lin JP, Kricheff II, Laguna J, et al. Brain tumors studied by computerized tomography. Advances in Neurology. 1976;**15**:175-199

[62] Kornienko VN, Pronin IN. Diagnostic Neuroradiology. Berline-Heidelberg: Springer-Verlag; 2009

[63] Kornienko VN, Pronin IN. Diagnostic neuroradiology. In: Tumors of the Skull Base. Vol. 4. Moscow: Alexeeva TM; 2012

[64] Kornienko VN et al. A study of brain tissue perfusion by computed tomography. Journal of Medical Imaging. 2007;**2**:70-81

[65] Miles K, Charnsangavej C, Cuenod C. Multi-Detector Computed Tomography in Oncology CT Perfusion Imaging. London: Informa Healthcare; 2007

[66] Lev M, Nichols S. Computer tomographic angiography and computed tomographic perfusion imaging of hyperacute stroke. Topics in Magnetic Resonance Imaging. 2000;**11**:283-287

[67] Konig M. Brain perfusion CR in acute stroke: Current status. European Journal of Radiology. 2003;**45**(1):11-22

[68] Pronin IN et al. The use of CT perfusion imaging in stereotactic biopsy of diffuse gliomas. In: Nevsky Radiological Forum. St Petersburg; 2005

[69] Dolgushin M et al. Use of CT perfusion to discriminate between brain metastases from different primaries. Clinical Imaging. 2015;**39**:9-14

[70] Dolgushin M et al. A CT perfusion method in the differential diagnosis of a secondary tumor lesions of the

brain. Journal of Medical Imaging. 2007;**4**:100-106

[71] Dolgushin MB et al. Perfusion CT in dynamic evaluation of the effectiveness of radiation therapy in secondary brain tumors. N.N. Blokhin Russian Cancer Research Centre. 2008;**19**(4):36-46

[72] Schellinger P, Meinck H, Thron A. Diagnostic accuracy of MRI compared to CCT in patients with brain metastases. Journal of Neuro-Oncology. 1999;**44**(3):275-281

[73] Barajas RF Jr, Cha S. Imaging diagnosis of brain metastasis. Progress in Neurological Surgery. 2012;**25**:55-73

[74] Seute T, Leffers P, ten Velde GP, et al. Detection of brain metastases from small cell lung cancer: Consequences of changing imaging techniques (CT versus MRI). Cancer. 2008;**112**:1827-1834

[75] Kruger S, Mottaghy FM, Buck AK, et al. Brain metastasis in lung cancer. Nuklearmedizin. 2010;**50**:101-106

[76] Seidl Z, Vymazal J, Mechl M, et al. Does higher gadolinium concentration play a role in the morphologic assessment of brain tumors? Results of a multicenter intraindividual crossover comparison of gadobutrol versus gadobenate dimeglumine (the MERIT study). American Journal of Neuroradiology. 2012;**33**:1050-1058

[77] Anzalone N, Essig M, Lee SK, et al. Optimizing contrast-enhanced magnetic resonance imaging characterization of brain metastases: Relevance to stereotactic radiosurgery. Neurosurgery. 2013;**72**:691-701

[78] Togao O, Hiwatashi A, Yamashita K, et al. Additional MR contrast dosage for radiologists' diagnostic performance in detecting brain metastases: A systematic observer study at 3T. Japanese Journal of Radiology. 2014;**32**:537-544

[79] Hoult DI, Lauterbur PC. The sensitivity of the zeugmatographic experiment involving human samples. Journal of Magnetic Resonance. 1979;**34**:425-433

[80] Ba-Ssalamah A, Nobauer-Huhmann IM, Pinker K, et al. Effect of contrast dose and field strength in the magnetic resonance detection of brain metastases. Investigative Radiology. 2003;**38**:415-422

[81] Krautmacher C, Willinek WA, Tschampa HJ, et al. Brain tumors: Full-and half-dose contrast-enhanced MR imaging at 3.0 T compared with 1.5 T-initial experience. Radiology. 2005;**237**:1014-1019

[82] Noebauer-Huhmann IM, Szomolanyi P, Kronnerwetter C, et al. Brain tumours at 7T MRI compared to 3T-contrast effect after half and full standard contrast agent dose: Initial results. European Radiology. 2015;**25**:106-112

[83] Deelchand DK, Van de Moortele PF, Adriany G, et al. In vivo 1H NMR spectroscopy of the human brain at 9.4 T: Initial results. Journal of Magnetic Resonance. 2010;**206**:74-80

[84] Kushnirsky M, Nguyen V, Katz JS, et al. Time-delayed contrast-enhanced MRI improves detection of brain metastases and apparent treatment volumes. Journal of Neurosurgery. 2016;**124**:489-495

[85] Yang S, Nam Y, Kim MO, et al. Computer-aided detection of metastatic brain tumors using magnetic resonance black-blood imaging. Investigative Radiology. 2013;**48**:113-119

[86] Szwarc P, Kawa J, Rudzki M, et al. Automatic brain tumour detection and neovasculature assessment with multiseries MRI analysis. Computerized Medical Imaging and Graphics. 2015;**46**:178-190

[87] Leenders W, Kusters B, Pikkemaat J. Vascular endothelial growth factor-A determines detectability of experimental melanoma brain metastasis in GD-DTPA-enhanced MRI. International Journal of Cancer. 2003;**105**:437-443

[88] Cascino T, Byrne T, Deck M, Posner JB. Intra-arterial BCNU in the treatment of metastatic brain tumors. Journal of Neuro-Oncology;**1**(3):211-218

[89] Roberts T. Physiologic measurements by contrast-enhanced MR imaging: Evaluate expectations and limitations. Journal of Magnetic Resonance Imaging. 1997;7:82-90

[90] Blouw B et al. The hypoxic response of tumors is dependent on their microenvironment. Cancer Cell. 2003;**4**:133-146

[91] Ostergaard L. Principles of cerebral perfusion imaging by bolus tracking. Journal of Magnetic Resonance Imaging. 2005;**24**(2):180

[92] Saremi F. Perfusion Imaging in Clinical Practice. A Multimodality Approach to Tissue Perfusion Analysis. New York: Wolters Klumer; 2015

[93] Tofts P. Quantitative MRI of the Brain. Chichester: Wiley; 2004

[94] Griffith B, Jain R. Perfusion in neuro-oncology basic techniques and clinical applications. The Journal of Pathology. 2015;**53**(3):497-511

[95] Grade M, Hernandez Tamames JA, Pizzini FB, et al. A neuroradiologist's guide to arterial spin labeling MRI in clinical practice. Neuroradiology. 2015;**57**:1181-1202

[96] Tourdias T, Rodrigo S, Oppenheim C, et al. Pulsed arterial spine labeling applications in brain tumors: Practical review. Journal of Neuroradiology. 2008;**35**:79-89

[97] Lowther E, Whitlow C, Maldjian J. Clinical applications of ASL brain perfusion imaging, chapter 14. In: Saremi F, editor. Perfusion Imaging in Clinical Practice. A Multimodality Approach to Tissue Perfusion Analysis. New York: Wolters Klumer; 2015

[98] Boxerman JL, Shiroishi MS, Ellingston BM, et al. Dynamic susceptibility contrast MR imaging in glioma: Review of current clinical practice. Magnetic Resonance Imaging Clinics of North America. 2016;**24**:649-670

[99] Sorensen A, Reimer P. Cerebral MR Perfusion Imaging: Principles and Current Applications. New York: Thieme; 2000

[100] Jones T, Rabiner EA, Company PETRA. The development, past achievements, and future directions of brain PET. Journal of Cerebral Blood Flow and Metabolism. 2012;**32**:1426-1454

[101] Li Z, Conti PS. Radiopharmaceutical chemistry for positron emission tomography. Advanced Drug Delivery Reviews. 2010;**62**:1031-1051

[102] Oriuchi N, Higuchi T, Ishikita T, Miyakubo M, Hanoka H, Iida Y, et al. Present role and future prospects of positron emission tomography in clinical oncology. Cancer Science. 2006;**97**:1291-1297

[103] Fischman AJ. PET imaging of brain tumors. In: Blake MA, Kalra MK, editors. Imaging in Oncology. Boston, MA: Springer; 2008

[104] Juhasz C, Dwivedi S, Kamson DO, et al. Comparison of amino acid positron emission tomographic radiotracers for molecular imaging of primary and metastatic brain tumors. Molecular Imaging. 2014;**13**:13

[105] Ohno Y, Koyama H, Nogami M, et al. Whole-body MR imaging vs FDG-PET: Comparison of accuracy of M-stage diagnosis for lung cancer patients. Journal of Magnetic Resonance Imaging. 2007;**26**:498-509

[106] Rohren EM, Provenzalle JM, Barboriak DP, et al. Screening for cerebral metastases with FDG PET in patients undergoing whole-body staging of non-central nervous system malignancy. Radiology. 2003;**226**:181-187

[107] Patronas NJ, Di Chiro G, Kufta C, et al. Prediction of survival in glioma patients by means of positron emission tomography. Journal of Neurosurgery. 1985;**62**:816-822

[108] Chao S, Suh JH, Raja S, et al. The sensitivity and specificity of FDG PET in distinguishing recurrent brain tumor from radionecrosis in patients treated with stereotactic radiosurgery. International Journal of Cancer. 2001;**96**:191-197

[109] Hutterer M, Nowosielski M, Putzer D, et al. [18F]-fluoro-ethyl-L-tyrosine PET: A valuable diagnostic tool in neuro-oncology, but not all that glitters is glioma. Neuro-Oncology. 2013;**15**:341-351

[110] Allen AM, Ben-Ami M, Reshef A, Steinmetz A, Kundel Y, Inbar E, et al. Assessment of response of brain metastases to radiotherapy by PET imaging of apoptosis with (1)(8) F-ML-10. European Journal of Nuclear Medicine and Molecular Imaging. 2012;**39**(9):1400-1408

[111] Chen W. Clinical applications of PET in brain tumors. Journal of Nuclear Medicine. 2007;**48**(9):1468-1481

[112] Brandao LA, Castillo M. Adult brain tumors: Clinical applications of magnetic resonance spectroscopy. Magnetic Resonance Imaging Clinics of North America. 2016;**24**:781-809

[113] Rapalino O, Ratai EM. Multiparametric imaging analysis: Magnetic resonance spectroscopy. Magnetic Resonance Imaging Clinics of North America. 2016;**24**:671-686

[114] De Edelenyi FS, Rubin C, Esteve F, et al. A new approach for analyzing proton magnetic resonance spectroscopic imaging of brain tumors: Nosologic images. Nature Medicine. 2000;**6**:1287-1289

[115] Fan G, Sun B, Wu Z, Guo Q, Guo Y. In vivo single-voxel proton MR spectroscopy in the differentiation of high-grade gliomas and solitary metastases. Clinical Radiology. 2004;**59**:77-85

[116] Ishimaru H, Morikawa M, Iwanaga S, Kaminogo M, Ochi M, Hayashi K. Differentiation between high-grade glioma and metastatic brain tumor using single-voxel proton MR spectroscopy. European Radiology. 2001;**11**:1784-1791

[117] Guzman-de-Villoria JA, Sanchez-Gonzalez J, Munoz L, et al. 1H MR spectroscopy in the assessment of gliomatosis cerebri. American Journal of Roentgenology. 2007;**188**:710-714

[118] Kuznetsov YE, Caramanos Z, Antel SB, et al. Proton magnetic resonance spectroscopic imaging can predict length of survival in patients with supratentorial gliomas. Neurosurgery. 2003;**53**:564-574

[119] Sjobakk TE, Johansen R, Bathen TF, et al. Metabolic profiling of human brain metastases using in vivo proton MR spectroscopy at 3T. BMC Cancer. 2007;**7**:141

[120] Murase K. Dynamic contrast-enhanced perfusion CT: Basic of mathematical tracer kinetic models and

applications. Chapter 4. In: Saremi F, editor. Perfusion Imaging in Clinical Practice. A Multimodality Approach to Tissue Perfusion Analysis. New York: Wolters Klumer; 2015. pp. 62-76

[121] Le Bihan D, Breton E. Imagieri de diffusion in-vivo par resonance magnetique. Comptes rendus de l'Académie des sciences. Série II. 1985;**15**:1109-1112

[122] Le Bihan D, Turner R, Mooner C, et al. Imaging of diffusion and microvasculation with gradient sensitization: Design, strategy and significance. Journal of Magnetic Resonance Imaging. 1991;**1**:7-28

[123] Chang S, Parney IF, McDermott M, et al. Perioperative complications and neurological outcome of first versus second craniotomy among patients enrolled in the Glioma outcomes project. Journal of Neurosurgery. 2003;**98**:1175-1181

[124] Deveaux BC, O'Fallon JR, Kelly PR. Resection, biopsy, and survival in malignant glial neoplasms: A retrospective study of clinical parameters, therapy, and outcome. Journal of Neurosurgery. 1993;**78**(5):767-775

[125] Fadul C, Wood J, Thaler H, et al. Morbidity and mortality for excision of supratentorial gliomas. Neurology. 1988;**38**:1374-1379

[126] Sawaya R, Hammoud M, Schoppa D, et al. Neurosurgical outcomes in a modern series of 400 craniotomies for treatment parenchymal tumors. Neurosurgery. 1998;**42**:1044-1055

[127] Mueller W. DTI for neurosurgeons: Cases and concepts. In: International Brain Mapping and Intraoperative Surgical Planning Society (IBMISPS) Brain, Spinal Cord Mapping and Image Guided Therapy Conference; 27 May 2010; Bethesda, MN. 2010

[128] Essayed WI, Zhang F, Unadkat P, Cosgrove GR, Golby AJ, O'Donnell LJ. White matter tractography for neurosurgical planning: A topography-based review of the current state of the art. NeuroImage: Clinical. 2017;**15**:659-672

[129] Wu JS, Zhou LF, Tang WJ, Mao Y, Hu J, Song YY, et al. Clinical evaluation and follow-up outcome of diffusion tensor imaging-based functional neuronavigation. Neurosurgery. 2007;**61**(5):935-949

[130] Duffau H et al. Intraoperative mapping of the subcortical language pathways using direct stimulations. Brain. 2002;**125**(1):199-214

[131] Berman JI. Advanced diffusion MR tractography for surgical planning. In: Pillai JJ, editor. Functional Brain Tumor Imaging. New York, NY: Springer; 2014. pp. 183-192

[132] Alexander AL, Hasan K, Kindlmann G, Parker DL, Tsuruda JS. A geometric analysis of diffusion tensor measurements of the human brain. Magnetic Resonance in Medicine. 2000;**44**(2):283-291

[133] Schilling KG, Janve V, Gao Y, Stepniewska I, Landman BA, Anderson AW. Histological validation of diffusion MRI fiber orientation distributions and dispersion. NeuroImage. 2018;**165**:200-221

[134] Grussu F, Schneider T, Yates RL, Tachrount M, Tur C, Newcombe J, et al. Quantitative histological validation of NODDI MRI indices of neurite morphology in multiple sclerosis spinal cord. Multiple Sclerosis Journal. 2015;**21**(S11):204-205

[135] Zhang H, Schneider T, Wheeler-Kingshott CA, Alexander DC. NODDI: Practical in vivo neurite orientation dispersion and density imaging of the human brain. NeuroImage.

2012;**61**(4):1000-1016 [Epub 2012/04/10]

[136] Jacobs B, Schall M, Prather M, Kapler E, Driscoll L, Baca S, et al. Regional dendritic and spine variation in human cerebral cortex: A quantitative golgi study. Cerebral Cortex. 2001;**11**:558-571

[137] Jacobs B, Driscoll L, Schall M. Life-span dendritic and spine changes in areas 10 and 18 of human cortex: A quantitative golgi study. The Journal of Comparative Neurology. 1997;**386**:661-680

[138] Evanglou N, Esiri MM, Smith S, Palace J, Matthews PM. Quantitative pathological evidence for axonal loss in normal appearing white matter in multiple sclerosis. Annals of Neurology. 2000;**47**:391-395

[139] Bruijn LI, Miller TM, Cleveland DW. Unraveling the mechanisms involved in motor neuron degeneration in ALS. Annual Review of Neuroscience. 2004;**27**:723-749

[140] Broad RJ, Gabel MC, Dowell NG, et al. Neurite orientation and dispersion density imaging (NODDI) detects cortical and corticospinal tract degeneration in ALS. Journal of Neurology, Neurosurgery, and Psychiatry. 2018

[141] Paula-Barbosa MM, Mota Cardoso R, Guimaraes ML, Cruz C. Dendritic degeneration and regrowth in the cerebral cortex of patients with Alzheimer's disease. Journal of the Neurological Sciences. 1980;**45**(1):129-134

[142] Jespersen SN, Bjarkam CR, Nyengaard JR, Chakravarty MM, Hansen B, Vosegaard T, et al. Neurite density from magnetic resonance diffusion measurements at ultrahigh field: Comparison with light microscopy and electron microscopy. NeuroImage. 2010;**49**:205-216

[143] Yoshihito K, Hirai T, Azuma M, Hattori Y, Khant ZA, Hori M, et al. Differentiation between glioblastoma and solitary brain metastasis using neurite orientation dispersion and density imaging. Journal of Neuroradiology. 2018. DOI: 10.1016/j.neurad.2018.10.005

[144] Caverzasi E, Papinutto N, Castellano A, Zhu AH, Scifo P, Riva M, et al. Neurite orientation dispersion and density imaging color maps to characterize brain diffusion in neurologic disorders. Journal of Neuroimaging. 2016;**26**(5):494-498. DOI: 10.1111/jon.12359 [Epub 2016/05/24]

[145] Maximov II, Tonoyan AS, Pronin IN. Differentiation of glioma malignancy using diffusion MRI. Physica Medica. 2017;**40**:24-32

[146] Yaeger KA, Nair MN. Surgery for brain metastases. Surgical Neurology International. 2013;**4**(Suppl 4):S203

[147] Patchell RA, Tibbs PA, Walsh JW, Dempsey RJ, Maruyama Y, Kryscio RJ, et al. A randomized trial of surgery in the treatment of single metastases to the brain. New England Journal of Medicine. 1990;**322**(8):494-500

[148] Yoo H, Kim YZ, Nam BH, Shin SH, Yang HS, Lee JS, et al. Reduced local recurrence of a single brain metastasis through microscopic total resection. Journal of Neurosurgery. 2009;**110**(4):730-736

[149] Ali A, Goffin JR, Arnold A, Ellis PM. Survival of patients with non-small-cell lung cancer after a diagnosis of brain metastases. Current Oncology. 2013;**20**(4):e300

[150] Vávra P, Roman J, Zonča P, Ihnát P, Němec M, Kumar J, et al. Recent development of augmented reality in

surgery: A review. Journal of Healthcare Engineering. 2017

[151] Wen R, Chui CK, Ong SH, Lim KB, Chang SKY. Projection-based visual guidance for robot-aided RF needle insertion. International Journal of Computer Assisted Radiology and Surgery. 2013;**8**(6):1015-1025

[152] Lapeer RJ, Jeffrey SJ, Dao JT, García GG, Chen M, Shickell SM, et al. Using a passive coordinate measurement arm for motion tracking of a rigid endoscope for augmented-reality image-guided surgery. The International Journal of Medical Robotics and Computer Assisted Surgery. 2014;**10**(1):65-77

[153] Besharati Tabrizi L, Mahvash M. Augmented reality-guided neurosurgery: Accuracy and intraoperative application of an image projection technique. Journal of Neurosurgery. 2015;**123**(1):206-211

[154] Mert A, Buehler K, Sutherland GR, Tomanek B, Widhalm G, Kasprian G, et al. Brain tumor surgery with 3-dimensional surface navigation. Operative Neurosurgery. 2012;**71**(suppl_2):286-295

[155] Badiali G, Ferrari V, Cutolo F, Freschi C, Caramella D, Bianchi A, et al. Augmented reality as an aid in maxillofacial surgery: Validation of a wearable system allowing maxillary repositioning. Journal of Cranio-Maxillofacial Surgery. 2014;**42**(8):1970-1976

[156] Madhavan K, Kolcun JG, Chieng L, Wang MY. Augmented-reality integrated robotics in neurosurgery: Are we there yet? Neurosurgical Focus FOC. 2017;**42**(5):E3

[157] Komarnicky LT, Phillips TL, Martz K, Asbell S, Isaacson S, Urtasun R. A randomized phase III protocol for the evaluation of misonidazole combined with radiation in the treatment of patients with brain metastases (RTOG-7916). International Journal of Radiation Oncology, Biology, Physics. 1991;**20**(1):53-58

[158] Sause WT, Scott C, Krisch R, Rotman M, Sneed PK, Janjan N, et al. Phase I/II trial of accelerated fractionation in brain metastases RTOG 85-28. International Journal of Radiation Oncology, Biology, Physics. 1993;**26**(4):653-657

[159] Phillips TL, Scott CB, Leibel SA, Rotman M, Weigensberg IJ. Results of a randomized comparison of radiotherapy and bromodeoxyuridine with radiotherapy alone for brain metastases report of RTOG trial 89-05. International Journal of Radiation Oncology, Biology, Physics. 1995;**33**:339-348

[160] Murray KJ, Scott C, Greenberg HM, Emami B, Seider M, Vora NL, et al. A randomized phase III study of accelerated hyperfractionation versus standard in patients with unresected brain metastases: A report of the radiation therapy oncology group (RTOG) 9104. International Journal of Radiation Oncology, Biology, Physics. 1997;**39**(3):571-574

[161] Tsao MN, Lloyd N, Wong RK, Chow E, Rakovitch E, Laperriere N, et al. Whole brain radiotherapy for the treatment of newly diagnosed multiple brain metastases. Cochrane Database of Systematic Reviews. 2012;**4**:1-106. DOI: 10.1002/14651858.CD003869.pub4

[162] Patchell RA, Tibbs PA, Regine WF, Dempsey RJ, Mohiuddin M, Kryscio RJ, et al. Postoperative radiotherapy in the treatment of single metastases to the brain: A randomized trial. JAMA. 1998;**280**(17):1485-1489

[163] Chang EL, Wefel JS, Hess KR, Allen PK, Lang FF, Kornguth DG, et al. Neurocognition in patients with brain metastases treated with radiosurgery or radiosurgery plus whole-brain irradiation: A randomised

controlled trial. The Lancet Oncology. 2009;**10**(11):1037-1044

[164] Kocher M, Soffietti R, Abacioglu U, et al. Adjuvant whole-brain radiotherapy versus observation after radiosurgery or surgical resection of one to three cerebral metastases: Results of the EORTC 22952-26001 study. Journal of Clinical Oncology. 2010;**29**(2):134-141

[165] Aoyama H, Tago M, Shirato H. For the Japanese radiation oncology study group 99-1 (JROSG 99-1) investigators. Stereotactic radiosurgery with or without whole-brain radiotherapy for brain metastases secondary analysis of the JROSG 99-1 randomized clinical trial. JAMA Oncology. 2015;**1**(4):457-464

[166] Kurtz JM, Gelber R, Brady LW, Carella RJ, Cooper JS. The palliation of brain metastases in a favorable patient population: A randomized clinical trial by the Radiation Therapy Oncology Group. International Journal of Radiation Oncology, Biology, Physics. 1981;7(7):891-895 [Epub 1981/07/01]

[167] Ogawa K, Yoshii Y, Nishimaki T, Tamaki N, Miyaguni T, Tsuchida Y, et al. Treatment and prognosis of brain metastases from breast cancer. Journal of Neuro-Oncology. 2008;**86**(2):231-238

[168] Mulvenna P, Nankivell M, Barton R, Faivre-Finn C, Wilson P, McColl E, et al. Dexamethasone and supportive care with or without whole brain radiotherapy in treating patients with non-small cell lung cancer with brain metastases unsuitable for resection or stereotactic radiotherapy (QUARTZ): Results from a phase 3, non-inferiority, randomised trial. Lancet. 2016;**388**(10055):2004-2014

[169] Brown PD, Ballman KV, Cerhan J, et al. N107C CEC.3: A phase III trial of post-operative stereotactic radiosurgery (SRS) compared with whole brain radiotherapy (WBRT) for resected metastatic brain disease. International Journal of Radiation Oncology. Biology. Physics. 2016;**96**:937

[170] Brown PD, Jaeckle K, Ballman KV, et al. Effect of radiosurgery alone vs radiosurgery with whole brain radiation therapy on cognitive function in patients with 1 to 3 brain metastases: A randomized clinical trial. JAMA. 2016;**316**:401-409

[171] Mehta MP, Rodrigus P, Terhaard CH, et al. Survival and neurologic outcomes in a randomized trial of motexafin gadolinium and whole-brain radiation therapy in brain metastases. Journal of Clinical Oncology. 2003;**21**:2529-2536

[172] Brown PD, Pugh S, Laack NN, et al. Memantine for the prevention of cognitive dysfunction in patients receiving whole-brain radiotherapy: A randomized, double-blind, placebo-controlled trial. Neuro-Oncology. 2013;**15**:1429-1437

[173] Rapp SR, Case LD, Peiffer A, et al. Donepezil for irradiated brain tumor survivors: A phase III randomized placebo-controlled clinical trial. Journal of Clinical Oncology. 2015;**33**:1653-1659

[174] Trifiletti DM, Lee CC, Kano H, Cohen J, Janopaul-Naylor J, Alonso-Basanta M, et al. Stereotactic radiosurgery for brainstem metastases: An international cooperative study to define response and toxicity. International Journal of Radiation Oncology, Biology, and Physics. 2016;**96**(2):280-288

[175] Koyfman SA, Tendulkar RD, Chao ST, Vogelbaum MA, Barnett GH, Angelov L, et al. Stereotactic radiosurgery for single brainstem metastases: The Cleveland clinic experience. International Journal of

Radiation Oncology, Biology, and Physics. 2010;**78**(2):409-414

[176] Muacevic A, Kreth FW, Horstmann GA, et al. Surgery and radiotherapy compared with gamma knife radiosurgery in the treatment of solitary cerebral metastases of small diameter. Journal of Neurosurgery. 1999;**91**:35-43

[177] Muacevic A, Wowra B, Siefert A, et al. Microsurgery plus whole brain irradiation versus gamma knife surgery alone for treatment of single metastases to the brain: A randomized controlled multicenter phase III trial. Journal of Neuro-Oncology. 2008;**87**:299

[178] Schöggl A, Kitz K, Reddy M, et al. Defining the role of stereotactic radiosurgery versus microsurgery in the treatment of single brain metastases. Acta Neurochirurgica. 2000;**142**:621

[179] O'Neill BP, Iturria NJ, Link MJ, et al. A comparison of surgical resection and stereotactic radiosurgery in the treatment of solitary brain metastses. International Journal of Radiation Oncology, Biology, Physics. 2003;**55**:1169-1176

[180] Rades D, Bohlen G, Pluemer A, Veninga T, Hanssens P, Dunst J, et al. Stereotactic radiosurgery alone versus resection plus whole-brain radiotherapy for 1 or 2 brain metastases in recursive partitioning analysis class 1 and 2 patients. Cancer. 2007;**109**:2515-2521

[181] Baschnagel AM, Meyer KD, Chen PY, et al. Tumor volume as a predictor of survival and local control in patients with brain metastases treated with gamma knife surgery. Journal of Neurosurgery. 2013;**119**:1139-1144

[182] Wolf A, Kvint S, Chachousa A, et al. BRAF V600E mutation and BRAF kinase inhibitors in conjunction with stereotactic radiosurgery for intracranial melanoma metastases. Journal of Neurosurgery. 2017;**126**:726-734

[183] Narayana A, Mathew M, Tam M, et al. Vemurafenib and radiation therapy in melanoma brain metastases. Journal of Neuro-Oncology. 2013;**113**:411-416

[184] Ahmed KA, Freilich JM, Sloot S, et al. LINAC-based stereotactic radiosurgery to the brain with concurrent vemurafenib for melanoma metastases. Journal of Neuro-Oncology. 2015;**122**:121-126

[185] Ahmed KA, Abuodeh YA, Echevarria MI, et al. Clinical outcomes of melanoma brain metastases treated with stereotactic radiosurgery and anti-PD-1 therapy, anti-CTLA-4 therapy, BRAF/MEK inhibitors, BRAF inhibitor, or conventional chemotherapy. Annals of Oncology. 2016;**27**:2288-2294

[186] Shin SM, Cooper BT, Chachoua A, et al. Survival but not brain metastasis response relates to lung cancer mutation status after radiosurgery. Journal of Neuro-Oncology. 2016;**126**:483-491

[187] Xu Z, Lee C, Ramesh A, et al. BRAF V600E mutation and BRAF kinase inhibitors in conjunction with stereotactic radiosurgery for intracranial melanoma metastases. Journal of Neurosurgery. 2017;**126**:726-734

[188] Patel KR, Chowdhary M, Switchenko JM, et al. BRAF inhibitor and stereotactic radiosurgery is associated with an increased risk of radiation necrosis. Melanoma Research. 2016;**26**:387-394

[189] Ly D, Bagsshaw HP, Anker CJ, et al. Local control after stereotactic radiosurgery for brain metastases of small diameter. Journal of Neurosurgery. 2015;**91**:35-43

[190] Kiess AP, Wolchok JD, Barker CA, et al. Stereotactic radiosurgery for melanoma brain metastases in patients receiving ipilimumab: Safety profile and efficacy of combined treatment.

International Journal of Radiation Oncology. 2015;**92**:368-375

[191] Cohen-Inbar O, Shih HH, Xu Z, et al. The effect of timing of stereotactic radiosurgery treatment of melanoma brain metastases treated with ipilimumab. Journal of Neurosurgery. 2017;**127**:1-8

[192] Barlesi F, Gervais R, Lena H, Hureaux H, Berard H, Paillotin D, et al. Pemetrexed and cisplatin as first-line chemotherapy for advanced non-small-cell lung cancer (NSCLC) with asymptomatic inoperable brain metastases: A multicenter phase II trial (GFPC 07-01). Annals of Oncology. 2011;**22**(11):2466-2470

[193] Dinglin XX, Huang Y, Liu H, et al. Pemetrexed and cisplatin combination with concurrent whole brain radiotherapy in patients with brain metastases of lung adenocarcinoma: A single-arm phase II clinical trial. Journal of Neuro-Oncology. 2013;**112**:461-466

[194] Robinet G, Thomas P, Breton JL, Léna H, Gouva S, Dabouis G, et al. Results of a phase III study of early *versus* delayed whole brain radiotherapy with concurrent cisplatin and vinorelbine combination in inoperable brain metastasis of non-small-cell lung cancer: Groupe Françcais de Pneumo-Cancéerologie (GFPC) Protocol 95-1*. Annals of Oncology. 2001;**12**(1):59-67

[195] Boogerd W, Dalesio O, Bais EM, et al. Response of brain metastases from breast cancer to systemic chemotherapy. Cancer. 1992;**69**:972-980

[196] Lin NU, Bellon JR, Winer EP. CNS metastases in breast cancer. Journal of Clinical Oncology. 2004;**22**:3608-3617

[197] Bobo RH, Laske DW, Akbasak A, Morrison PF, Dedrick RL, Oldfield EH. Convection-enhanced delivery of macromolecules in the brain. Proceedings of the National Academy of Sciences of the United States of America. 1994;**91**:2076-2080

[198] Walter KA, Tamargo RJ, Olivi A, Burger PC, Brem H. Intratumoral chemotherapy. Neurosurgery. 1995;**37**:1128-1145

[199] Lieberman DM, Laske DW, Morrison PF, Bankiewicz KS, Oldfield EH. Convection-enhanced distribution of large molecules in gray matter during interstitial drug infusion. Journal of Neurosurgery. 1995;**82**:1021-1029

[200] Bodell WJ, Giannini DD, Singh S, Pietronigro D, Levin VA. Formation of DNA adducts and tumor growth delay following intratumoral administration of DTI-015. Journal of Neuro-Oncology. 2003;**62**:251-258

[201] Ramsay GS. Interstitial irradiation of the pituitary. Proceedings of the Royal Society of Medicine. 1960;**53**:641-644

[202] Chase NE, Atkins HL, Correll JW. Interstitial irradiation of brain tumors with iridium 192. Radiology. 1961;**77**:842-843. DOI: 10.1148/77.5.842

[203] Hosobuchi Y, Phillips TL, Stupar TA, Gutin PH. Interstitial brachytherapy of primary brain tumors. Preliminary report. Journal of Neurosurgery. 1980;**53**:613-617

[204] Ware ML, Larson DA, Sneed PK, Wara WW, McDermott MW. Surgical resection and permanent brachytherapy for recurrent atypical and malignant meningioma. Neurosurgery. 2004;**54**: 55-63. Discussion 63-54

[205] Vitaz TW, Warnke PC, Tabar V, Gutin PH. Brachytherapy for brain tumors. Journal of Neuro-Oncology. 2005;**73**:71-86

[206] Wernicke AG, Smith AW, Taube S, Yondorf MZ, Parashar B, Trichter S, et al. Cesium-131 brachytherapy for

recurrent brain metastases: Durable salvage treatment for previously irradiated metastatic disease. Journal of Neurosurgery. 2017;**126**(4):1212-1219

[207] Wernicke AG, Yondorf MZ, Peng L, Trichter S, Nedialkova L, Sabbas A, et al. Phase I/II study of resection and intraoperative cesium-131 radioisotope brachytherapy in patients with newly diagnosed brain metastases. Journal of Neurosurgery. 2014;**121**:338-348

[208] Xia Y, Mashouf LA, Baker BR, et al. Outcomes of metastatic brain lesions treated with radioactive Cs-131 seeds after surgery: Experience from one institution. Cureus. 2018;**10**(7):e3075

[209] Hawasli AH, Bagade S, Shimony JS, Miller-Thomas M, Leuthardt EC. Magnetic resonance imaging-guided focused laser interstitial thermal therapy for intracranial lesions: Single-institution series. Neurosurgery. 2013;**73**:1007-1017

[210] Carpentier A, McNichols RJ, Stafford RJ, Itzcovitz J, Guichard JP, Reizine D, et al. Real-time magnetic resonance-guided laser thermal therapy for focal metastatic brain tumors. Neurosurgery. 2008;**63**:ONS21-ONS28

[211] Ahluwalia M, Barnett GH, Deng D, Tatter SB, Laxton AW, Mohammadi AM, et al. Laser ablation after stereotactic radiosurgery: A multicenter prospective study in patients with metastatic brain tumors and radiation necrosis. Journal of Neurosurgery. 2018;**130**:804-811

[212] Ashraf O, Patel NV, Hanft S, Danish SF. Laser-induced thermal therapy in neuro-oncology: A review. World Neurosurgery. 2018;**112**:166-177

[213] Kipnis J. Multifaceted interactions between adaptive immunity and the central nervous system. Science. 2016;**353**:766-771

[214] Berghoff AS et al. Density of tumor-infiltrating lymphocytes correlates with extent of brain edema and overall survival time in patients with brain metastases. Oncoimmunology. 2016;**5**:e1057388

[215] Berghoff AS et al. Characterization of the inflammatory response to solid cancer metastases in the human brain. Clinical and Experimental Metastasis. 2013;**30**:69-81

[216] Wyler L et al. Brain metastasis in renal cancer patients: Metastatic pattern, tumour-associated macrophages and chemokine/chemoreceptor expression. British Journal of Cancer. 2014;**110**:686-694

[217] Berghoff AS et al. Tumor infiltrating lymphocytes and PD-L1 expression in brain metastases of small cell lung cancer (SCLC). Journal of Neuro-Oncology. 2016;**130**:19-29

[218] Duchnowska R et al. Immune response in breast cancer brain metastases and their microenvironment: The role of the PD-1/PD-L axis. Breast Cancer Research. 2016;**18**:43

[219] Pardoll D. The blockade of immune checkpoints in cancer immunotherapy. Nature Reviews. Cancer. 2012;**12**:252-264

[220] Brochez L et al. The rationale of indoleamine 2,3-dioxygenase inhibition for cancer therapy. European Journal of Cancer. 2017;**76**:167-182

[221] Ferris RL et al. Nivolumab for recurrent squamous-cell carcinoma of the head and neck. The New England Journal of Medicine. 2016;**375**:1856-1867

[222] Borghaei H et al. Nivolumab versus docetaxel in advanced nonsquamous nonsmall-cell lung cancer. The New England Journal of Medicine. 2015;**373**:1627-1639

[223] Motzer RJ et al. Lenvatinib, everolimus, and the combination in patients with metastatic renal cell carcinoma: A randomised, phase 2, open-label, multicentre trial. The Lancet Oncology. 2015;**16**(5):1473-1482

[224] Herbst RS et al. Lung master protocol (Lung-MAP)—A biomarker-driven protocol for accelerating development of therapies for squamous cell lung cancer: SWOG S1400. Clinical Cancer Research. 2015;**21**(7):1514-1524

[225] Seiwert TY, Burtness B, Mehra R, et al. Safety and clinical activity of pembrolizumab for treatment of recurrent or metastatic squamous cell carcinoma of the head and neck (KEYNOTE-012): An open-label, multicentre, phase 1b trial. The Lancet Oncology. 2016;**17**(7):956-965

[226] Robert C, Schachter J, Long GV, Arance A, Grob JJ, Mortier L, et al. Pembrolizumab versus ipilimumab in advanced melanoma. The New England Journal of Medicine. 2015;**372**:2521-2532

[227] Robert C, Long GV, Brady B, Dutriaux C, Maio M, Mortier L, et al. Nivolumab in previously untreated melanoma without BRAF mutation. The New England Journal of Medicine. 2015;**372**:320-330

[228] Tawbi HA, Forsyth PA, Algazi A, Hamid O, Hodi FS, Moschos SJ, et al. Combined nivolumab and ipilimumab in melanoma metastatic to the brain. The New England Journal of Medicine. 2018;**379**(8):722-730

[229] Caponnetto S, Draghi A, Borch TH, Nuti M, Cortesi E, Svane IM, et al. Cancer immunotherapy in patients with brain metastases. Cancer Immunology, Immunotherapy. 2018;**67**(5):703-711

[230] Kanai O, Fujita K, Okamura M, Nakatani K, Mio T. Severe exacerbation or manifestation of primary disease related to nivolumab in non-small-cell lung cancer patients with poor performance status or brain metastases. Annals of Oncology. 2016;**27**(7):1354-1356

[231] Goldman JW, Crino L, Vokes EE, Holgado E, Reckamp K, Pluzanski A, et al. P2.36: Nivolumab (nivo) in patients (pts) with advanced (adv) NSCLC and central nervous system (CNS) metastases (mets): Track: Immunotherapy. Journal of Thoracic Oncology. 2016;**11**(10S):S238-S239

[232] Mellman I, Coukos G, Dranoff G. Cancer immunotherapy comes of age. Nature. 2011;**480**:480-489

[233] Hodi FS, O'Day SJ, McDermott DF, Weber RW, Sosman JA, Haanen JB, et al. Improved survival with ipilimumab in patients with metastatic melanoma. The New England Journal of Medicine. 2010;**363**(8):711-723

[234] Margolin K, Ernstoff MS, Hamid O, Lawrence D, McDermott D, Puzanov I, et al. Ipilimumab in patients with melanoma and brain metastases: An open-label, phase 2 trial. The Lancet Oncology. 2012;**13**(5):459-465

[235] Long GV, Atkinson V, Menzies AM, Lo S, Guminski AD, Brown MP, et al. A randomized phase II study of nivolumab or nivolumab combined with ipilimumab in patients (pts) with melanoma brain metastases (mets): The anti-PD1 brain collaboration (ABC). In: Abstract from the American Society of Clinical Oncology (ASCO) Annual Meeting. 2017

[236] Haanen J, Hwu WJ, Martín-Algarra S, Hodi FS, Bhatia S, Slingluff CL, et al. Efficacy and safety of nivolumab (NIVO) alone or combined with ipilimumab (IPI) in patients with melanoma (MEL) metastatic to the brain in a phase 1 study. In: Poster from the Society for Melanoma Research Annual Meeting. 2016

[237] Silva IP, Johnpulle RAN, Banks PD, Grass GD, Smith JL, Everett AS, et al. Incidence, features and management of radionecrosis (RN) in melanoma patients (pts) treated with cerebral radiotherapy (RT) and anti-PD-1 antibodies (PD1). In: Abstract from the American Society of Clinical Oncology (ASCO) Annual Meeting. 2017

[238] Zang YW, Gu XD, Xiang JB, Chen ZY. Clinical application of adoptive T cell therapy in solid tumors. Medical Science Monitor. 2014;**20**:953-959. Epub 2014/06/11

[239] Weber JS. At the bedside: Adoptive cell therapy for melanoma-clinical development. Journal of Leukocyte Biology. 2014;**95**(6):875-882

[240] Hong JJ, Rosenberg SA, Dudley ME, Yang JC, White DE, Butman JA, et al. Successful treatment of melanoma brain metastases with adoptive cell therapy. Clinical Cancer Research. 2010;**16**(19):4892-4898

[241] Rosenberg SA, Restifo NP. Adoptive cell transfer as personalized immunotherapy for human cancer. Science. 2015;**348**:62-68. A comprehensive review of the clinical development and potentially transformative impact of adoptive T-cell therapy on cancer by one of its pioneers; see also ref. [42]

[242] Mehta GU, Malekzadeh P, Shelton T, et al. Outcomes of adoptive cell transfer with tumor-infiltrating lymphocytes for metastatic melanoma patients with and without brain metastases. Journal of Immunotherapy. 2018;**41**(5):241-247

[243] Mullinax JE, Hall M, Prabhakaran S, et al. Combination of ipilimumab and adoptive cell therapy with tumor-infiltrating lymphocytes for patients with metastatic melanoma. Frontiers in Oncology. 2018;**8**:44. This is an interesting study and its design is a little similar to that of phase I study. The results showed that combination of ipilimumab and tumor-infiltrating lymphocytes was well tolerated and the efficacy is higher than those of any of the regimen itself in contrast to historical control

[244] Valiente M et al. The evolving landscape of brain metastasis. Trends in Cancer. 2018;**4**:176-196

[245] Cheng X, Hung MC. Breast cancer brain metastases. Cancer Metastasis Reviews. 2007;**26**:635-643

[246] Leyland-Jones B. Human epidermal growth factor receptor 2-positive breast cancer and central nervous system metastases. Journal of Clinical Oncology. 2009;**27**:5278-5286

[247] Bendell JC et al. Central nervous system metastases in women who receive trastuzumab-based therapy for metastatic breast carcinoma. Cancer. 2003;**97**:2972-2977

[248] Melisko ME, Glantz M, Rugo HS. New challenges and opportunities in the management of brain metastases in patients with ErbB2-positive metastatic breast cancer. Nature Clinical Practice. Oncology. 2009;**6**:25-33

[249] Lin NU et al. Phase II trial of lapatinib for brain metastases in patients with human epidermal growth factor receptor 2-positive breast cancer. Journal of Clinical Oncology. 2008;**26**:1993-1999

[250] Lin NU et al. Multicenter phase II study of lapatinib in patients with brain metastases from HER2-positive breast cancer. Clinical Cancer Research. 2009;**15**:1452-1459

[251] Bachelot T et al. Lapatinib plus capecitabine in patients with previously untreated brain metastases from HER2-positive metastatic breast cancer (LANDSCAPE): A single-group

phase 2 study. The Lancet Oncology. 2013;**14**:64-71

[252] Cameron D, Casey M, Press M, Lindquist D, Pienkowski T, Romieu CG, et al. A phase III randomized comparison of lapatinib plus capecitabine versus capecitabine alone in women with advanced breast cancer that has progressed on trastuzumab: updated efficacy and biomarker analyses. Breast Cancer Research and Treatment. 2008;**112**(3):533-543

[253] Kaufman B, Crown J, Chan A, Campone M, Viens P, Davidson N, et al. A phase III randomized comparison of lapatinib plus capecitabine versus capecitabine alone in women with advanced breast cancer that has progressed on trastuzumab: Updated efficacy and biomarker analyses. Breast Cancer Research and Treatment. 2008;**112**:533-543

[254] Freedman RA et al. Translational breast Cancer research consortium (TBCRC) 022: A phase II trial of neratinib for patients with human epidermal growth factor receptor 2-positive breast cancer and brain metastases. Journal of Clinical Oncology. 2016;**34**:945-952

[255] Kennecke H, Yerushalmi R, Woods R, Cheang MC, Voduc D, Speers CH, et al. Metastatic behavior of breast cancer subtypes. Journal of Clinical Oncology. 2010;**28**:3271-3277

[256] Helleday T. The underlying mechanism for the PARP and BRCA synthetic lethality: Clearing up the misunderstandings. Molecular Oncology. 2011;**5**:387-393

[257] Anders CK, Winer EP, Ford JM, Dent R, Silver DP, Sledge GW, et al. Poly(ADP-ribose) polymerase inhibition: "Targeted" therapy for triple-negative breast cancer. Clinical Cancer Research. 2010;**16**:4702-4710

[258] Lane AA, Chabner BA. Histone deacetylase inhibitors in cancer therapy. Journal of Clinical Oncology. 2009;**27**:5459-5468

[259] Langer CJ, Mehta MP. Current management of brain metastases, with a focus on systemic options. Journal of Clinical Oncology. 2005;**23**:6207-6219

[260] Palmieri D, Lockman PR, Thomas FC, Hua E, Herring J, Hargrave E, et al. Vorinostat inhibits brain metastatic colonization in a model of triple-negative breast cancer and induces DNA double-strand breaks. Clinical Cancer Research. 2009;**15**:6148-6157

[261] Qian Y, Hua E, Bisht K, Woditschka S, Skordos KW, Liewehr DJ, et al. Inhibition of polo-like kinase 1 prevents the growth of metastatic breast cancer cells in the brain. Clinical and Experimental Metastasis. 2011;**28**:899-908

[262] Liu Z, Sun Q, Wang X. PLK1, a potential target for cancer therapy. Translational Oncology. 2017;**10**(1): 22-32. Epub 2016/11/27

[263] Holohan C et al. Cancer drug resistance: An evolving paradigm. Nature Reviews. Cancer. 2013;**13**:714-726

[264] Albritton JL, Miller JS. 3D bioprinting: Improving in vitro models of metastasis with heterogeneous tumor microenvironments. Disease Models and Mechanisms. 2017;**10**(1):3-14

[265] Shi W, Lawrence YR, Choy H, Werner-Wasik M, Andrews DW, Evans JJ, et al. Vorinostat as a radiosensitizer for brain metastasis: A phase I clinical trial. Journal of Neuro-Oncology. 2014;**118**:313-319

[266] Ricciardi S, de Marinis F. Multimodality management of non-small cell lung cancer patients with

brain metastases. Current Opinion in Oncology. 2010;**22**(2):86-93

[267] Slotman BJ, Mauer ME, Bottomley A, Faivre-Finn C, Kramer GW, Rankin EM, et al. Prophylactic cranial irradiation in extensive disease small-cell lung cancer: Short-term health-related quality of life and patient reported symptoms: Results of an international phase III randomized controlled trial by the EORTC radiation oncology and lung cancer groups. Journal of Clinical Oncology. 2009;**27**:78-84

[268] Cagney DN et al. Incidence and prognosis of patients with brain metastases at diagnosis of systemic malignancy: A population-based study. Neuro-Oncology. 2017;**19**:1511-1521

[269] Iuchi T et al. Frequency of brain metastases in nonsmall-cell lung cancer, and their association with epidermal growth factor receptor mutations. International Journal of Clinical Oncology. 2015;**20**:674-679

[270] Lynch TJ, Bell DW, Sordella R, Gurubhagavatula S, Okimoto RA, Brannigan BW, et al. Activating mutations in the epidermal growth factor receptor underlying responsiveness of non-small-cell lung cancer to gefitinib. New England Journal of Medicine. 2004;**350**(21):2129-2139

[271] Porta R et al. Brain metastases from lung cancer responding to erlotinib: The importance of EGFR mutation. The European Respiratory Journal. 2011;**37**:624-631

[272] Iuchi T et al. Phase II trial of gefitinib alone without radiation therapy for Japanese patients with brain metastases from EGFR-mutant lung adenocarcinoma. Lung Cancer. 2013;**82**:282-287

[273] Wu YL et al. Erlotinib as second-line treatment in patients with advanced non-small-cell lung cancer and asymptomatic brain metastases: A phase II study (CTONG-0803). Annals of Oncology. 2013;**24**:993-999

[274] Heon S, Yeap BY, Britt GJ, Costa DB, Rabin MS, Jackman DM, et al. Development of central nervous system metastases in patients with advanced non-small cell lung cancer and somatic EGFR mutations treated with gefitinib or erlotinib. Clinical Cancer Research. 2010;**16**:5873-5882

[275] Mok TS et al. Osimertinib or platinum-pemetrexed in EGFR T790M-positive lung cancer. The New England Journal of Medicine. 2017;**376**:629-640

[276] Metro G et al. CSF concentration of crizotinib in two ALK-positive non-small-cell lung cancer patients with CNS metastases deriving clinical benefit from treatment. Journal of Thoracic Oncology. 2015;**10**:e26-e27

[277] Kim DW et al. Brigatinib in patients with crizotinib-refractory anaplastic lymphoma kinase-positive non-small-cell lung cancer: A randomized, multicenter phase II trial. Journal of Clinical Oncology. 2017;**35**:2490-2498

[278] Gadgeel SM et al. Pooled analysis of CNS response to alectinib in two studies of pretreated patients with ALK-positive non-small-cell lung cancer. Journal of Clinical Oncology. 2016;**34**:4079-4085

[279] Bafaloukos D, Gogas H. The treatment of brain metastases in melanoma patients. Cancer Treatment Reviews. 2004;**30**:515-520

[280] Long GV et al. Dabrafenib in patients with Val600Glu or Val600Lys BRAF-mutant melanoma metastatic to the brain (BREAK-MB): A multicentre, open-label, phase 2 trial. The Lancet Oncology. 2012;**13**:1087-1095

[281] Davies MA et al. Dabrafenib plus trametinib in patients with BRAF(V600)-mutant melanoma brain metastases (COMBI-MB): A multicentre, multicohort, open-label, phase 2 trial. The Lancet Oncology. 2017;**18**:863-873

[282] McArthur GA et al. Vemurafenib in metastatic melanoma patients with brain metastases: An open-label, single-arm, phase 2, multicentre study. Annals of Oncology. 2017;**28**:634-641

[283] Flaherty KT, Puzanov I, Kim KB, Ribas A, McArthur GA, Sosman JA, et al. Inhibition of mutated, activated BRAF in metastatic melanoma. The New England Journal of Medicine. 2010;**363**:809-819

[284] Long GV, Kefford RF, Carr PJ. Phase 1/2 study of GSK2118436, a selective inhibitor of V600 mutant (MUT) BRAF kinase; evidence of activity in melanoma brain metastases (METS). Annals of Oncology. 2010;**21**(Suppl. 8):viii12

[285] Jain KK. Applications of Biotechnology in Oncology. New York: Springer; 2014

[286] Jain KK. Recent advances in nanooncology. Technology in Cancer Research & Treatment. 2008;**7**:1-13

[287] LeBrun A, Zhu L. Magnetic nanoparticle hyperthermia in cancer treatment: History, mechanism, imaging-assisted protocol design, and challenges. In: Shrivastava D, editor. Theory and Applications of Heat Transfer in Humans. Hoboken, NJ: Wiley; 2018:631-667

[288] Son KH, Hong JH, Lee JW. Carbon nanotubes as cancer therapeutic carriers and mediators. International Journal of Nanomedicine. 2016;**11**:5163-5185

[289] Al-Jamal WT, Kostarelos K. Liposomes: From a clinically established drug delivery system to a nanoparticle platform for theranostic nanomedicine. Accounts of Chemical Research. 2011;**44**:1094-1104

[290] Bozzuto G, Molinari A. Liposomes as nanomedical devices. International Journal of Nanomedicine. 2015;**10**:975-999

[291] Hamill RJ. Amphotericin B formulations: A comparative review of efficacy and toxicity. Drugs. 2013;**73**:919-934

[292] O'Brien MER. Reduced cardiotoxicity and comparable efficacy in a phase III trial of pegylated liposomal doxorubicin HCl (CAELYXTM/Doxil®) versus conventional doxorubicin for first-line treatment of metastatic breast cancer. Annals of Oncology. 2004;**15**:440-449

[293] Rafiyath SM, Rasul M, Lee B, et al. Comparison of safety and toxicity of liposomal doxorubicin vs. conventional anthracyclines: A meta-analysis. Experimental Hematological Oncology. 2012;**1**:10

[294] Gabizon A, Goren D, Horowitz AT, et al. Long-circulating liposomes for drug delivery in cancer therapy: A review of biodistribution studies in tumor-bearing animals. Advanced Drug Delivery Reviews. 1997;**24**:337-344

[295] Zhigaltsev IV, Maurer N, Akhong QF, et al. Liposome-encapsulated vincristine, vinblastine and vinorelbine: A comparative study of drug loading and retention. Journal of Controlled Release. 2005;**104**:103-111

[296] Danhier F, Feron O, Préat V. To exploit the tumor microenvironment: Passive and active tumor targeting of nanocarriers for anti-cancer drug delivery. Journal of Controlled Release. 2010;**148**:135-146

[297] Torchilin VP. Passive and active drug targeting: Drug delivery to

tumors as an example. In: Handbook of Experimental Pharmacology. Vol. 197. Berlin, Heidelberg: Springer; 2010. pp. 3-53

[298] Passero FC, Grapsa D, Syrigos KN, Saif MW. The safety and efficacy of Onivyde (irinotecan liposome injection) for the treatment of metastatic pancreatic cancer following gemcitabine-based therapy. Expert Review of Anticancer Therapy. 2016;**16**:697-703

[299] Gaillard PJ, Appeldoorn CCM, Dorland R, van Kregten J, Manca F, Vugts DJ, et al. Pharmacokinetics, brain delivery, and efficacy in brain tumor-bearing mice of glutathione pegylated liposomal doxorubicin (2B3-101). PLoS One. 2014;**9**(1):e82331

[300] Linot B, Campone M, Augereau P, Delva R, Abadie-Lacourtoisie S, Nebout-Mesgouez N, et al. Use of liposomal doxorubicin-cyclophosphamide combination in breast cancer patients with brain metastases: A monocentric retrospective study. Journal of Neuro-Oncology. 2014;**117**(2):253-259

[301] Akbarzadeh A, Rezaei-Sadabady R, Davaran S, et al. Liposome: Classification, preparation, and applications. Nanoscale Research Letters. 2013;**8**:102

[302] Stummer W, Pichlmeier U, Meinel T, Wiestler OD, Zanella F, Reulen HJ, et al. Fluorescence-guided surgery with 5-aminolevulinic acid for resection of malignant glioma: A randomised controlled multicentre phase III trial. The Lancet Oncology. 2006;7(5):392-401

[303] Roy M, Niu CJ, Chen YH, McVeigh PZ, Shuhendler AJ, Leung MK, et al. Estimation of minimum doses for optimized quantum dot contrast-enhanced vascular imaging in vivo. Small. 2012;**8**:1780-1792

[304] Zhou RH, Li M, Wang SL, Wu P, Wu L, Hou XD. Low-toxic Mn-doped ZnSe/ZnS quantum dots conjugated with nano-hydroxyapatite for cell imaging. Nanoscale. 2014;**6**:14319-14325

[305] Li ZS, Xu W, Wang YT, Shah BR, Zhang CL, Chen YJ, et al. Quantum dots loaded nanogels for low cytotoxicity, pH-sensitive fluorescence, cell imaging and drug delivery. Carbohydrate Polymers. 2015;**121**:477-485

[306] Lee J, Kang HJ, Jang H, Lee YJ, Lee YS, Ali BA, et al. Simultaneous imaging of two different cancer biomarkers using aptamer-conjugated quantum dots. Sensors. 2015;**15**:8595-8604

[307] Sureshkumar S, Jothimani B, Sridhar TM, Venkatachalapathy B. Synthesis and characterization of gadolinium doped ZnSe quantum dots for fluorescence imaging of cancer cells. RSC Advances. 2016;**6**:16081-16086

[308] Karamanos Y, Pottiez G. Proteomics and the blood-brain barrier: How recent findings help drug development. Expert Review of Proteomics. 2016;**13**:251-258

[309] Huang N, Cheng S, Zhang X, Tian Q, Pi JL, Tang J, et al. Efficacy of NGR peptide-modified PEGylated quantum dots for crossing the blood-brain barrier and targeted fluorescence imaging of glioma and tumor vasculature. Nanomedicine. 2017;**13**:83-93

[310] Wu CF, Hansen SJ, Hou Q, Yu JB, Zeigler M, Jin YH, et al. Design of highly emissive polymer dot bioconjugates for in vivo tumor targeting. Angewandte Chemie (International Edition). 2011;**50**:3430-3434

[311] Maguire AM et al. Age-dependent effects of RPE65 gene therapy for Leber's congenital amaurosis: A phase 1 dose-escalation trial. Lancet. 2009;**374**:1597-1605

[312] Marks WJ Jr et al. Gene delivery of AAV2-neurturin for Parkinson's disease: A double-blind, randomised, controlled trial. Lancet. 2010;**9**:1164-1172

[313] Green NK, Seymour LW. Adenoviral vectors: Systemic delivery and tumor targeting. Cancer Gene Therapy. 2002;**9**:1036-1042

[314] Ostertag D, Amundson KK, Espinoza FL, Martin B, Buckley T, Galvao da Silva AP, et al. Brain tumor eradication and prolonged survival from intratumoral conversion of 5-fluorocytosine to 5-fluorouracil using a nonlytic retroviral replicating vector. Neuro-Oncology. 2012;**14**(2):145-159

[315] Perez OD et al. Design and selection of Toca 511 for clinical use: Modified retroviral replicating vector with improved stability and gene expression. Molecular Therapy. 2012;**20**:1689-1698

[316] Hickey MJ, Kasahara N, Mueller BM, Kruse CA. Combining cellular and gene therapy approaches for treatment of intracranial tumors. Oncoimmunology. 2013;**2**(10):e25989

[317] Reinshagen C, Bhere D, Choi SH, Hutten S, Nesterenko I, Wakimoto H, et al. CRISPR-enhanced engineering of therapy-sensitive cancer cells for self-targeting of primary and metastatic tumors. Science Translational Medicine. 2018;**10**(449)

[318] Cooper ML, Choi J, Staser K, Ritchey JK, Devenport JM, Eckardt K, et al. An 'off-the-shelf' fratricide-resistant CAR-T for the treatment of T cell hematologic malignancies. Leukemia. 2018;**32**(9):1970-1983

[319] Mukherjee S. The Emperor of All Maladies: A Biography of Cancer. New York: Simon & Schuster; 2010

[320] Siegel RL, Miller KD, Jemal A. Cancer statistics, 2018. CA: A Cancer Journal for Clinicians. 2018;**68**(1):7-30

[321] Tabouret E, Chinot O, Metellus P, Tallet A, Viens P, Goncalves A. Recent trends in epidemiology of brain metastases: An overview. Anticancer Research. 2012;**32**(11):4655-4662

[322] Gordon RJ. Why has economic growth slowed when innovation appears to be accelerating? CEPR Discussion Papers 13039, C.E.P.R. Discussion Papers. 2018

[323] Scannell JW, Blanckley A, Boldon H, Warrington B. Diagnosing the decline in pharmaceutical R&D efficiency. Nature Reviews. Drug Discovery. 2012;**11**(3):191-200

[324] Dubois P, de Mouzon O, Scott-Morton F, Seabright P. Market size and pharmaceutical innovation. The RAND Journal of Economics. 2015;**46**(4):844-871

[325] Prasad V, Mailankody S. Research and development spending to bring a single cancer drug to market and revenues after approval. JAMA Internal Medicine. 2017;**177**(11):1569-1575

[326] Shambaugh J, Nunn R, Breitwieser A, Liu P. The state of competition and dynamism: Facts about concentration, start-ups, and related policies. The Hamilton Project. 2018:1-36

[327] Vaishampayan UN. Changing face of metastatic prostate cancer: The law of diminishing returns holds true. Current Opinion in Oncology. 2017

Section 7

Nutritional Support

Chapter 15

A Nutrition Perspective on the Ketogenic Diet as Therapy for Malignant Brain Cancer

Meredith Morgan

Abstract

Glioblastoma multiforme is the most deadly primary brain tumor. Current therapies have not demonstrated improved outcomes for patients; generally the median life expectancy is 8–15 months. Due to brain tumor cells dependence on glucose as a sole energy source, there is potential to target treatments towards glucose metabolism. The ketogenic diet (KD) is a high fat, low carbohydrate diet that has proven successful in the animal model. However, human studies are limited and there currently is not enough research to conclude the KD is an effective therapy. A few aspects need to be addressed for inclusion in protocols of future studies: (1) when to initiate the KD during treatment; (2) how much carbohydrate per day to provide to patients; (3) how to ensure patient compliance to diet; (4) the optimum duration of the diet; (5) how to mitigating patient weight loss. In addition, the registered dietitian nutritionist (RD or RDN) is a vital, and underutilized, member of the health care team. The inclusion of a RD to future KD protocol, as well as oncology practices, can enhance patient outcomes and help future patients overcome barriers when adhering to the KD.

Keywords: nutrition, ketogenic diet, glioblastoma multiforme, registered dietitian nutritionist, brain cancer

1. Introduction

In 2013, it was estimated that there were 23,130 cases of primary brain cancer in the United States and 14,080 deaths from the disease [1]. One type of tumor is glioblastoma multiforme (GBM), which is the most deadly primary brain tumor in children and adults [2]. Most cases of GBM occur in patients over the age of 50 years old [3]. Current median life expectancy for these patients is 8–15 months; 1 year survival is 34.6% and 5 year survival is less than 5% [1, 3]. Standard treatment is typically palliative in nature and includes surgery (maximal tumor resection), radiation, as well as chemotherapy [2, 3]. While there are new therapies, which include gene therapy, immune modulating therapy and anti-angiogenic therapy, these have not demonstrated improved outcomes for this disease [4]. Overall, the current aims of therapies are to increase life expectancy and enhance quality of life [3].

Patients with cancer often have a "wide range of nutrition related problems" [5]. These nutritional issues may occur anywhere along the digestive tract-from salivary dysfunctions to changes in stooling and often involve weight loss [5]. Other

IntechOpen

patients may be at higher risks of developing morbidities such as "diabetes, adipositas, hyperlipidemia or cardiovascular disease" related to cancer therapies [5]. Patients with head and neck cancers have a high risk of mortality (50%) and many of these patients suffer from malnutrition [6]. This is often a result of the malignancy and may be attributed to loss of appetite, difficulties eating, weight loss as well as fatigue [6]. Malnutrition is an issue as it may cause setbacks in healing, such as weakened immune system, longer treatment times and increased complications along with the cancer [6].

When it comes to medical nutrition therapy (MNT), cancer patients are often "under-recognized and undertreated" as a patient population [5]. Data constantly demonstrates that patients with cancer that do not receive MNT have decreased likelihood of responding to therapies and success may be lower [5]. A registered dietitian nutritionist (RD or RDN) is trained to deliver nutrition facts as well as scientifically based nutrition education and counseling, while also considering educational levels and "psycho-oncological" influences [5]. Current nutrition recommendations correspond generally to patients with head and neck cancer, and there are no specific nutrition recommendations for patients with GBM. The ketogenic diet (KD) has shown promising results in the animal model for malignant brain tumors, but as of 2015, very few studies detail the treatment of primary brain tumors with the KD [1]. Currently, the data is limited whether the KD is effective for patients with GBM for improving outcomes and extending longevity. In addition, the question remains: should health professionals recommend the KD as a therapeutic treatment for patients with GBM?

2. Brain cell metabolism

The brain is a "metabolically active organ" that is almost completely dependent on glucose as its exclusive energy source [7]. Without the ability to locally store glucose, the brain relies on tight homeostasis of blood glucose to ensure adequate energy supplies [7]. Blood glucose concentrations are considered normal between 70 and 144 mg/dL, while any concentration over 200 mg/dL is considered hyperglycemic [7].

For patients with GBM, blood glucose concentrations have been found to average 459 mg/dL [7]. In part, this may be due to high dose of glucocorticoids to help with peritumor associated edema [8, 9]. Glucocorticoids usage results in impaired glucose transport and high plasma glucose [8]. In addition, glucose metabolism is higher in environments with poor blood supply, such as acidic and hypoxemic environments [7]. This may be attributed to the Warburg effect. This effect is part of the aberrations observed in cancer cell metabolism; it involves a switch from oxygen dependent oxidative phosphorylation to "glucose intensive" anaerobic glycolysis for ATP production [7]. This results in the production of essential proteins, lipids and nucleic acids required for cell growth under hypoxic conditions [7]. Tumors in microenvironments are negative indictors of "therapeutic response" and overall survival [7]. Previous work has demonstrated that cancer cells have enhanced aptitude to defy damage from radiation when in hyperglycemic environments [10]. Unfortunately, due to high mortality rate, and decreased likelihood of patients developing diabetes in the long term, hyperglycemia is not managed by intensive therapies; rather, the goal is to avoid acute complications [8]. However, previous studies have demonstrated that higher amounts of glucose in the brains of cancer patients is correlated to a shorter survival [7, 8]. Other reports have demonstrated that the higher the glucose levels, the faster the tumor growth [9]. Glioma cells have previously been shown to display a "threefold increase" in the rate of glycolysis compared to normal astrocytes and when glucose is removed; this leads to apoptosis in tumor cells, compared to normal cells [11].

When the brain has decreased access to glucose, it is able to metabolize ketone bodies (acetoacetate and β-hydroxybutyrate) for energy [9]. This occurs as the liver transforms fat into ketone bodies and fatty acids. The ketone bodies then circulate to the brain and substitute glucose as the brain's energy source [4]. The benefit is that as brain tumor cells are completely dependent on glucose to perform glycolysis, they are unable to metabolize ketones. The latter is due to impaired mitochondria [2]. Another benefit is that ketones may be toxic to some tumor cells by decreasing free radicles from oxygen and improving metabolism in healthy cells [9]. Therefore, focusing anti-tumor treatments on glucose metabolism may be beneficial for GBM patients' outcomes [2].

2.1 The ketogenic diet

The ketogenic diet (KD) was established in the 1920s and consists of a high fat content while providing a low carbohydrate content [2, 10]. It is best executed under medical supervision; it has been effective for treating children with epilepsy and may be successful in neurodegenerative diseases such as Alzheimer's and Parkinson's [2, 12]. The diet is successful as it mimics the fasting state by increasing the level of ketones circulating in the blood, while decreasing circulating glucose; this diet also avoids malnutrition in patients [2, 10]. The KD typically consists of 90% fat, with the remaining 10% contributed by both protein and carbohydrate [13]. Protein is indispensable in the diet, but too much protein can result in the transformation to glucose via gluconeogenesis and act metabolically as a carbohydrate [13]. It has previously been demonstrated that extremely malnourished oncology patients that were given a diet consisting of 44 kcal/kg, where medium chain triglycerides provided 70% of the macronutrient content, had no significant changes in nitrogen balance or protein synthesis [13].

Using the KD as a therapeutic approach for malignant brain cancer rests on the assumption that brain tumors do not have the necessary enzymes to oxidize ketones, and are based on successful rodent studies [4]. However, a recent study contradicted previous findings and reported that rodent brain tumors were able to metabolically change and the "up regulation of the ketone body monocarboxylate transporter," which "facilitated the update and oxidation of ketone bodies in the gliomas" [4]. To date, there are very few human studies and most of them have small sample sizes [4]. Using the KD as the sole treatment or part of the treatment may be effective against GBM, and has been suggested and discussed in previous literature [3, 9, 14].

Another idea worth noting is that the treatment of GBM with the KD may be enhanced by a calorie restriction; this idea has been shown to prevent tumor progress in a range of models [15]. Schwartz et al. provided a calorie restriction after calculating energy needs based on ideal body weight, then providing 20–25 kcals/kg with a 20% restriction in kcals per day [1]. A calorie restriction typically provides a 20–40% reduction in daily calories. During calorie restriction, serum levels of glucose and insulin decrease while fat breakdown increases. This eventually activates peroxisome proliferator-activated receptor-α (PPAR-α), which hinders glycolysis and fatty acids production. PPAR-α also stimulates transcription of enzymes that promote ketogenesis and fatty acid oxidation in the mitochondria and peroxisome [13]. For the tumor cells, which lack the enzymes needed to metabolize ketones, energy in the form of adenosine triphosphate (ATP) can no longer be produced via glycolysis; the cells also lack the ability to compensate via oxidative phosphorylation, which deprives the cell of ATP and means for growth [13]. A calorie restriction may be a beneficial aspect along with the KD, but is not consistently explored in KD studies. A few concerns should be addressed when considering the KD as a therapeutic treatment for patients with GBM: carbohydrate content of diet; compliance to diet; when to initiate the diet; duration of diet; quality of life, and involving a RD with the treatment protocol to improve outcomes.

2.2 Exploring best practices

While the KD typically provides 90% fat, the amount of carbohydrate permitted during treatment tends to vary with each study [13]. In the human studies investigated, the carbohydrate content ranged from 10 grams (g) per day, up to 70 g per day [2, 16]. Previous studies using the animal model have demonstrated that by restricting carbohydrates to <50 g/day, ketone levels ≥1 millimoles per liter (mmol/L) enhances the expression of monocarboxylic acid transporters in the brain; this results in the movement of ketones through the blood brain barrier [13]. An issue with very restrictive dietary carbohydrate is that patients with malignant tumors have been documented to have higher rates of gluconeogenesis, which decreases the body's stores of lean mass and hurts the patient [16]. Therefore, cancer patients may benefit from slightly more carbohydrate, and not risk leaving ketosis [16]. In addition, more carbohydrate options increases the types of food that can be eaten, which helps with compliance [16]. Best practice may be to allow patients to eat around 50 g of carbohydrate per day, which may improve adherence to the prescribed diet and improve treatment outcomes.

Compliance to the KD is an issue as it requires a lifestyle change, which may be difficult for some patients [16]. It is not uncommon for studies to report that some participants had low compliance [4, 16]. However, a few participants found the KD was tolerable: the diet was rated as good by seven patients, moderate by three patients and poor by only one patient [16] and was reported to be "relatively well tolerated" [15]. One patient was reported to strictly adhere to the KD and a calorie restricted diet for 56 days [2]. For patients following the KD, it is important for strict adherence to the diet. For those with strict compliance to the KD, it was reported there was a partial response to treatment, and ketone bodies were found in the normal appearing white matter 8 months after starting the diet; although, this response was attributed to bevacizumab therapy and not the KD [4]. However, there may be other barriers that exist that hinder patients from strictly adhering to the diet. To help mitigate these barriers, the addition of a RD to the treatment team would be best practice; this will be discussed later in the chapter.

Having patients test their own ketone and glucose levels may help them to comply with the diet, as they can see if their levels are in goal range. The goal for GBM therapy is to have blood glucose ranges between 55 and 65 milligram per deciliter (mg/dL) for maximum therapeutic implications [2]. To measure compliance to the KD, ketones are measured via urine analysis; however, there is evidence to show that urine concentrations are not reflective of the concentrations of ketones available to the brain for consumption [4]. Artzi et al. reported only three incidences where ketones were found in the brain using magnetic resonance spectroscopy (MRS): two times in the normal appearing white matter, at 4 and 25 months after starting KD, and one in the tumor area 13 months after starting KD; it was noted that participant compliance to the KD was low [4]. Compliance to the KD was measured either by urine analysis or by blood analysis. The goal for urine ketones was set >2, while blood ketone goals were between 3 and 8 mmol/L [1, 4]. It was reported that 92% of patients that tested urine ketones 2–3 times per week achieved ketosis at least one during the study [15]. Schwartz et al. went further and also had their participants test their blood glucose at least two times per day. Goals for blood glucose were between 50 and 70 mg/dL, which is a suggested best practice for maximum therapeutic effect [1]. A benefit to testing ketones via the blood is that the patient can also test blood glucose and have measureable results. While the goal for blood glucose is 50–70 mg/dL, it is important that patients keep track of blood glucose to avoid hypoglycemic events, which is defined as blood glucose <45 mg/dL [2]. Hypoglycemia is a concern because if it goes untreated it can lead to coma and death [17]. However, it has been reported that while following the KD, there was no issue with hypoglycemic events, and that patients that had elevated blood glucose prior to the study, ended up with normal levels after starting the KD [2, 16]. There is valid concern that ketosis, defined by urine or blood concentrations, may not be indicative of the brain and tumor usage of ketones. However, MRS may not be a tool available for all patients and providers. Best practice would be to have patients test blood glucose and ketones 2–3 times per day to help with measurable goals, help encourage compliance and to avoid any hypoglycemic events.

While the KD has been promising in the mouse model, the studies in human clinical trials have yet to clearly demonstrate that the KD is effective as a sole intervention. Part of the issue is that the KD has not been consistently used an isolated therapy and many of the studies use KD concomitantly with other treatments; therefore, the studies have not able to conclude if the KD was an effective therapy [1, 2, 4, 16]. However, the KD may be most effective when used in combination with chemotherapy. Rieger et al. found that patients that received the KD and received bevacizumab had a median progression free survival of 20.1 weeks while patients receiving bevacizumab and not on the KD had a median progression free survival of 16.1 weeks [15].

The duration of the KD ranged greatly amongst the studies, and there does not appear to be a pattern for best practice. However, it has previously been reported that effects of the KD cannot be ascertained until after 8 weeks on the diet [16]. As mentioned previously, a case study reported on a patient following the KD and a calorie restriction for 56 days, then discontinued the KD and followed a low calorie diet for 5 months and was found to be disease free at that follow up [2]. Artzi et al. had dietary components that lasted from 2 months up to 31 months, although not all patients were able to follow the KD strictly [4]. Meanwhile, Reiger et al. had a median duration of 36 days for diet adherence and reported that patients followed the diet for 6.8 days out of the week. Schwartz et al. reported two participants followed the KD for 12 weeks, but there was no benefit to stopping tumor growth [1]. Meanwhile, there was evidence that the KD could be effective for longer "progression free survival;" in patients with stable ketosis, the median overall survival was 32 weeks, with a range from 6 to 86+ weeks [15]. Current recommendations state that dietary interventions should be started before cancer treatments then continue along with and after treatments; it also may be more successful of an intervention if a registered dietitian is an active part of the treatment team [18].

Nutrition status and quality of life have a positive relationship and both are associated with survival [10, 19]. While most patients with GBM have a short life expectancy, it is important that their quality of life is maximized, and the quality of their diet is an important factor. Food is one of the few aspects of health that both patients and care givers continue to have control over, and is both a "mental and social act" that has many external influences [5]. Schmidt et al. investigated the quality of life for patients with different types of cancer on the KD. Quality of life was initially low for participants due to stage of tumor progression, but the KD was found to increase their quality of life over time. Symptoms of fatigue, pain and dyspnea amplified over time, but emotional function and insomnia improved. Previous side effects reported on the KD have included vomiting, fatigue, hunger and constipation; however, the study reported no incidence of hunger, meanwhile nausea and vomiting were reported as infrequent [16]. In addition, the KD has been found to have no adverse neurological or physiological impacts for patients [2].

Another aspect of quality of life is weight loss. Ten to eighty-three percent of patients with cancer may have unwanted weight loss [5]. The KD in theory should mimic the benefits of long term fasting, while avoiding weight loss in the "oncological setting" [10]. The KD is intended to meet the energy and nutrition requirements of oncology patients while also stimulating lean body mass recovery [13]. From a nutrition perspective, unintentional weight loss is defined as ≥5% in 1 month or ≥10% in 6 months [18]. In the few studies that investigate the KD, most reported that participants lost weight [1, 2, 15, 16]. Zuccoli et al. reported on a patient that received the KD along with a calorie restriction and after 20 days had experienced a 13.4 pound (9.5%) weight loss, which is nutritionally significant based on malnutrition criteria [2, 20]. It is to be noted that this patient was on a calorie restriction of 600 calories per day [2]. Meanwhile, Rieger et al. reported a statistically significant weight loss of 2.2% overall for patients on the KD [15]. While the KD, especially if paired with a calorie restriction, may cause weight loss, one of the goals during cancer treatment is preventing malnutrition. Significant weight loss is one of the criteria used to diagnose malnutrition. Malnutrition has been found to be the leading reason for interrupted treatments [6].

Overall, the KD appears relatively safe for patients with GBM, and may help increase longevity, although excessive weight loss may be a concern. It is important that patients following the KD have a balance of food choices to increase quality of life and mitigate weight loss while also adhering to the KD for best treatment outcomes.

2.3 Role of registered dietitian in cancer treatment

It is essential for patients with head and neck cancers to follow nutrition advice for best "treatment and health outcomes" [6]. Patients that participated in a nutrition intervention during treatment were able to "maintain or improve nutritional status" as well as improving the rate of treatments completion, decreasing hospital visits, length of hospital stays and decreasing the amount of weight lost during treatment [6]. Unfortunately, patients with head and neck cancer are not always compliant with dietary advice, especially if dietary is not considered an essential part of the treatment by patients [6]. It has previously been reported that more participants received nutrition counseling after treatment (60.7%) compared to during cancer treatment (47.4%) [5].

When considering diet therapy in combination with anti-tumor treatments, it would be best practice to consult a registered dietitian. A registered dietitian nutritionist (RD or RDN) is a food and nutrition expert with a bachelor and/or master degree from an accredited university, and has taken coursework that has been approved by the Accreditation Council for Education in Nutrition and Dietetics. In addition, the RD has completed a 1200 hour supervised practice with rotation concentrations in clinical, community and food service management, and passed a national credentialing exam. RDs have to take continuing education credits, regarding up-to-date food and nutrition information, to maintain RD credentials. RDs also have the option to become certified in specific areas of practice; one such area is oncology [21]. RDs are trained to do assessments and give detailed nutrition educations. As part of the assessment, the RD assesses current weight and discusses weight history, discusses current nutrition symptoms, assesses diet history, and calculates protein and energy needs [22]. RDs use the nutrition care process, which is an internationally validated and accepted tool, which makes nutrition care more visible amongst the health profession and ensures access of information to qualified professionals [5].

The RD is an integral part of the health care team, and may be an underutilized resource. Maschke et al. found that cancer patients were more likely to receive nutrition advice from a dietitian if they were between ages 45–70 years old, and those patients between ages 27–45 years old received nutrition information from the internet, nurse or doctor. It would have been beneficial for more patients to see a dietitian as the most often reported questions was regarding a "healthy diet" as well as issues with fatigue and weakness [5]. Kiss et al. found that when the dietitian clinic was located separately from the oncology clinic, the RD was not included as part of the multidisciplinary team and patients did not attend the dietitians' clinic. When the RD team was moved to be a part of the oncology team, it was found to improve communication amongst team members, resulting in the ability to quickly identify nutrition complications and reduce hospital admissions [22].

In regards to the studies administering the KD to patients, a RD was mentioned in a few studies as part of the protocol. Benefits of adding the RD as a part of the study protocol team is the ability to check in on patients more often, either via the phone or in the clinic, answer questions and refer patients to the doctor if there are medical treatment issues that arise. This can help take part of the burden off of the doctors [1]. In addition, it has been reported that when patients visited with a RD regularly, the percent of patients admitted to the hospital for nutrition related issues decreased from 12 to 4.5% and that hospital days decreased from 199 to 62 days [22]. The RD has the expertise and the experience to calculate energy and protein needs as well as diet plans to fit patient's individual needs, which has some benefit [4]. To best highlight this, it is best to discuss the studies that do not involve a RD. For the two studies that did not provide patients with a RD, the study provided patients with instructions or a diet manual with a list of foods, the nutrition contents of foods, recipes and rules to follow when on the KD. Patients were left to their own devices to prepare meals and only one of the studies provided a daily menu [15, 16]. This could be one of the barriers that prevented patients from strictly adhering to the KD. Previous findings have shown that individualized diet counseling based on patients' normal food preferences, along with head and neck cancer treatments, is a very successful way to improve patients' nutrition status, nutrition intake and quality of life [19]. Maschke et al. reported that over half of their study respondents wanted nutrition information, which suggested there is a need for providing consistent and evidenced based MNT. In addition, they suggested that there is the potential for a strong partnership between RDs and oncologists to meet the "informational needs" of patients [5]. The majority of the cancer patients that followed a special diet reported they adhered to it after receiving education from a registered dietitian [5].

3. Conclusion

GBM is a deadly primary brain tumor and patients with this diagnosis have a limited life expectancy. The ketogenic diet has shown promising results in the animal model and in theory should work to target brain tumor cells' glucose metabolism. However, it is difficult to draw conclusions on the effectiveness of the diet due to the limited number of studies, small sample sizes, and the inability to use the KD as an isolated therapy. More studies need to be performed before the KD can be recommended as a sole therapy for GBM, and using the KD as a therapy should occur only with direct medical supervision. Future research needs to include a standardized protocol for including KD in studies. Based on the current literature, best practice would include: (1) initiate KD prior to chemotherapy and continue concomitantly with chemotherapy; (2) KD composed of 50 grams of carbohydrate per day; (3) patients test blood levels of ketones and glucose daily for compliance and to prevent hypoglycemia; (4) continue the KD for at least 8 weeks; (5) minimize patient weight loss. In addition, it would be best practice to include a registered dietitian nutritionist with the protocol to improve patient outcomes, educate patients on the KD, monitor patient progress, calculate energy needs and help patients overcome potential barriers while following the KD.

Conflict of interest

No conflict of interests.

Notes

At time of publication, Meredith Morgan, is completing her supervised practice, and is anticipated to be a Registered Dietitian upon the completion of her dietetic internship.

Thanks

A special thanks to Dr. Morgan for constantly sharing his passion for oncology, and for his appreciation for medical nutrition therapy as a vital piece of healthcare.

Author details

Meredith Morgan
DEKK-TEC, New Orleans, Louisiana, USA

*Address all correspondence to: meredithpmorgan@gmail.com

References

[1] Schwartz K, Chang HT, Nikolai M, Pernicone J, Rhee S, Olson K, et al. Treatment of glioma patients with ketogenic diets: Report of two cases treated with an IRB-approved energy-restricted ketogenic diet protocol and review of the literature. Cancer & Metabolism. 2015;**3**:3

[2] Zuccoli G, Marcello N, Pisanello A, Servadei F, Vaccaro S, Mukherjee P, et al. Metabolic management of glioblastoma multiforme using standard therapy together with a restricted ketogenic diet: Case report. Nutrition and Metabolism. 2010;**7**:33

[3] Weeks HD, Weidman-Evans E. Adjuvant metabolic therapy for glioblastoma multiform. Clinical Nutrition ESPEN. 2017;**19**:70-72

[4] Artzi M, Liberman G, Vaisman N, Bokstein F, Vitinshtein F, Aizenstein O, et al. Changes in cerebral metabolism during ketogenic diet in patients with primary brain tumors: 1H-MRS study. Journal of Neuro-Oncology. 2017;**132**(2):267-275

[5] Maschke J, Kruk U, Kastrati K, Kleeberg J, Buchholz D, Erickson N, et al. Nutritional care of cancer patients: A survey on patients' needs and medical care in reality. International Journal of Clinical Oncology. 2017;**22**(1):200-206

[6] Britton B, McCarter K, Baker A, Wolfenden L, Wratten C, Bauer J, et al. Eating as treatment (EAT) study protocol: A stepped-wedge, randomised controlled trial of a health behaviour change intervention provided by dietitians to improve nutrition in patients with head and neck cancer undergoing radiotherapy. BMJ Open. 2015;**5**(7):e008921

[7] Flavahan WA, Wu Q, Hitomi M, Rahim N, Kim Y, Sloan AE, et al. Brain tumor initiating cells adapt to restricted nutrition through preferential glucose uptake. Nature Neuroscience. 2013;**16**(10):1373-1382

[8] Derr RL, Ye X, Islas MU, Desideri S, Saudek CD, Grossman SA. Association between hyperglycemia and survival in patients with newly diagnosed glioblastoma. Journal of Clinical Oncology. 2009;**27**(7):1082-1086

[9] Seyfried TN, Marsh J, Shelton LM, Huysentruyt LC, Mukherjee P. Is the restricted ketogenic diet a viable alternative to the standard of care for managing malignant brain cancer? Epilepsy Research. 2012;**100**(3):310-326

[10] Klement RJ, Champ CE. Calories, carbohydrates, and cancer therapy with radiation: Exploiting the five R's through dietary manipulation. Cancer Metastasis Reviews. 2014;**33**(1):217-229

[11] Chaichana KL, McGirt MJ, Woodworth GF, Datoo G, Tamargo RJ, Weingart J, et al. Persistent outpatient hyperglycemia is independently associated with survival, recurrence and malignant degeneration following surgery for hemispheric low grade gliomas. Neurological Research. 2010;**32**(4):442-448

[12] Prins ML. Cerebral metabolic adaptation and ketone metabolism after brain injury. Journal of Cerebral Blood Flow and Metabolism. 2008;**28**(1):1-16

[13] Bozzetti F, Zupec-Kania B. Toward a cancer-specific diet. Clinical Nutrition. 2016;**35**(5):1188-1195

[14] Noorlag L, De Vos FY, Kok A, Broekman MLD, Seute T, Robe PA, et al. Treatment of malignant gliomas with ketogenic or caloric restricted diets: A systematic review of preclinical and early clinical studies. Clinical Nutrition. 2018. Available from: http://www.sciencedirect.com/science/article/pii/S0261561418325196

[15] Rieger J, Bähr O, Maurer GD, Hattingen E, Franz K, Brucker D, et al. ERGO: A pilot study of ketogenic diet in recurrent glioblastoma. International Journal of Oncology. 2014;**44**(6):1843-1852

[16] Schmidt M, Pfetzer N, Schwab M, Strauss I, Kämmerer U. Effects of a ketogenic diet on the quality of life in 16 patients with advanced cancer: A pilot trial. Nutrition and Metabolism. 2011;**8**:54

[17] Mahan LK, Escott-Stump S, Raymond JL, Krause MV, editors. Krause's Food & the Nutrition Care Process. 13th ed. St. Louis, MO: Elsevier/Saunders; 2012. 1227 p

[18] van den Berg MGA, Rasmussen-Conrad EL, Wei KH, Lintz-Luidens H, Kaanders JHAM, Merkx MAW. Comparison of the effect of individual dietary counselling and of standard nutritional care on weight loss in patients with head and neck cancer undergoing radiotherapy. The British Journal of Nutrition. 2010;**104**(6):872-877

[19] Ravasco P, Monteiro-Grillo I, Vidal PM, Camilo ME. Impact of nutrition on outcome: A prospective randomized controlled trial in patients with head and neck cancer undergoing radiotherapy. Head & Neck. 2005;**27**(8):659-668

[20] White JV, Guenter P, Jensen G, Malone A, Schofield M. Consensus statement: Academy of Nutrition and Dietetics and American Society for Parenteral and Enteral Nutrition. Journal of Parenteral and Enteral Nutrition. 2012;**36**(3):275-283

[21] What is a Registered Dietitian Nutritionist [Internet]. 2019. Available from: https://www.eatrightpro.org/about-us/what-is-an-rdn-and-dtr/what-is-a-registered-dietitian-nutritionist

[22] Kiss NK, Krishnasamy M, Loeliger J, Granados A, Dutu G, Corry J. A dietitian-led clinic for patients receiving (chemo)radiotherapy for head and neck cancer. Supportive Care in Cancer. 2012;**20**(9):2111-2120